EAT CHOCOLATE, LOSE WEIGHT

NEW SCIENCE PROVES YOU SHOULD EAT CHOCOLATE EVERY DAY

WILL CLOWER, PhD

RODALE.

To my sweet mom.
Thank you for everything;
I love you.

Direct exclusive edition will be published by Rodale Inc. in January 2014.

© 2013 by Will Clower, PhD

Rodale books may be purchased for business or promotional use or for special sales.
For information, please write to:
Special Markets Department, Rodale Inc., 733 Third Avenue, New York, NY 10017
Printed in the United States of America

Rodale Inc. makes every effort to use acid-free ♾, recycled paper ♻.

Book design by Elizabeth Neal

Library of Congress Cataloging-in-Publication Data is on file with the publisher.
ISBN 978–1–62336–127–3 hardcover

Distributed to the trade by Macmillan
2   4   6   8   10   9   7   5   3   1   hardcover

We inspire and enable people to improve their lives and the world around them.
rodalebooks.com

Contents

Acknowledgments

I would like to acknowledge the fact that there are people I love who have all contributed in ways, large and small, visible and invisible, to this work. I so appreciate the opportunity to express the gratitude I feel and that all too often goes unspoken.

I would not be who I am and do what I do if it were not for the family love that surrounds me every day with the friendship and affection, the laughter and love, that defines who we are together. Thank you, Ben, Grace, and Dottie for my life.

I am grateful to friends and coworkers who help me keep my head on my shoulders and have provided critical support while writing this book: Rita Madden, Laura Todd, and Anthony McKee.

Thank you to my friend Paul Morrison, whose keen actuarial eye combined with his own cooking skill helped focus my recipes into vastly better products.

Finally, let me say that I cannot imagine working with a better editor. Lora Sickora has been positive and supportive and has helped to keep me from rambling when I ramble and prodded me to provide detail where needed. Thank you.

Introduction

What is a "health food"? Normally, this question conjures up thoughts of broccoli, brussels sprouts, celery sticks, etc. But have you noticed that chocolate never makes the list? The reason for this is that we've been coached by our culture to think about healthy foods in a completely wrongheaded way. For example, you commonly hear that chocolate is a guilty pleasure that is "bad for you." Of course, that doesn't stop you: You eat it anyway, absorbing all that guilt with all that pleasure. So how did something as deliciously wonderful as chocolate get to be the bad guy? Why have we come to believe that everything fabulous must be unhealthy and that "good for your soul" must mean "bad for your body"?

I do not accept that notion. Believe it or not, chocolate is an amazing health food that is as good for your physical heart as it is for your emotional heart—and, yes, it can even be good for your waistline, too!

CHOCOLATE and the "PR" Problem

Chocolate doesn't exude malevolent health waves into the air, requiring a culinary version of a Geiger counter to sniff out the chocolaty particles before they sicken you. Nor will it make you unhealthy if you eat a milligram of it, or even a gram of it. And just as healthy people all over the earth have encouraged chocolate consumption for thousands of years, we should promote this amazing health food as a staple element of any diet.

Does that mean chocolate is a miracle food that you can eat buckets of and still be superthin and healthy? Of course not. Chocolate, like everything else, becomes bad for you when it's eaten with abandon: brilliant for you at one volume, awful for you at another. And the good news is that the volume of chocolate consumed, which determines whether it swings from good for you to bad for you, is completely up to you.

The bottom line is that we have a serious cultural "PR" problem, and that stands for "personal responsibility." For the past 40 years, we've been told that eating eggs was going to kill us.[1] Now we know that having about one egg per day is actually great for us.[2] We were told that butter was bad, that carbs were bad, that wine was bad, that beer was bad, that pizza was bad, and on and on and on. But wine actually has wonderful resveratrols, beer has beneficial B vitamins, pizza is composed of the same veggies (with all of their vitamins)—tomatoes with beneficial lycopenes, and the crust with its fiber—recommended by the USDA, and even butter has vitamins A and E and selenium (which doctors prescribe for heart health).

So while you've been told that these foods were unhealthy for you, that's not necessarily true. Food doesn't become good or bad for you until you eat it in a way that's either in control or out of control. And that is especially true of chocolate. Of course, this basic fact leads to a logical conclusion that is both good news and bad news at the same time: Whether your chocolate helps you live 10 extra years or makes you pack on 10 extra pounds is totally up to you. Many will see this as great news, because you get to be in control and determine if chocolate will be a health food. However, this also means that any weight gain brought about by chocolate has zero to do with the chocolate and everything to do with how it was eaten.

So don't have a PR problem. Own your health by taking responsibility for your eating behavior. This requires that we think differently about our food. Forget the advice of this disordered culture of health that says you're a food victim. Instead of an *abstinence approach* (avoid all chocolate because it can make you fat), we are going to adopt a *responsibility approach*: Eat the right kind of chocolate, in control. When you do this, you will get all the health benefits without eating so much that you make it bad for you.

Own Your Own Health with **CHOCOLATE**

Now is the time to finally *own your own health,* and chocolate is the perfect food to practice with. But to do that, we must have the courage to confront our culture of health, which defines what we believe about food and feeding, home and hearth, cooking and consumption. In nearly every ad and article, our culture encourages the confusion of volume and value; pushes cost-cheap, nutrient-cheap foods at us; and confuses the love of food with the love of consumption. As a result, we end up way overfed and way undernourished. Managing this roil of influences is like going for a dip in Class V rapids: Before you even know what has happened, you are lifted and tumbled and turned right over the dietary cliff.

Swimming against this chaotic cultural current isn't easy, because it hits you everywhere: in public ads, private language, and even our official health guidelines. As a consequence, we end up avoiding foods that are healthy and consuming foods that aren't. We've forgotten the eating traditions that worked for us when our country wasn't overweight, and we now lurch after the glitzy new fad diets that come at us every January: low fat, low carb, food combining, caveman, eat every 3 hours, glycemic index–based, grapefruit diet, peanut butter diet, blood type diet, cabbage soup diet, and on and on and on. Unfortunately, the direction we've received from nutrition science has been all over the map and seems as haphazard as the diet fads. If you've been paying attention to the official diet advice over the past 20 years, you know this intuitively. Remember the cholesterol that was going to kill us? Now we're told that we actually need to eat more of the (good) cholesterol foods that we were once told to avoid. On the other end of the stick, that margarine we were told to eat to "save our hearts" had the hydrogenated oils that were actually killing our hearts the entire time—contributing to up to 100,000 heart attack deaths every year.[3] That's dead people—and all because we did what we were told.

It seems like everything we thought we knew about dieting gets reversed every 5 years or so. Nuts were bad; now they're great. Coffee used to cause cancer,[4] and now it helps prevent cancer![5] The zero-calorie soft drinks we were coached to drink to prevent obesity are actually linked to weight gain: Drink $\frac{1}{2}$ to 1 can per day and your obesity risk increases by 37.5%; drink 1 to 2 cans per day and your risk increases by 54.5%; drink more than 2 cans per day and that risk increases by 57.1%![6]

Given this nutritional weirdness and absolutely Olympic-caliber flip-flopping, is anyone really surprised that the old ideas have turned out to be utterly wrong? And that brings us right back to chocolate, which is a perfect poster child for the stupendous failure of our ever-changing culture of health. This culture told you that chocolate is fattening, that its saturated fats are going to clog your arteries, that its sugars are going to make you a diabetic—and mercy, don't even get near it if you're on a diet. This is what we've always heard.

So when I say, "Of course you can eat chocolate and lose weight," you channel the messaging that's been drilled into your head, thinking that this must be some kind of 30-days-to-thinner-thighs infomercial claim to magically melt fat away. But the reason the idea of chocolate weight loss sounds so smarmy has exactly zero to do with the chocolate itself and everything to do with those crazy ways our culture of health has programmed you to think about it.

How many times have you heard chocolate called an indulgence and a decadence? You've been told to hate that you love it! And like the Class V rapids that whoosh you into the dietary abyss, this attitude encourages you to eat chocolate as a reward only after you've "been good." But being good typically means suffering through some species of low-carb, low-fat, low-flavor cardboard that's less satisfying, less delicious, and far less wonderful than chocolate. Eating chocolate is the 5 minutes of heaven you're allotted after going through diet hell.

Well now there's good news, followed immediately by more good news. First of all, nutrition science is finally catching up to common sense. The food that we were told was a dietary vice is actually a massive virtue, and not just for your heart either, but also for your weight. Write that down. Second, what everyone said was a guilty pleasure is actually just . . . a pleasure. You can subtract "guilty" altogether. In other words, you don't have to suffer to get your reward anymore, or to eat Styrofoam-tasting "food products" to lose weight.

It's funny, too, because research has discovered that chocolate is filled with molecules that are beneficial for some cardiovascular parameter. Whatever. People don't eat chocolate because they are trying to boost their biorhythms and certainly don't give it up because they aren't convinced of its antioxidant oomph. They eat chocolate because it is sensual, is delicious, makes you feel better, and goes with almost anything. And they give it up because someone convinced them that it'd make them fat.

Listen, we're turning that page. Not only can you get all the scientifically proven health benefits of this wonderful food, but also you can do it in a way that makes you lose weight in the process. You can eat chocolate every day and still lose weight. What's the trade-off? Well, you just trade in that angst and self-loathing for a smaller pair of pants. It's that simple.

Of course, I fully expect pushback from our standard health culture. I expect it to keep trying to sell the idea that chocolate is a candy: bad for you, unhealthy, and fattening. But remember that this is the very same Class V rapids culture of health that had you eating margarine (hydrogenated oil) and low-fat food products (high fructose corn syrup). And the consumption of these foods had us tumbling over the cliff the entire time.

So you actually have a choice. You can certainly just go with the standard line. Follow the fad. Tumble down the rapids, bobbing along wherever the cultural current carries you. Or you can swim sideways against the undertow of thoughts and gimmicks that has led to the most massive increase in weight and health problems the world has ever known. Whatever you want to do. (By the way, if you decide to confront this unhealthy culture of health, chocolate is the perfect place to start!)

Your Chocolate Eating Lessons

Eat Chocolate, Lose Weight consists of a six-step plan based on the Mediterranean dietary approach that I currently provide for people around the world. Based on this program, I offer principles of healthy eating, not molecule micromanagement. In other words, every time you put food in your mouth, you won't have to calculate the proportion of fats (saturated, monounsaturated, polyunsaturated) and carbohydrates (the good ones, the bad ones, the high-glycemic ones, the low-glycemic ones) as a percentage of the 2,000-calorie-per-day diet that the USDA tells us we have to consume. No healthy culture specifies that level of overt detail. None of them. And you shouldn't have to either.

In fact, tens of thousands of people have followed my approach to learn what real food really is. And in case you're wondering, chocolate is definitely a real food and it *can* help you lose weight (which you'll hear over and over again in the success stories shared throughout this book from real people who have followed my program and found success!). However, to keep that real food really healthy, you are also going to learn the healthy eating behaviors that keep you from eating so much that you make it bad for you by your own overconsumption. And to help you do this, I've included a section called "The Cocoa Q&A" in each chapter to answer the most common questions that I receive throughout my program. Sound good? Let's do this!

Here are the six steps:

Step 1: Choose the weight-*loss* chocolate, not the weight-*gain* chocolate.

Step 2: Determine the right amount of daily chocolate.

Step 3: Use chocolate to lose your sweet tooth.

Step 4: Discover *how* to eat chocolate.

Step 5: Avoid stress-induced overconsumption of chocolate.

Step 6: Use chocolate to boost your workouts.

During this process, you're going to learn *why* chocolate on the brain is actually a very good thing, *which* chocolate provides the most weight loss, *how much* is the right amount, and *how* to control consumption through your chocolate-eating behavior. And by learning how to eat chocolate, you'll also be better able to make healthy selections for all of your foods. Once you learn these "Chocolate Eating Lessons," you'll be better able to stop the chronic consumption that frustrates your weight-loss efforts. You'll lose your sweet tooth, reduce your hunger at each meal (resulting in less consumption), and help solve portion distortion. Logically, then, because eating chocolate is the poster child for your other dietary eating habits, and because it can help lead the way out of your weight problems, we should practice eating chocolate every day. Bummer, eh? Work, work, work.

Before we move forward, I need to address an issue that may be the biggest hurdle standing between you and chocolate-induced weight loss: perception. Because we've been coached by our culture to believe that chocolate is bad for you, anyone suggesting that you can eat it and still lose weight is seen as selling snake oil—a faddish hoaxer cynically hawking promises without substance or foundation of any kind. This is a valid concern. After all, new fad diets pop up year after year and promise you the moon and the stars and whatever else you want to hear. Dieters try—again—to turn promises into reality and just fail, again. It's dispiriting.

Now, here comes a book that your culture of health tells you is literally unbelievable: *Eat Chocolate, Lose Weight*. What are you to make of the seemingly surreal claim of the title itself? Too good to be true?

I can promise you this: You and I have to unlearn many of the things that our culture of health has programmed us to believe. But once you do that, "chocolate weight loss" becomes realistic, attainable, and practical in your daily life. Is it effortless? No. You've got some homework and practice to do. Can you eat all the chocolate you want all the time? Of course not. You're going to train your physiology to move in a healthy direction, and that takes actual effort on your part. But there is a middle ground. And this is the ground on which you and I can finally have an adult conversation about weight and health.

It's All in the Science

Eat Chocolate, Lose Weight is built on a foundation of research and experience. I apply my neuroscience training to inform our understanding *and implementation* of eating behavior. It applies the mind-body connection to your diet. I've provided these principles for tens of thousands of people, and those accumulated data will be revealed throughout this book.

Finally, this is the most well-researched book you will find on eating behavior as it relates to chocolate. I'll dig into the data for you and break them down into what you really need to know to succeed with this plan. Moreover, all the interviews conducted with scientists have been done to make sure my sense of the research literature is spot-on.

So open your heart and mind to the new paradigm in *Eat Chocolate, Lose Weight*. When you do, you will realize, as I did, that chocolate is not the end of weight control. It's the means.

THE COCOA Q&A

Q: These six steps sound good, but how does this all work together?

A: I have put together a structured meal plan in Chapter 9 to show you how chocolate should be applied, when it should be eaten, and what outcomes you can expect from it. Plus, the wealth of recipes in Chapter 10 shows you how to add chocolate into your life in a healthful way every day.

Chapter 1

There's Chocolate and There's "Chocolate"

Remember the rule: There's nothing so wonderful in this world, so marvelous and perfect, that someone can't come along and totally screw it up. And chocolate is a great example: It can be used as a tool to lose weight, control consumption, and live a very healthy lifestyle. But not all chocolates will do this for you, because not all of them are created equal. There are as many versions and perversions of chocolate as there are of bread and butter. And just because you pick up a wrapper that has the word "chocolate" slapped on the label doesn't mean it has a place in your new healthy lifestyle.

So the very first step for you to take in the direction of chocolate-induced weight loss is to choose the type of chocolate that will help you lose weight and to avoid the kind that will pack on the pounds. To help you understand what's good chocolate, what's average chocolate, and what's complete nastiness, this chapter will walk you through the elements of normal real chocolate, how it's made, why it's good for you, and which "chocolates" you need to avoid completely.

CHOCOLATE versus "Chocolate"

If you want to eat chocolate and lose weight doing it, you are going to have to begin with this first lesson: There's good chocolate and there's bad chocolate. The same rule applies to everything, actually. Remember when we were told that all fat was bad? By the late 1970s and early 1980s, the low-fat dogma had become entrenched and was promoted by physicians, the federal government, the food industry, and the media. We all jumped on board, even though empirical evidence that it actually led to weight loss just wasn't there.[1] Then the health advice was reversed, and we were told that some fats were actually good for you, but other fats were completely off-limits.

Next came the low-carb revolution. The Atkins-style diets became the fab fave diets du jour, and we were coached to believe that all carbs were bad. As a result, millions of people ate bacon, egg, and cheese omelets every day while avoiding the evil carbohydrate-laden items like fruit. After the perhaps predictable demise of that overly simplistic notion, even the most enthusiastic supporters of low-carb diets amended their advice: "Oops, sorry. Yes, actually there are also good carbs and bad carbs." And bread lovers all over the world breathed a collective sigh of relief. Do you see the theme yet? People make broad, sweeping generalizations, then have to eat their overportioned words. They tell us that we have to avoid every speck of some specific type of food, only to later backpedal from absolute value to nuance, from simplistic to realistic.

Cholesterol is a more recent example. That great dietary Darth Vader of the nutritional dark side turned out to have a softer side, too. At first, we were told to limit all cholesterol—yes, all of it. Now we've learned that advice was probably terrible, because cholesterol is all Jekyll-and-Hyde as well, just like the fats and the carbs that have a good side and a bad side. Right now, before you read on, I want you to guess what they're going to say about the new advice on cholesterol: There's good cholesterol (high-density lipoprotein, or HDL) and there's bad cholesterol (low-density lipoprotein, or LDL). You actually need good cholesterol. Welcome to the world of nutritional nuance.

What makes this all so confusing for ordinary people simply trying to live a healthy lifestyle is just how confident the voices are, every single time. Whether they're telling you to eat or not eat the margarine, to avoid eggs or not, to eat bread or avoid it like the plague, it's all stated with absolute conviction. The fact that their advice has been dead wrong in the past seems to have no bearing on the certainty they show now.

This same pattern of overstatement, followed by the inevitable graded retraction, will turn out to be just as true for chocolate. Chocolate is not bad. Chocolate is not something you should avoid. Chocolate is not your problem. In fact, it's your solution. The key to this distinction, just as with your carbs, fats, and cholesterol, is in knowing which is the good kind and which is the bad kind.

Although, I have to say, even the phrase "there's good chocolate and there's bad chocolate" is misleading, because all real chocolate is good chocolate. It only becomes bad when someone takes wonderful, delicious, healthful chocolate and diddles with it to the point that it has cheapened nutrition, dishwater flavor, and zero weight-loss potential. So, to sort all this out and get to the difference between chocolate and "chocolate," this chapter will cover the good, the bad, and the just plain ugly.

The Best Chocolates

All the amazing weight-loss and health benefits of chocolate come from one place and one place only: cocoa. That's all. High cocoa content equals high health benefits. Low cocoa content equals low health benefits. So, when you're browsing the zoo of chocolate choices spilling off your grocery store shelves, make sure to maximize the cocoa and minimize the rest.

Even though it sounds simple, it's about as easy as picking out a healthy breakfast cereal (which is nearly impossible). Why? Because so many brands spike plain, wonderful foods with ingredients designed to make it sound all sexy and supercharged—like when they put omega-3 fatty acids in your butter, squirt docosahexaenoic acid (DHA) in your milk, and lace faux-food fillers like synthetic sweeteners, colors, and oils into all the processed products that we're told to eat. But remember that regardless of the clever, artful, gorgeous ad campaigns, the health benefits of chocolate are not a function of these additions, but rather of the cocoa itself. So, to help you out in your struggle for chocolate-induced weight loss, here are three simple rules for finding the healthiest chocolate bar on planet Earth. Write these down, and be sure to put them in this order:

1. Darker is better.
2. Darker is better.
3. Darker is better.

Why is darker better? It's simple: You get darker chocolate when you choose versions that also have a higher cocoa content. The nice thing about this rule is that the percentage of cocoa found in chocolate is not something that marketers can gloss over. They have to be honest about the ingredients. In other words, the wrapper may say that a product will instantly turn you into a bombshell babe or a sexy stud muffin. However, the ingredient list on the back must be stated correctly by law. Therefore, find out the cocoa percentage of the chocolate product and opt for the darker (higher-cocoa) choices.

Some Solid (Chocolate) Health Advice

If you smear thin, waxy milk chocolate over a long, sugary wafer, you'll get a candy that's popular today. If you pour a veneer of the same anemic confection over caramel, you'll get another one; and over nougat, another one. But the nougat is awful for you, the caramel is just sugar concentrate, and there is nothing whatsoever about that wafer that is important for your health.

This is one of the confusions that our culture of health has created for us by dropping a small amount of something wonderful (like chocolate) into a vat of something else that happens to be terrible for you. The strawberry doesn't redeem the gummy candy, the blueberry doesn't make the

The Health Benefits of Cocoa Stand the Test of Time

This is an amazing story: W. Jeffrey Hurst, a researcher at the Hershey Company, made an incredible discovery. He found that 80-year-old cocoa powder and 116-year-old cocoa beans still retained very high levels of antioxidant activity through their flavonol content.[2] And it's not just the beans but even the cocoa itself: Hershey's cocoa powder from 80 years ago has an antioxidant value of 55.5, 50-year-old cocoa powder still retains a value of 52.7, 30-year-old cocoa powder weighs in at 56.6, and a container you would pick up from the store shelves today averages 60.2. Note: All of these values are statistically the same. In other words, cocoa powder from the Great Depression era still has the very same antioxidant power as the cocoa you could pull off the shelf at your neighborhood grocery store this afternoon! So even after all that time, the cocoa is still exceptionally good for you! To find out what happened here, I called Dr. Hurst and spoke with him over the phone.

How does a biochemist at Hershey get his experimental hands on 116-year-old cocoa beans? It turns out that he was asked to give a lecture on chocolate and cocoa at the Field Museum in Chicago. While there, the organizer mentioned that he had some cocoa beans from 1893! They had been saved from the original World's Columbian Exposition in Chicago. But there's another reason why this is so cool: These beans, which Dr. Hurst brought back to analyze in Hershey, Pennsylvania, were taken from the very same Columbian Exposition that had changed Milton Hershey's life and led to the most amazing dissemination of chocolate the world has seen.

Most people know that Milton Hershey visited the 1893 Columbian Exposition, where he witnessed the complete chocolate manufacturing operation in action. Inspired to bring this process to the world on a massive scale, he opted *not* to try to re-create it back home. Instead, he simply purchased the entire assembly, as is, and had it shipped to Lancaster, Pennsylvania, as soon as the exposition closed. Apparently he did not, however, purchase all the beans, because some of those beans remained in Chicago, at the museum, until 116 years later, when Dr. Hurst finally brought them back to analyze in the laboratories that Milton Hershey made possible in the first place.

What's the take-home message? You know how there's an exception to every rule (except the rule that there's an exception to every rule)? If your food has so many preservatives in it that it will never go bad (think Twinkies and fast-food hamburger buns), that means that bacteria won't even eat it! And a great rule of thumb is that you shouldn't eat it either, as it has got to be unhealthy for you. However, there's even an exception to this rule. And, as Dr. Hurst discovered, that exception turns out to be the cocoa in chocolate!

toaster pastry okay, and the cherry flavoring doesn't mean that cola should be used for anything other than cleaning grease stains off your driveway (the phosphoric acid in colas will actually do that for you).

This seems so rational, but it's amazing how many people are sold on a product because there's an iota of health food in it. They're sold on the good part on the front end, but left dealing with the hefty consequences of the bad part on the back end, so to speak.

So, if you really want to eat chocolate and actually lose weight doing it, don't eat wafers, caramel, or nougat. Instead, follow a simple rule: Just eat chocolate—solid dark chocolate.

Look at the chocolate you might have at home or at work. If it amounts to shellacked sugar slathered over a confection that's awful for you, put it down, step away from the vending machine, and go find some real chocolate. What I do not want is for you to use this book as your excuse to eat the overt sugars that harm your health, push you toward diabetes, and make you buy larger pants. Listen, I want you in smaller pants. So, again, just eat chocolate—solid dark chocolate.

That's not to say certain ingredients that are added to plain chocolate can't be healthy for you. For example, some solid chocolates have hazelnuts in them, and hazelnuts are great for you. Some solid chocolates have blueberries, or chile peppers, or cherries, or walnuts in them. These are perfectly acceptable additions. Why? Because they're great to eat on their own. They're real foods in their own right. For example, say you picked up a walnut, a hazelnut, or a blueberry and asked me, "Dr. Clower, is it okay for me to eat this?" I'd pause for a minute and then tell you, "Yes, of course you can. It's food. Eat it! Why are you asking me silly questions?"

However, if you asked me whether you should eat a spoonful of caramel or a nougat or wafer, I'd respectfully tell you to put the spoon down and step away from your kids' Halloween stash. In other words, if the addition to your chocolate is something that is a real food all by itself, it's okay to include as a chocolate additive. Otherwise, leave it out.

So, in case you're still bewildered by the zoo of chocolate choices out there and what you need to put into your mouth in order to eat chocolate and lose weight, there's that easy rule for you to follow: Just eat chocolate—solid dark chocolate.

What about Cocoa?

Choosing healthy cocoa should be simple because cocoa powder comes from the cocoa bean, which is definitely not a faux food. The reason we have to talk about cocoa is because our industrially produced methods have messed with normal, natural, wonderful cocoa to the point that some versions are no longer good for your health. As with fats, carbs, and cholesterol, there are even good cocoas and not-so-good cocoas. So how do you know which kinds to grab?

Don't Go Dutch

When you get plain unsweetened cocoa from the store (note: not cocoa syrup, cocoa candies or confections, or cocoa-licious breakfast cereal), the better variety is the kind that doesn't have the word "Dutch" any-where on the container: Dutch cocoa, Dutch method, Dutch shoes, Dutch flowers, going Dutch for lunch . . . nothing. Why is that? Well, if your cocoa has gone Dutch, that means that the manufacturer has taken the normal chocolate liquor and added some species of alkali to it. Alkali, chemically, is the opposite of an acid. For example, vinegar is acidic and has a very low pH. By contrast, ammonia is alkaline and has a very high pH. They're on opposite sides of the chemical coin. That said, they have the same basic effect on you—alkalis will burn your skin just like acids will, despite the fact that it will occur for opposite chemical reasons.

Normal chocolate is slightly acidic, with a pH of about 5.5 or so. When it gets all "Dutched up" with alkali, the pH rises to about 7 or 8. The question is: Why on earth would they change chocolate in the first place? It's been flawless for thousands of years—since the ancient Mesoamerican civilizations (the Aztecs and Mayans) cultivated the cocoa bean for their people and even their kings. In fact, the great Aztec king Montezuma himself reportedly drank about 50 cups of cocoa every single day. Why would our modern manufacturers mess with perfection?

I know this may surprise you, but it's not done for your benefit. I know this may stun you to your very core, but it's not done to improve chocolate's flavor, savor, or even health properties. Cocoa is altered to make it easier for the manufacturer to produce it in mass quantities. And it all started with a Dutch chemist whose name has a gracious overabundance of vowels, Coenraad Van Hoeten, who invented this process almost 300 years ago to help make the chocolate paste mix better with water. But for you to truly understand this process, first I have to explain how normal chocolate is made.

You've often heard that money doesn't grow on trees, but that's not actually true. Cocoa beans grow inside pods that are shaped like little skinny footballs and that bud right off the side of the cocoa tree trunks and limbs. And those same cocoa beans were used as currency by the Aztecs to purchase food (a small rabbit was 30 cocoa beans; a large tomato, 1 cocoa bean) and to pay wages (a porter could earn 100 beans per day). So ubiquitous was the use and utility of cocoa beans that they could even be traded for any manner of services. In fact, when the Aztecs conquered tribes, they extracted payment in cocoa beans![3]

To get to those beans in the first place, one must take them out of the football-shaped pods. Then they must be dried out in the hot Central American sun. Once they're dry, they must be fermented. (You know what's weird, though? Cocoa bean fermentation is just like sourdough bread fermentation. In both cases, during the first 24 hours all the growth is dominated by yeast. After this period, lactic acid bacteria move in to take over the process.)

Once the yeast and bacteria have had their way with your beans, they're cleaned, dried, and roasted. Up to this point, cocoa beans are treated just like their bitter cousins, coffee beans. And both types of beans need to be ground in order to expose and liberate the flavors.

Unlike coffee beans, however, cocoa beans happen to contain about 50% cocoa butter (by comparison, coffee beans contain only about 10% fat). So when you grind up the cocoa beans, the oils inside heat up. Under the high temperature of the milling process, the oils then melt and mix with the rest of the solid matter, resulting in a viscous paste. You may have heard of this paste: It's called chocolate liquor.

Now, getting that paste to combine with water was a problem for the wonky food chemists because of chocolate's high percentage of cocoa butter. That whole "oil and water don't mix" thing made it hard to mass-produce the chocolate liquor paste into the small candies you sneak from the office candy bowl.

To fix this "problem," our Dutch chemist Coenraad Van Hoeten soaked the roasted cocoa beans in alkali chemicals (either potassium or sodium carbonates) to blunt their natural acidity. In the process, he also discovered that this weakened the taste, making the chocolate liquor blander in flavor and darker in color. How much blander? Well, it didn't make the chocolate taste like chalky plastic, and you wouldn't spit it onto the floor, but the natural flavors of a paste made from simply fermented and roasted cocoa beans were lost when he chemically altered the beans with alkali.

I have to say, though, that some people like milder tastes and can't tolerate stronger tastes. So if that's you, and you're not all that into flavor, then Dutch-processed chocolate is a great solution for you. On the other hand, if you want more flavor in your chocolate, you'll want un-Dutched cocoa. And the same is true from a health perspective. Dutch-processed chocolate is still good for you, but the un-Dutched variety is just much, much better.

The Reduced Health Benefits of Dutch Cocoa

In addition to lowering the (chocolate) bar on taste, Dutch-processed cocoa has health consequences that Van Hoeten couldn't have anticipated. For example, when you dumb down the flavor, you also dramatically reduce perhaps the single most important health property of chocolate: its antioxidants.[4] In fact, in a study published in the *Journal of Agricultural and Food Chemistry,* scientists analyzed a slew of cocoa powders and chocolates to compare their levels of antioxidants.[5] Even better, they looked to see what effect, if any, mass production processing had on those antioxidant levels.

The scientists reported that the highest levels of antioxidants can be found in unripe cocoa beans. The specific form of those antioxidants in chocolate are the flavonols known as catechins and epicatechins, which are the same types of antioxidants found in other heart-healthy foods, such as tea and coffee. The next highest level of these antioxidants can be found in ripe cocoa beans, followed by unfermented cocoa beans. Fermenting and roasting the beans lowers the catechins and epicatechins by just a tad more, but once alkali is added, they are dramatically reduced.

Here are the data. Before Dutching, normal cocoa powders contain about 34 milligrams of these healthy flavonols per gram of cocoa powder, making cocoa the heart-healthiest superfood on the planet. However, according to this study, processing it with alkali can cause the antioxidant catechin and epicatechin levels in the final chocolate product to plummet by more than 90%, leaving you with only 10% of, again, the most important elements needed for your chocolate-induced weight loss.

So, if you want to lose weight, you'll need to eat chocolate that includes these particular antioxidants, which means you're more likely to be successful by not going Dutch with your cocoa. If you don't want to lose weight, don't sweat it; just keep eating the smeary, schlocky "chocolate" products.

One more reason to find chocolate that hasn't been all "Dutched up" is because the Dutching process can vary. The amount of alkali added to cocoa can vary from "light" to "medium" to "heavy," depending on the goals of the chocolate maker, and you'll have no idea which amount you're getting. We need to know this, though, because antioxidants and alkali are like buckets in a well—when one goes up, the other goes down. Lightly Dutched chocolate will shed 60% of its catechin content, medium Dutching will eat up 75%, and heavily Dutched cocoa loses a whopping 90% of its antioxidant levels.[6]

And actually, there are two forms of catechin—a "minus" form and a "plus" form (also known as its chirality). But all you need to know is that your body is better able to absorb the minus form than the plus form. And when cocoa is processed with alkali, the wonderful healthy catechins go from being mostly minus (your body can absorb them) to being more plus (your body is far less likely to absorb them). The wonderful antioxidants are still there—you're just unable to use them as efficiently. Bottom line? Look for cocoa powder and chocolates that have not been Dutched up. And you can easily find them—all you have to do is look on the label.

The Worst Chocolates: A Dietary Detective Story

You may think that the idea of chocolate-induced weight loss is impossible, but it won't be if you choose the healthy chocolates and avoid the unhealthy ones. To know the difference, start by avoiding sweeter chocolates and those with a scant amount of cocoa. Think about it. Even the phrase "white chocolate" is an oxymoron. White? Chocolate? I don't even get that. There's no cocoa in it. Do you need a diet rule that can't fail? Here's one: Don't eat oxymorons. Fat-free half-and-half? What would that even be?

As far as white chocolate goes, the actual amount of its healthy antioxidants can be rounded down to zero. The same is true of its ability to provide cocoa's beneficial properties, like lowering blood pressure.[7] Zero. So darker is definitely better. And the less milky your chocolate is, the better it is as well.

All that added milk and sugar in lighter, sweeter chocolates isn't just taking up space that should be occupied by more cocoa. Research shows that milk and sugar can actually make chocolate less healthy by blocking the body's ability to absorb the antioxidant power of cocoa itself.[8]

(continued on page 14)

What's in My Chocolate?

Since you're going to be looking at the labels on your chocolate and cocoa, we should talk about the ingredients, so you know exactly what you're getting. The list below includes the ingredients that you should expect to find in normal chocolate, along with an explanation of what they are and where they come from.

✓ **CHOCOLATE LIQUOR:** The seeds of the cocoa tree are quite bitter. You can't just pluck them and pop them into your mouth like berries. As we've discussed, those beans have to be dried out, fermented, and then roasted before they develop the chocolate flavors you love. Finally, the shell has to be taken off to get at what's called the cocoa nib. Those pieces and parts are then ground into a paste. During the process, the paste becomes liquefied so it can be poured. And that pourable stuff? That's called chocolate liquor. (It's not alcoholic, though, so no worries there.)

✓ **COCOA BUTTER:** The chocolate liquor paste is quite rich. In fact, it consists of between 50% to 58% cocoa butter, which is the vegetable oil naturally present in the bean. If you eat chocolate (and most people do), then you're going to want it to have cocoa butter, which really increases the flavor and improves the texture. Unfortunately, many manufacturers use cheaper oils like coconut and palm oil as a substitute for the cocoa butter. If you ever put a piece of chocolate in your mouth and it doesn't melt very well or it has a waxy taste and feel, it's likely been made with a cheaper cocoa butter substitute.

Some manufacturers reduce the amount of cocoa butter without adding substitute oils, but then end up with a chemical conundrum on their hands. The chocolate still has to be pourable when melted so it can be made into the shapes you expect to see in your local store's candy aisle. So, they add an emulsifier known as polyglycerol polyricinoleate (PGPR), which is a yellow liquid composed of polyglycerol esters of castor oil fatty acids.[9] Keep in mind that PGPR hasn't been found to be harmful; it just undermines the taste and dilutes the health properties of the final product.

✓ **SUGAR:** Typically, the sugar used is some form of liquid sugar, like cane or beet. It's in liquid form so it dissolves easily into the mix.

✓ **LECITHIN:** This is a natural substance (a phospholipid) found in many plants and animals. Chocolate manufacturers extract it, typically from soybeans, and put it in your chocolate so all the ingredients of the concoctions they're concocting blend together better—and also simply to make the chocolate less thick. But can we take a step back for a second? On a scale of 1 to totally whacked, how crazy is it that we put soybean extract into chocolate?

I can't imagine the Mayan and Aztec Indians stymied in their chocolate making because they just couldn't find a soybean to grind in with their mortars and pestles. Modern chocolate makers could simply use cocoa butter to thin chocolate down, but they don't because it's cheaper to use lecithin. You get the very same thinning with lecithin as you do with cocoa butter, and it takes less lecithin to achieve the same target viscosity.

So, should you avoid this food additive? Lecithin isn't harmful on its own, unless you happen to have a specific allergy to soy. However, chocolate made without lecithin will be more expensive and have a much better mouthfeel (meaning, it will be smoother and melt more easily).

✓ **VANILLA OR VANILLIN:** Isn't it funny that chocolate and vanilla are typically seen as opposite flavors? But vanilla was actually cultivated by the ancient Mesoamerican people specifically as the original flavoring additive for chocolate. (They also added spices such as chili, coriander, sage, and the petals of certain local flowers to their chocolate products.)

But what people want to know is whether we should insist on real vanilla, or whether a synthetic version is okay. To answer this question, let me just gross you out for a second. Most synthetic vanillin comes from processes using a chemical called guaiacol, which is a greasy yellow liquid that comes from wood creosote. Nice, eh?

All you have to do is mix the yellowy greasy guck with glyoxylic acid and poof—you have synthetic vanillin. Mmmm, just like Mama used to make. Sounds like something you'd like to dip strawberries into, doesn't it? Actually, even though the mad-scientist method of making vanillin has a massive *eww* factor to it, the final product is the identical molecule to that of natural vanilla and the flavor is said to be identical as well. I don't know, myself, because I'd just as soon put synthetic vanilla in my mouth as chew on a tree. But that's just me.

Dr. Mauro Serafini at Italy's National Institute for Food and Nutrition Research in Rome wanted to find out just how less healthy milk chocolate is. So he had subjects consume either plain dark chocolate, plain dark chocolate with 200 milliliters of milk, or plain milk chocolate. He made sure to insert additional antioxidants (epicatechins) into the milk chocolate to match their level in the dark chocolate. That way, he could tell how much the subjects absorbed from each. Even better, this experimental design allowed him to see how much the milk might block the antioxidant uptake.

The results were amazing. Over the next 4 hours of digestion, subjects absorbed five times more of the antioxidants from the dark chocolate as they did from the milk chocolate! In other words, any healthy aspect of milk chocolate won't even be absorbed by your body. It goes to waste (and also goes to your waist). And what about the effect of drinking a glass of milk along with your dark chocolate? The milk reduced the amount of antioxidants that subjects absorbed by about half! Why would this be?

The scientists suggested that this happened because the milk proteins bonded with the antioxidants, partially blocking the body's ability to absorb them. But if you are Sherlock, the dietary detective, you might wonder if it's the milk that's blocking the absorption of healthy antioxidants or if it's something in the dark chocolate that's boosting it. With your deductive powers, you would surmise that you needed to look at some non–dark chocolate form of cocoa to see if milk blocked the absorption of those antioxidants as well! Logically, you would put cocoa in both milk and water, and then give that to people to drink. Then you would measure the amount of antioxidants in their blood before and after they drink it and determine how much that milk blocks the absorption.

Perhaps, surprisingly, the cocoa that you and Watson dissolve in milk gets absorbed into your bloodstream pretty well—almost as well as cocoa dissolved in water.[10] In other words, milk does block antioxidant absorption, but only a little bit. Back to the drawing board!

What if we're thinking about it the wrong way? What if milk chocolate actually does lower the healthy antioxidants, but not because the milk is blocking your body from absorbing them? What if there is something extra in dark chocolate that's boosting the antioxidants? In other words, instead of it being a negative statement about the milk in milk chocolate, maybe there's just something very positive about dark chocolate that we have not considered!

Dark chocolate may provide such a higher level of antioxidants to your body because it happens to contain more cocoa butter. Yes, the very same fats we have been told to avoid actually assist in the uptake of cocoa's antioxidants![11] When animals are given a known quantity of these antioxidants, some amount makes it into their bloodstream. But when those same animals are given the same amount of the same antioxidants, but this time with added fats, the body absorbs more of them—a whopping 50% more!

In other words, there's a little bit of both going on: The milk in milk chocolate blocks your body's ability to absorb antioxidants. But that milk chocolate also has less of the cocoa butter that can boost absorption. So it's a double-whammy lose-lose scenario that leaves you with far more calories than it does nutrition.

So the case of the cocoa conundrum is now solved. And what you really need to know is that darker chocolates are great, cocoa in milk is still good, but milk chocolates are not.

Before we close this case, however, there's one more bit of bad news for milk chocolate lovers. In your chocolate bar, sugar and cocoa act as direct opposites. When one goes up, the other goes down, which means that high-cocoa chocolate contains lower amounts of sugar while low-cocoa chocolate contains higher amounts of sugar. And when you eat the versions with added sugar, it destabilizes your insulin and can create hypoglycemia, which causes you to become tired and hungry in about an hour and a half. As a result, you begin moving less and eating more, which is, of course, a recipe for weight gain.

(continued on page 18)

Defining Chocolate

I wonder what the ancient Mayans would think about us. For them, chocolate was what you get when you dry cocoa beans, let them ferment in the sun, and grind them into a paste that's whipped into a frothy drink for your neighborhood emperor sun god. But we've taken something so natural and simple and altered it with so many additions that you cannot even legally call them chocolate. In fact, our Food and Drug Administration set forth a legal definition to prevent marketers from labeling anything that happens to be brown as "chocolate." Hence, federal regulations specify how much cocoa butter, which additives, which alkalies, and so on, can be added to the confection and still have it qualify as a chocolate. How strange is it that we have to use such bizarre specificity? These regulations are every bit as contorted as chocolate is simple.

CFR—CODE OF FEDERAL REGULATIONS TITLE 21

Sec. 163.111 . . . Chocolate liquor.

(A) DESCRIPTION.

(1) Chocolate liquor is the solid or semiplastic food prepared by finely grinding cacao nibs. The fat content of the food may be adjusted by adding one or more of the optional ingredients specified in paragraph(b)(1) of this section to the cacao nibs.

    Chocolate liquor contains not less than 50 percent nor more than 60 percent by weight of cacao fat. . . .

(2) Optional alkali ingredients specified in paragraph (b)(2) of this section may be used as such in the preparation of chocolate liquor. . . .

(3) Optional neutralizing agents specified in paragraph (b)(3) of this section may be used as such in the preparation of the chocolate liquor. . . .

(4) Chocolate liquor may be spiced, flavored, or seasoned with one or more of the ingredients listed in paragraphs (b)(4), (b)(5), and (b)(6) of this section.

(B) OPTIONAL INGREDIENTS.

The following safe and suitable ingredients may be used:

(1) Cacao fat and cocoas (breakfast cocoa, cocoa, or lowfat cocoa);

(2) Alkali ingredients. Ammonium, potassium, or sodium bicarbonate, carbonate, or hydroxide, or magnesium carbonate or oxide, added as such, or in aqueous form;

(3) Neutralizing agents. Phosphoric acid, citric acid, and L-tartaric acid, added as such, or in aqueous solution;

(4) Spices, natural and artificial flavorings, ground whole nut meats, ground coffee, dried malted cereal extract, and other seasonings that do not either singly or in combination impart a flavor that imitates the flavor of chocolate, milk, or butter;

(5) Butter or milkfat; or

(6) Salt.

(C) NOMENCLATURE.

The name of the food is "chocolate liquor", "chocolate", "unsweetened chocolate", "bitter chocolate", "baking chocolate", "cooking chocolate", "chocolate coating", or "unsweetened chocolate coating".

(1) When any optional alkali ingredient specified in paragraph (b)(2) of this section is used, including those used in the preparation of the cacao nibs and cocoas from which the chocolate liquor was prepared, the name of the food shall be accompanied by the statement "Processed with alkali" or "Processed with _____", the blank being filled in with the common or usual name of the specific alkali ingredient used in the food.

(2) When any optional neutralizing agent specified in paragraph (b) (3) of this section is used, including those used in the preparation of the cacao nibs and cocoas from which the chocolate liquor was prepared, the name of the food shall be accompanied by the statement "Processed with alkali" or "Processed with _____", the blank being filled in with the common or usual name of the specific alkali ingredient used in the food.

(3) When one or more spices, flavorings, or seasonings specified in paragraphs (b)(4) and (b)(5) of this section are used in the chocolate liquor, the label shall bear an appropriate statement, e.g., "Spice added", "Flavored with _____", "Seasoned with _____", or "With _____ added", the blank being filled in with the common or usual name of the spice, flavoring, or seasoning used, in accordance with 101.22 of this chapter.

(4) When two or more of the statements in this paragraph are required, such statements may be combined in a manner that is appropriate, but not misleading.

(5) Whenever the name of the food appears on the label so conspicuously as to be easily seen under customary conditions of purchase, the statements prescribed in this section, showing optional ingredients used, shall precede or follow the name without intervening printed or graphic matter.

(D) LABEL DECLARATION.

Each of the ingredients used in the food shall be declared on the label as required by the applicable sections of parts 101 and 130 of this chapter.

So when people say that chocolate contributes to plus-size pants, it's not actually the cocoa that's doing it. It's the sugar. That's how cheap hyper-sweetened chocolates undermine your weight-loss efforts. So remember: If you want to eat chocolate and lose weight doing it, follow the rules and eat the right kind of chocolate: Solid. Dark. Chocolate.

TAKE THE
Chocolate Challenge

There are many chocolate challenges in this book for you to step up to. Some will be exactly what you need to work on, and others may be only slightly applicable. For example, if you don't have a sweet tooth, and sweets have just never been a problem for you, then the "losing your sweet tooth" challenge in Chapter 3 may be something you do for a week or so and then let go. You may pick up the exercise challenge and then put it down once you've met your goal.

But if you want to eat chocolate in a way that will help you lose weight, you *must* first challenge yourself to eat clean. Remove the additive products that are sabotaging your efforts to control your weight and health. You do that by exchanging the chocolates that increase your weight for those that help you decrease your weight.

WHAT DO I DO?

Eat clean. Start by purging your pantry of those unhealthy, weight gain–promoting chocolates so that you're only eating chocolate with the real ingredients listed in this chapter. If you are doing this chocolate challenge, the first step is to make sure you're not undermining your own efforts.

HOW DO I DO THIS?

Throw away the schlock. Let it go. Do not think to yourself, *Oh, I see, so I'll just eat my way to the bottom of this bag . . . and then I'll start being good.*

Go cold turkey. And when you are at the store, find the large rectangular bars and choose the solid dark variety.

Read the ingredient list. If you see any additive sugars, wafers, nougat, or caramel, I want you to realize that these are your little helpers en route to plus-size britches. The only exception to this rule is when your solid dark chocolate has something in it that is actually good for you on its own (such as almonds, dried cherries, chile pepper, etc.).

WHAT CAN I EXPECT WHEN I DO THIS?

Week 1: Your tastes will accommodate to the healthier chocolates. If you haven't already been eating this kind of chocolate, expect there to be an adjustment period as your body and brain transition your mouth's flavor expectations to the taste of the healthier chocolates.

How long will this transition last? There's no simple answer to that, because each person is different. The physiology of your sugar cravings, the psychology of your affections for confections, and the sociology of your environment (your spouse/co-workers/friends) all conspire to keep you locked into your old pattern of eating. And the ease with which this pattern can be broken varies from person to person. All that said, the first week is the most important, as your old patterns and preferences must be broken and new ones must be established during this time.

Weeks 2–4: The flavor of the healthier chocolates will eventually establish itself as the new normal for you. The texture will be less waxy, the flavor will be less overtly sweet, and you will actually notice an aroma! We will cover every aspect of the physical sensuality of chocolate in the following chapters, but here's what you need to look for during these next 3 weeks: Don't expect some big "aha" moment when a light switch turns on and you look to the person beside you on the subway and exclaim that there's a chocolate party going on inside your mouth. The flavor accommodation will be gradual and steady, as long as you are consistent. During these weeks, do not go back to the nasty confections you were eating before. Make the investment in your health during this important time when you're resetting your tastes.

Weeks 5–8: The longer-term effects will be stunning to you. As you continue to eat only healthy chocolate, two changes will happen during Weeks 5 to 8 that will fundamentally change your life. During this time, you will alter your tastes for the better so that you will end up making healthier choices. And you will do this not because I told you to or you're following some diet, but because you now crave healthier foods. This is absolutely key to living a healthy lifestyle.

Even better, this improvement in your taste preferences will spill over into other foods as you learn the art of discriminating good food from bad food. In Weeks 5 to 8, expect to begin seeking out other higher quality foods, just as you sought out higher-quality chocolates. And when you start choosing healthier foods because you've fundamentally shifted your tastes in a healthy direction, then you're just living a healthier life . . . for life!

HOW DO I HELP MYSELF?

See how far you've come. After the 4th week of eating healthy chocolates, check in with your tastes to see just how they've changed by using one of the cheap chocolates you used to like as a probe. First, taste the same solid dark chocolate you've enjoyed over the past 4 weeks. Take your time. Love on it. Eat it in the way you will have learned to in the remaining chapters of this book.

Then, taste the cheap chocolate you used to eat. Leave it in your mouth and note the following:

- How does the texture compare to that of the dark chocolate?

- Is it like wax, or does it melt easily in your mouth?

- How sweet is it: garishly sweet or only lightly sweet?

- How does it taste?

- Can you taste any actual cocoa, or is it totally masked by the additives?

- Does it have even an aroma of cocoa?

This is your "aha" moment. This is when you get it. Schlocky chocolate is gross, and always has been. You just never knew it before because your tastes had been so bludgeoned by sweeteners and additives that you couldn't actually taste the chocolate itself. And now that you know what good chocolate tastes like, you simply cannot "un-know" that; you cannot go back to unhealthy chocolate, because you have taken charge of your own cravings and sculpted them in a healthy way.

One more very important "aha" for you: Once you take this chocolate challenge, you'll realize how much control you can have over your cravings. You can create them, and in the process, you can finally take charge of your own health. This is a freedom from feeling like your health happens to you and you are powerless to do anything about it. In fact, knowing how much control you actually have empowers you to make the change and to keep the change for life.

When that happens, you win.

HOW CHOCOLATE SAVES YOUR DIET

As we've discussed above, "high-quality" chocolate is just another way of saying "normal chocolate": without the added fillers and junk and synthetic ingredients that make it easier for manufacturers to produce a cheap, stripped-down version with bland flavor and blunted health properties. The same principle is true for all your food, though. If you want to eat chocolate that promotes weight loss, you're going to need to be as selective about all of your food as you are about your chocolate.

So, use chocolate as an example for all of your other foods. Do a total purge of your pantry, just like you have done a purge of your schlocky, additive-laden chocolates. Find the faux foods laden with artificial stuff, and get the junk out of your chocolate, out of your cupboard, out of your diet, and out of your life. On a practical level, the downstream effect for you is that your body responds without those constant cravings for salt and sugar. Without those cravings, you get out of your body's own way, and it can "right the ship" en route to better health and those smaller pants.

Just as unadulterated chocolate (without Dutch-processed cocoa) has between 60% and 90% more of the antioxidants that are beneficial to your heart and weight than chocolates that contain heavily processed cocoa, every single other unadulterated food is better for your heart and your weight than any of the invented new "miracle" food products that show up on grocery store shelves every year.

Let's take a look at a few different foods and what happens to them when they become synthesized. We can synthesize anything in a lab, but if that thing is abstracted from the original food that it came from, it will certainly lose its health benefits. Check out the chart below, which includes a few examples of normal items versus their synthetic counterparts.

	NORMAL VERSIONS	SYNTHETIC VERSIONS
Sugar	Darker sugars have minerals that are wonderful for your heart.	Artificial sweeteners have zero health properties. They are only sweet. That's all.
Oil	Olive oil has more than 200 nutrients, improves vascular function, and is linked to diabetes control.	Hydrogenated oils have no additional health benefits and are actually linked to heart disease.
Vanilla	Vanilla contains about 200 organic compounds, all with positive health properties.	Tastes like vanilla. It's the same molecule, but contains zero health properties.

So, if you want both flavor and better health, check the ingredients list of chocolate (and all your other food) for the word "artificial" or "imitation." If you see it on the label, get something else. And this leads me to one more diet rule: Don't eat inventions. We are not invented, and if a company tries to convince you that it invented something that is healthier for you than the normal foods that grow from the earth, which our

Eat Chocolate, Lose Weight

physiology has adapted to for the past million years, then it's just selling something.

Over the next 8 weeks of this plan, resolve to eat clean! Why 8 weeks? I've found that when participants in my corporate wellness programs stick to eating real food for this period of time, they quite naturally continue to eat less sugar, less sodium, and zero synthetics. You can do this, too! And in the process, your tastes will adapt to the healthier choices, and you will eventually favor and even crave these real foods over your formerly favorite faux foods. And to think: It all starts with chocolate!

THE COCOA Q&A

Q: Now that I know how to choose normal chocolate, how can I apply this to all of my food choices?

A: People ask me what kind of milk I drink, and I respond, "Normal milk."

- What kind of butter? **Normal.**
- What kind of coffee? **Normal.**
- What kind of meat? **Normal.**

But what is "normal" food anymore? "Weird" food seems to have become the new normal, even though it is hyper-processed, modified, tainted, or enhanced. Great examples of "weird" include low-fat food products, low-carb food products, eggs without yolks, dairy without fats, and the food products that have unpronounceable chemical additives that won't even come up on your spell-checker. By contrast, normal food was alive at some point, had a mother and a father, will eventually spoil, or is something that humans have typically consumed for the past 100 years. Just eat normal food.

You get the picture. When you eat normal food, you automatically have more beneficial nutrients that come prepackaged in the things that just happen to grow right here on this very planet to be eaten by animals like us.

There's Chocolate and There's "Chocolate" 23

SUCCESS STORY
Michele Fennell

AGE: 38

POUNDS LOST: 105

CHOCOLATE TIP: *"Now I'm a little more creative with my food. I mix melted coconut oil, dark chocolate, and stevia and pour the mixture over frozen raspberries. Then I refreeze the raspberries and after they're frozen, I break them apart to eat. My family calls it 'Raspberry Crinkle.'"*

AFTER

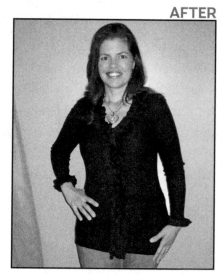

Michele Fennell had a bad history with diets. After developing type 1 diabetes in college, she yo-yo dieted for years. "None of the other plans I tried were sustainable, no matter how committed I was or how much willpower I had. I was so confused about what to eat," Michele admits. "Nothing worked—the more I dieted, the more weight I gained. I just wanted someone to tell me what to eat."

Michele especially struggled with her sugar cravings, saying that her sweet tooth ruled her life. "I couldn't go more than an hour or two without that sugar fix," she says. Fortunately, this all changed when her mother invited her to try a new program where participants actually used chocolate to help promote weight loss. A huge chocolate lover, Michele was intrigued by the idea that chocolate was not only permitted but actually encouraged in the plan.

BEFORE

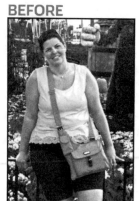

"I've always loved, loved, loved chocolate," she exclaims. "And I always felt sad because chocolate didn't seem to love me back. I actually blamed chocolate for a lot of the weight gain: the Snickers bars, the ice cream, the chocolate cake. I had a love/hate relationship with chocolate. (I even began the first day of the program with a Snickers bar in my purse.) So when I learned I could have chocolate on this plan, I was all over it."

Immediately after starting the program, Michele was surprised by how much she enjoyed the healthier, dark chocolate. "When I tasted that first bit of quality dark chocolate, I was hooked—and satisfied by it, too. It helped so much during the first few weeks of the plan, because even though I couldn't buy the Snickers bars, I could browse the dark chocolate bars, and that was a good transition. I then progressed to including chocolate in my meals," she says. In fact, Michele credits her ability to fight cravings to the piece of dark chocolate she eats at the end of each meal.

"When I would eat my chocolate 'ender,' it felt like closure. Now I could go and do other things without thinking about food," she says. And in addition to feeling satisfied, Michele also began to see other improvements. "Within the first week, I had a significant drop in my blood sugar levels. And around Week 3, I realized this was so much more than just a 'diet.'" Michele's healthy new lifestyle certainly paid off—by Week 8, she discovered she had already lost 20 pounds!

In addition to using chocolate to finally lose her sweet tooth, Michele found that consuming other "real foods" (i.e., unprocessed) further ensured her success. She explains, "I was blown away when I learned about real food versus fake food, and it changed my whole paradigm about what to eat. Instead of being so confused, I finally knew what to eat. Before I started this plan, I would think about food all the time. And now I know it was because I was depriving myself by eating processed foods with no nutrition."

And Michele's friends and family have taken note of her new diet. "They've seen the changes and my family has adopted this new lifestyle as well! My mother had some issues with her cholesterol that have settled down because she now eats according to this plan. We've simply changed the way we eat. If it's not real food, we won't eat it—it's just as simple as that."

Today, Michele is more than 100 pounds lighter, dropping from 275 pounds to 170 pounds and going from a size 22 to a size 12. In addition, her lowered blood sugar has remained stable. "When I started this plan, my A1c was 12.0 or higher. Within a year, it was down to 5.0, and I've been able to maintain that." Motivated by the positive changes in her own health and inspired to share her new paradigm with others, Michele recently returned to school to complete her degree in wellness and fitness. In addition, she went on to become a certified personal trainer.

Michele found success on the Eat Chocolate, Lose Weight plan—and notes that it's not a diet, but a lifestyle. "This plan turned my life around—I can't remember the last time I craved a candy bar!" she smiles. "Extreme diets aren't sustainable. And if anyone tells you that you have to take that pleasure component out of your food, they're missing an essential element of nutritional food. And by eating chocolate, you get to experience the process of eating that is pure pleasure."

Chapter 2

How Much Is Too Much?

Size matters. Our culture of health has amazing problems with portion control, as we're constantly coached to confuse "better" with "more." But the *only* reason these totally independent variables are conflated for you is to sell you more food products.

This chapter provides guidelines on the amount of chocolate you should be eating. And actually, these recommendations have less to do with the amount of chocolate that you'll be eating than the amount of cocoa that comes in your chocolate. But before we get started parsing your portion problems, I have to confront our bizarre culture of health.

How many times have you heard and read that chocolate makes you fat? That attitude is absurd. Chocolate does not make you fat. Overeating makes you fat. And this is true regardless of what you eat. Whether you consume high volumes of potatoes or bread or butter or carrots or rice or chili or lasagna or pizza or pasta or olives or chicken tetrazzini, you'll get fat. Are olives fattening? Is chicken fattening? Is rice fattening? Of course not. No food, on its own, sitting on your counter, outside your body, is fattening. Not one. And it's not the food's fault that you get fat from eating too much of it. I love you, but I have to tell you straight up that we simply can't blame the thing we're overeating for the fact that we're overeating.

Need a principle that works for everything from cocoa to coconuts and chocolate to chili? Eat small, be small. Eat big, be big. If you remember this one simple principle, it will help you keep your calorie consumption in control in the short term, and then help you train your physiology to expect a more appropriate amount in the long term. That's why this is a critical element. So, write that on a napkin, scribble it on your forehead, or just make a magnet to put on your refrigerator.

Now say this back to me: Chocolate doesn't make you fat. Eating too much chocolate will make you fat; eating an amount that is healthful for you will not make you fat. Thus, if you eat chocolate and get fat, it likely has very little to do with the wonderful food called chocolate and everything to do with you. In other words, chocolate is not the bad guy. Chocolate is the very, very good guy.

This means that you and I are ultimately responsible for our weight and health. You must own that responsibility, too—and not only with your chocolate but also with anything else you put in your mouth.

And I think we all know, at least intuitively, that quantity is the real issue. Having a little chocolate is fine, and we know that. But just how do you keep from eating your way to the bottom of an entire sleeve of chocolate cookies? And what is the tipping point at which the amount of healthy chocolate you consume becomes so great that it then becomes unhealthy for you?

In this chapter, we're going to discuss where that line is and exactly how much chocolate you can have each day. And just as important, you'll also learn how that amount can change based on the kind of chocolate you're eating! Because in order to eat chocolate and lose weight doing it, the daily volume needs to be a function of the species of chocolate you choose.

Your Daily Dose of **CHOCOLATE**

So let's break it down. There are two ways to look at the daily volume of chocolate you should be eating to achieve and sustain weight loss: First, you will begin by determining the appropriate amount of chocolate to eat in each bite, which will establish the amount consumed at each sitting.

Then, based on this information, you'll set the optimal amount that you should have throughout an entire day.

Allow me to be the bearer of good news: There's nothing wrong with having chocolate as a part of every single meal. In fact, I recommend it! And making this wonderful superfood a part of your daily diet is even easier when you use cocoa to flavor your cooking and when you break out a hot cocoa to warm your chilly winter evenings. Just remember that in order to keep chocolate working for weight loss, and not weight gain, the amount you have at each meal should be limited. But what does "limited" mean?

To get this amount right, we have to be very clear about which species of chocolate we're eating. Think about it: There are roughly a billion chocolate products on the shelves, in every stripe imaginable, from high-cocoa chocolate to milk chocolate to chocolate syrup to candy-coated chocolate to chocolate-covered bacon, and everything in between. There's simply no way I could give you a single rule about quantity that would apply to every confection configuration out there, and no way I could list every single product and tell you how much of each one you can have in a day.

The solution to dealing with that crazy diversity of chocolate choices, then, is to boil it all down to the lowest common denominator of chocolate health. And that element is the cocoa itself. So we have to reframe the question from "How much chocolate can I have?" to "How much cocoa can I have?"

Read the Label

When you need a chocolate fix for your chocolate cravings, check the labels and choose the item with the most cocoa. Those that are best for you will disclose how much cocoa they contain right on the front of the label. In that way, good chocolate is a lot like most healthy food. Take chicken, for example. If the chicken is free-range, it will say so right on the front of the package. If the tomato is organic or the beef is grass-fed, you won't be able to miss the notification. However, if the label says nothing more than "CHICKEN" in big giant letters, you know it was raised in a cage the size of your fist and force-fed hormone-, antibiotic-, and steroid-filled super-chicken pellets morning, noon, and night. (How do you think that Franken-chicken got that big?)

The same is true for chocolate. You can count on those that are actually awful for you to *not* tell you how much cocoa they have, because it's probably about a total of 3 micrograms. By contrast, those choices with higher levels of healthy cocoa will trumpet that right on the front of the wrapper. This is a very easy principle to follow.

Choose Your Percentage

Once you've identified the chocolates that tell you how much cocoa they contain, the next question to ask is "What percentage cocoa should I have?" With all the options, it can be hard to know which is the right choice: Is it 50%? Maybe 70%? Or 86%? Or even 100%?

Well, none of these choices is the right answer, because there is no "right" answer. None of these cocoa percentages will instantly, magically deliver better health and smaller pants. But to move toward better health, you should move up higher on the cocoa scale. (If you want to move your health in the opposite direction, then choose chocolate with less cocoa.) So your goal, then, is to get as high up on that scale as your current tastes allow. Over time you'll be able to train your tastes so that you prefer chocolates that are even darker and healthier.

If you need a target amount, though, aim to work your way up to about 70% cocoa. If you can go higher than 70%, that's better. But whatever your current cocoa tolerance, slowly work your way up from there until you reach a cocoa content of 70% or above.

Actually, that amount—70% cocoa—is becoming the standard definition of a healthy cocoa concentration because of nutrition research. It's not that nutrition science has discovered that chocolate with 70% or more cocoa makes people healthy and chocolate with 69% or less cocoa makes them unhealthy. The 70% cocoa amount is becoming the standard simply because it is the percentage that researchers often choose to use in their studies. As a matter of fact, we now hear news stories about dark chocolate and about the research showing the amazing list of benefits you can get from eating it (like heart health,[1] lower blood pressure,[2] reduced risk of diabetes,[3] improved cognitive performance,[4] brain health,[5] and so on). The latest nutrition science research provides overwhelming evidence that dark chocolate is the most amazing health food for your head, your heart, and your soul.

Again, though, keep in mind that 70% cocoa is not magic. It's just an arbitrary recommendation. I come back to this because people often ask me, "What amount of cocoa should I eat to be healthy?" They're looking for a digital answer to an analog question. They want one simple number that, when they plug it in (*pling!*), makes them instantly healthy—and with the skin, metabolism, energy, and pant size of a younger person. However, there is no one single cocoa percentage level that suddenly makes you healthy. There is no *pling!* Instead, there is a very simple principle to remember: More cocoa equals more health; less cocoa equals less health.

So let's just take the 70% cocoa chocolate as an example and ask the question again. If this is the amount of cocoa in my solid dark chocolate, *how much chocolate should I eat in order to lose weight and increase my overall health?*

Let me give you a quick example from some data. The amount of 70% cocoa chocolate you need to eat to decrease your blood pressure as you increase your heart health ranges from 6.3 grams to a whopping 100 grams daily.[6] In layman's terms, that's between 1 and 20 tablespoons of straight, 100% cocoa every day! And the woman on record as living longer than any person on earth, ever, was a Frenchwoman named Jeanne Calment. She lived to be an amazing 122 years old and ate about 2 pounds of dark chocolate per week! That's just a bit more than one entire chocolate bar (3.5 ounces, or 100 grams) a day.

Does that mean eating that much chocolate makes you live a longer, healthier life? Not necessarily, as this is simply a really interesting correlation. That said, eating such an amount of chocolate obviously didn't hurt her. But what if you're a typical person living a typical life? Some of us are more likely to eat Nesquik by the spoon than pure cocoa, and we're not likely to down more than one entire chocolate bar every day either. So how can we translate these interesting data to the real-world? And more important, how much of that will help you lose, rather than gain, even more pounds?

A research group from the University of San Diego, headed by Dr. Beatrice Golomb, looked at this exact question to correlate the amount of chocolate people consumed with their weight. They analyzed the food records of 975 men and women with an average body mass index (BMI) of 28, which would categorize a person as overweight but not quite obese. On average, this group of people ate about 1 ounce of chocolate two to five times per week. But when the researchers looked at the patterns of chocolate-eating behavior, they found that the participants who ate chocolate on a regular basis were actually thinner (had a lower BMI) than those who didn't, and it was the consistency of that consumption that was associated with a lower BMI. In fact, those who ate chocolate at least five times a week had a BMI that was, on average, a full point lower than those who didn't eat any chocolate. It didn't matter whether the subjects were male or female, how much they exercised, or even what age they were! The key weight-control factor turned out to be the consistency of chocolate consumption.

Dr. Golomb looked at these data and pointed out that even though chocolate has calories, it can also increase your basal metabolic rate. She suggested that perhaps the lower BMI in those who consistently consumed chocolate could be explained by the fact that the increase in metabolism could more than make up for any calories in the chocolate itself.[7]

This is an incredibly cool scientific question, but not all scientists are on board with this conclusion. In fact, I interviewed Dr. Lone Brinkmann Sørensen about her work showing that high-cocoa chocolate can control appetite more than low-cocoa chocolate. She wrote me with *the exact opposite conclusion* as Dr. Golomb's, stating: "I would never recommend anyone to use dark chocolate to curb their appetite, as the amount of energy they would get from the chocolate would exceed the amount of energy saved by decreasing appetite and thereby eating less food."

So perhaps it's the combination of increase in metabolism and better appetite control that explains the finding that consistent chocolate consumption is associated with a lower BMI. In other words, a higher metabolic calorie burn coupled with controlled consumption would, over time, produce the kind of BMI reduction observed. In fact, we will discuss how making use of both of these chocolate-induced benefits can help you manage your weight.

But again, it is the consistency of controlled chocolate consumption that is associated with weight control. And isn't that the way it is for everything? Consistency is what turns your well-meaning dietary intentions into healthy behaviors. For example, taking one single 30-minute stroll honestly doesn't do a great deal for your fitness level. But if you do that stroll daily, the very same amble becomes amazingly good for your fitness level, heart, and brain.[8] The same thing is true, according to the data above, regarding chocolate consumption.

So what does one full BMI point even mean? For those of you who don't do BMI calculations in your head all the time, let me give you a sense of the magnitude of this chocolate-induced change. If you are between 5 and 6 feet tall, a one-point reduction from a BMI of 30 (obese) down to a BMI of 29 (not obese) is equivalent to a 10- to 15-pound drop. So if you think about the weight you're carrying around every day, 10 to 15 extra pounds off your back, off your creaking joints, off your belly, turns out to be a lot. That, my friend, is when you get the smaller pants.

And lest you think that this is just an anecdotal finding, an October 2013 study published in the journal *Nutrition* also shows that consuming chocolate is associated with lower weight.[9] This time, however, the focus was on adolescents.

In the new study, Dr. Magdalena Cuenca García of the Department of Medical Physiology in Granada University's School of Medicine analyzed the food records of approximately 1,500 adolescents to see (1) what they were eating, and (2) how that compared to their BMIs and body fat percentages. She discovered that those who consumed the most chocolate (approximately 42 grams/day, or 1.5 ounces) also had BMIs that averaged 1.2 points lower than those who consumed the least amount of chocolate (4.7 grams/day, or 0.16 ounce). Moreover, those higher chocolate consumers also had an average of 4.6% *less* body fat. Now here's the really incredible news: This result was independent of sex, age, the amount of saturated fat consumed, the amount of fruits and vegetables consumed, and even the amount of physical activity completed by participants! So what does that mean? Basically, we can deduce that chocolate consumption may be an active driver of weight loss and actually help reduce the percentage of body fat you carry around.

And in case you haven't reached your fill, here's some even better news: For ordinary people like you and me, eating that amount (1 to 1.5 ounces of chocolate per day) just sets an amount we *know* is associated with thinness. Study participants who ate *at least* this amount of chocolate daily weighed the least and had the least body fat. Of course, this raises the next question: Just how much could you eat and still lose weight? That "upper limit" study has not been done, so we really don't know.

Honestly though, the biggest worry most people have about eating chocolate isn't that they just *can't* get themselves to eat enough of it. They're way more concerned that they might not be able to stop eating and eating and eating before they eat themselves into dietary oblivion. So when I share the data above (people who ate 1 full ounce every single day lost the most weight), I hear the giddy giggle from chocolate lovers, despite their secret fear that 1 ounce will quickly turn into one bucket, followed quickly by plus-size pants.

Self-control is the real concern. To prevent that problem, in later chapters you'll be coached on how to eat your chocolate so that you do not overconsume it. We'll talk in detail about the "how" of eating in Chapter 4. But for now, let's talk about the volume of chocolate you should shoot for and how the chocolate itself helps you control that consumption.

How Much **CHOCOLATE** You Can Eat ... in a Bite

Control consumption. Got it? Everybody hears that. Everybody knows that. But how do you *do* it, especially with chocolate? First of all, controlling portion distortion may start at your plate, but it continues in your mouth. In other words, larger portions on your plate can lead to larger bite sizes, which can lead to drastic overconsumption. Welcome to weight problems.

An interesting study shows what happens to your bite size when you're confronted by larger portions on your plate.[10] It seems as though large portions on the plate translate to bite sizes of anaconda proportions. In this study on the eating habits of children, researchers discovered that doubling the portions increases the total energy intake by 25%. That's not surprising, except that those increases were entirely due to the increased bite size taken.

With adults, the impact of bite size is amazingly similar. Research shows that adults who take big bites as opposed to small bites (three times smaller) consume approximately 25% more food.[11] So, clearly, we need a principle to follow so we can control bite size, and therefore also control eating volume, and calories, and ultimately our weight. But how does this all start with chocolate?

By determining the amount of chocolate you can have in a bite, you'll also learn how much food you should be eating in each bite you take during your meals. So how big should your bite size of chocolate be? When choosing your piece of solid dark chocolate, select one that's smaller than a golf ball but bigger than the head of a tee. Go for a piece that's just a bit smaller than a quarter but larger than a nickel. Basically, a good rule of thumb is to look at the end joint of your thumb.

How Much You Can Eat ... in a Day

Every piece of chocolate you eat has good parts and bad parts, like angels and demons, or yin and yang. These opposites coexist and duke it out in delicious unity. The good stuff is the cocoa itself, because it can help increase your sleepy metabolism[12] and reduce your food cravings.[13] As a result of these two factors, weight can be controlled in the process. The bad stuff is the sugar, because it can destabilize your insulin levels, create food cravings, and, as a result, increase your weight in the end.

If you want to increase the amount of chocolate you can have in a day, you must have more of the chocolate angels and fewer of the chocolate demons. You can have more high-cocoa dark chocolate in a day because the yin and the yang (the cocoa and the sugar) are reciprocal: When one goes up, the other goes down. Higher cocoa means lower sugar. Thus, high-cocoa chocolate maximizes the ratio between the good stuff and the bad stuff, helping to control your hunger cravings, and therefore your consumption, your calories, and your weight. It's the best of all possible chocolaty worlds.

The Chocolate "Rule of Thumb"

Here's your bite-size rule of thumb, which you should use not only for chocolate but also for all other foods.[14]

1. Standing in front of a mirror, hold up your right hand, and give yourself the thumbs-up sign.

2. Bend the top joint of your thumb down and tilt your hand back so that the tip of your thumb is facing the ceiling.

3. Lightly place your top teeth on the tip of your thumb and your bottom teeth below your bent thumb joint.

4. Now, without adjusting your bite, remove your thumb and look in the mirror. Notice how wide open your mouth is. It's huge! If you had to open your mouth any wider, you'd practically have to unhinge your jaws like an anaconda.

So this is your rule: The size of your piece of solid dark chocolate should match the end joint of your thumb. Throughout this book, I'll refer to you having one or two "thumb-size pieces" to remind you to control your bite size, which we now know leads to smaller portions.[15]

The opposite of that optimal situation is when you have low-cocoa, high-sugar milk chocolate. And if you want to eat these kinds of confections, you are allowed to eat fewer of them. That's because the good stuff (cocoa) plummets as the bad stuff (sugar) increases. If you were to write a prescription for the "how to" of weight gain, that would be it. So listen, if you are serious about getting to a healthy weight, you cannot eat these sugary confections. You must replace them with the darker varieties. Otherwise, this just won't work.

As with all things, the right amount boils down to balance: the balance between the chocolate angels and the chocolate demons. Because high-cocoa chocolate has so much more cocoa than it does sugar, it's wicked healthy for you. It's almost like a vitamin—let's call it vitamin Ch—that you need to have every day. The low-cocoa, sugary, milky chocolate has so little cocoa and so much sugar that it's terrible for you. Therefore, if you really want to lose weight, you're going to have to let those go.

The Cocoa Tipping Point

So at what cocoa level does the balance of the good stuff outweigh the detriment of the bad? The table below provides an estimate of your chocolate consumption recommendations as a function of cocoa content.

% COCOA	MAXIMUM DAILY AMOUNT	THUMB-SIZE EQUIVALENT: 1 THUMB ≈ 0.12 OUNCE
100% cocoa powder	1 cup, or ≈ 85 grams	The cocoa powder will mainly be used in cooking and not eaten on its own.
100% bar	1.5 ounces	12 thumb-size pieces
85% bar	1.25 ounces	10 thumb-size pieces
70% bar	1 ounce	8 thumb-size pieces
60% bar	0.5 ounce	4 thumb-size pieces
50% bar	0.25 ounce	2 thumb-size pieces
‹50% bar	0	0

Eat Chocolate, Lose Weight

Here's the good news. Eating delicious high-cocoa chocolate with very little sugar definitely works in your favor. So, if you want more chocolate in your life, you can have it. But you have to work your way up the scale in the table listed here to optimize your ratio of good stuff to bad stuff. But here's what you cannot do—and this is why the table is so important. You can't game the system by thinking, "Oh, I see. I need to eat more cocoa to lose weight. So, if I eat lower-cocoa milk chocolates, with less cocoa in each piece, well, then I will just have to eat *more* pieces so the total amount of cocoa will be higher!" This is a perfect strategy for weight gain and larger pants, because with your very first bite, you're getting more bad stuff than good stuff. You will lose that weight-loss battle because with every additional bite, the chocolate becomes worse and worse for your weight and your health.

That's why, according to the table, you can have more chocolate only when you have healthier chocolates with higher cocoa content. If you want to lose weight by eating chocolate, you have to increase the percentage of cocoa in your chocolate. Doing so also increases the cocoa-to-sugar ratio, which helps reduce your cravings, your calorie intake, and your weight.

THE COCOA Q&A

Q: Is there a time of day that's best for eating chocolate?

A: Not really. The effects of chocolate on weight loss are not immediate but rather a result of consistent consumption. So, in that sense, eating in the morning is no better or worse than eating in the evening or in the middle of the day. There's really no reason to be concerned about the time of day you choose to eat your chocolate. Why? Well, eating in the morning doesn't rev your metabolism, so don't think you have to eat your chocolate at that time. Likewise, the idea that you have to eat early in the evening may not be the silliest idea on earth, but it's definitely in the top five. Eating later in the evening is most common in cultures that have historically low weight, while eating early in the evening is common in the United States. So there you go.

How Much Is Too Much?

Keep in mind that the value represents the maximum you should have in a day. That doesn't mean that you *have* to eat that much. It only means you should eat no more than that amount. Likewise, if you get burned out on having chocolate with your daily meals, don't feel like you can't skip it for a day.

The issue of total chocolate volume is critical, because throughout this book we will learn a number of ways to apply that chocolate wonderfulness to your life: to control portion distortion, chronic consumption, stress-induced overeating, and your sweet tooth, and even to help with your workout. There are so many ways to make chocolate a healthy part of your diet and lifestyle that you could easily go over your daily allotment, but you have to be careful to keep the total amount under control. Otherwise, the same chocolate that is so very good for you may become bad for you in the end.

Straight 100% Unsweetened Cocoa Powder

Obviously you get the most angels and the fewest demons from 100%, un-Dutched, unsweetened, high-test, high-octane cocoa powder. That's why you can have up to 1 cup of it per day. The trouble is that most people don't eat straight cocoa powder, because it's a chalky, bitter mess. So, to dose up on cocoa, you'll have to put it into other foods that you prepare. (See Chapter 10 for recipes that are laser-focused on giving you every opportunity to increase your cocoa content.)

As we discussed, high-cocoa chocolate can increase your heart and brain health by increasing the catechin antioxidants. But where you're going to experience the impact of cocoa and high-cocoa chocolate in your day-to-day life is in your between-meal food cravings and the amount of food you desire at any given meal. Fortunately, cocoa contains elements that can help control your cravings, which is another key reason why increasing your cocoa content helps you control your weight.

How Cocoa Controls Consumption

Cocoa Protein

When you eat chocolate with your meal, it adds something very important: protein. I know you probably think of high-protein foods as relics of the low-carb phase we suffered through like we did with the embarrassing 1980s shoulder pads and feathered hair. But there actually is a massive amount of protein in cocoa! How much? Plain cocoa powder has 1 gram of protein in every tablespoon. And based on the Institute of Medicine's recommendation that adult men consume about 56 grams of protein and adult women consume 46, you may be surprised to hear what that means for your overall diet.[16] Just half a cup of cocoa provides 14% of the protein men need in a day and 17% of the protein women need. If we boil this down to a currency we all understand, a standard bar of 70% dark chocolate has between 8 and 9 grams of protein. And all of that is derived from the cocoa itself.

Increasing the protein in your chocolate is important because it increases your levels of satiety.[17] This results in reduced cravings between meals, which obviously helps you control your weight.[18] The protein in cocoa can also help reduce cravings by stimulating satiety neurohormones such as cholecystokinin, which drift up to your brain and act as the "off switch" of hunger. Neurohormones tell your brain that you're full, so you don't make it all the way to the bottom of that bag of fat-free Newtons.[19]

The above conclusions are all based on research studies, but the people who've gone through high-protein diets typically report the same thing: They're just far less hungry at meals and throughout the day. The protein content of their meals is one principal reason.

Cocoa Butter

When you say the words "cocoa butter," many people reflexively assume that it's unhealthy because we've been coached to believe that all kinds of butter are bad for your weight and your heart. In Chapter 3, we'll put that tired idea back to bed, tuck it in, and say good night for good. For now, though, let me just give you the bottom line: Cocoa butter is not unhealthy for your heart. Of course, if you eat too much of it (or of any food at all, for that matter), it will become bad for you. But that wouldn't be because of the food. It would be because you ate too much of it.

In addition, cocoa butter can promote health because it helps stimulate the satiety hormones that turn off the hunger signals in your brain. As with protein, healthy fats like cocoa butter can also stimulate anti-hunger hormones like cholecystokinin. And when you're eating less food volume and you feel satiated on fewer calories, you lose weight. This is simple math.

And the great part about this effect (besides the fact that you're getting it while eating chocolate) is that it can train your body over time to expect less food in the long term. In other words, every time you eat, you train your brain and body on that amount of food. It's as if every meal is a training event. And when you train your body on high-quality food like high-cocoa chocolate, it leads to controlled consumption in the long term. This brings the amount you're hungry for in line with the amount your physiology actually needs. In that way, the consumption of vegetable oils like cocoa butter is a part of a long-term solution to your weighty bottom-line issues.

Cocoa Fiber

You know you're supposed to have more fiber in your diet. In fact, the Institute of Medicine recommends that kids get around 10 to 15 grams per day, adult men anywhere from 30 to 38, and grown women anywhere from 21 to 25.[20] (Caveat: Women who are pregnant or lactating need a little more.)

Why is this important? Because you can reduce your risk of colon cancer by about 10% for every 10 grams of fiber you consume.[21] Plus, if you double your fiber consumption, you can lower your risk of colon cancer by 40%.[22]

And if white beans are commonly portrayed as the fiber king—

because you get 19 grams in just 1 cup—the fiber emperor is plain cocoa. That's because 1 cup of plain powdered cocoa has a whopping 32 grams of fiber. It's amazing to me that you don't hear more about this. When people are talking about beans and grains, they should also say, "Honey, you need to sprinkle cocoa throughout your life to get more of the fiber you need."

Even though the concentrated fiber found in 100% cocoa is diluted down when it's made into chocolate bars, they still offer a wonderful amount of fiber: approximately 6 grams per serving in 85% cocoa chocolate bars and about 4 grams in 70% cocoa chocolate bars.

In addition to lowering your risk of colon cancer, this also matters for your weight. Why? Because high-fiber foods increase your feeling of satiety, so you feel full before you overconsume whatever it is you're eating.[23]

Want a principle for general weight control? Add fiber-rich foods to control calories. Here are the data: If you add 14 grams of fiber per day to your diet for more than 2 days, the total daily calorie decrease is around 10%. According to this research, that works out to 4.2 pounds in just 1 month! And the heavier you are, the greater the impact that fiber can have in controlling your calories.[24]

So one of the explanations for chocolate's impact on weight control may be due to the fiber in the cocoa. This fact also reiterates the point that when you choose high-cocoa chocolate, you boost your weight-loss potential.

TAKE THE
Chocolate Challenge

Here's a chocolate challenge for you: Don't be a goldfish.

Many of us cannot say no to food. We're like goldfish in that if there's food in front of us, we eat it. "Oh look, food." And then we go hand to mouth, hand to mouth, hand to mouth until that food is gone. Why is that like a goldfish? The number-one cause of death in goldfish is the overconsumption that happens when someone spills too much food in front of them. If there's too much food in front of them, they eat it until they hurt themselves.

As for us, as smart as we are, as advanced as we like to think ourselves, overconsumption threatens to overtake tobacco as the number-one cause of preventable death. In that way, we are no smarter than goldfish.

We all know this phenomenon as the "clean your plate problem." You may have learned to eat everything in sight because you grew up in a family of 12 kids and the last one to start just didn't get any food. Or perhaps you had it drilled into you from Day 1 that eating everything on your plate somehow helped the starving children in third-world countries (I never understood that one).

Whatever the stimulus, the response is the same. Our culture of health has coached us to act like goldfish and eat for no other reason than that the food is in front us. But here's some good news:

A. We can fix this.

B. We can do it together.

C. We can do it with chocolate.

WHAT DO I DO?

First, realize that the clean-your-plate problem is nothing more than a psychological reflex. It's analogous to the physical reflex response that happens when a doctor taps your knee with a little rubber mallet and your leg lurches upward. In this case, though, the sight of food generates an internal urgency to grab it and put it in your mouth.

Unlike the physical reflex that will always be there (unless you have some kind of neurological problem), the psychological reflex is more malleable. You can change that one by either strengthening it or by weakening it. Think of it like this: Your physical reflex is *hardware,* but your psychological reflex is the *software.* You can rewrite the code.

HOW DO I DO THIS?

I'm a big believer that we can correct these psychological reflexes, not by running away from them, but by confronting them head-on. You do this by putting yourself in the condition that elicits the reflex response you're trying to break—in this case, the habit of eating mindlessly. It sounds dangerous, but here's the difference. You're going to take this challenge on your own terms and play by your own rules.

After you've had your lunch and your dinner, eat your high-cocoa chocolate to finish your meal, as usual. However, for this challenge, if you normally have two thumb-size bites of chocolate, add one more piece.

If you want to break the clean-your-plate pattern, here's what you do. Set your thumb-size pieces of chocolate out in front of you and take your time eating the first two pieces, as you normally would. You break your psychological reflex by taking that last piece and leaving it on your plate in front of you for 5 minutes after you've finished your second piece.

Just leave it there at your desk (if you're at work) or at your table (if you're at home). You don't have to stare at it or anything—just finish up your meal, talk to those around you, drink up your wine or whatever. After those 5 minutes have passed, put the third piece away, out of your sight and reach. This is the procedure.

At first, you'll do this by rote. It'll be nothing more than a mechanistic routine ("Okay, first I eat my normal amount of chocolate, then I put my "bonus" piece away, back where it belongs"). However, as you follow this procedure during the week, each and every time you intentionally leave chocolate in front of you in order to *not* eat it, you wear away at the reflex that has been determining your behavior and pushing your buttons to create the overconsumption that drives your weight problems. You break it, and it no longer breaks you.

This is how you regain control of your choices. This is how you take control of your own health again. You'll do this at first because it's nothing more than a series of items on your to-do list. But the overt series of steps will become fluid and natural over time—just as with learning to dance.

In fact, when I work with dieters in my corporate wellness programs, we find that this process creates freedom. It releases you from the drive to consume when you don't want to, and it places you in control again. The peace that comes with being in control of your food, instead of being controlled by your food, is transformational.

WHAT CAN I EXPECT WHEN I DO THIS?

How soon until you are free? How soon until you can look at food and not be driven by your own inner urges to eat yourself from here to self-loathing and back?

The reflex is more variable than the knee-jerk reaction. As I said, the knee-jerk is hardware, whereas the clean-your-plate problem is software. Because of person-to-person variability, it's really impossible to say when you will be released from it. I can tell you, though, that some people let go of it in 1 week. For others, it takes 2 or even 3 weeks.

So you are your own baseline here. Trust yourself. Keep practicing the behavioral habit of leaving something on your plate, on purpose, only to put it away at the end of the meal (in this case, you'll be doing it with chocolate).

You'll know you are close when you find yourself in a situation that would normally trigger goldfishlike eating but instead you realize that the drive is suddenly manageable. You look at the chocolate (or the food, for that matter) and find that the urge to eat and eat and eat simply isn't overwhelming anymore. You are finally getting the better of it.

You'll know you're there when the presence of food doesn't, on its own, stimulate feeding. Then you are truly free and do not have to have your decisions determined by the mere presence of chocolate.

HOW DO I HELP MYSELF?

Recognize that you are better than your urges and that you are in fact smarter than a goldfish. The psychological reflexes that drive the mindless overconsumption that frustrates your efforts are not immutable. Just as they were formed at some time in your past, they can be broken. And the angle to take in breaking them is a direct one: head-on.

HOW CHOCOLATE SAVES YOUR DIET

If you take this chocolate challenge, you will break the psychological reflex that leads you to eat so very much of this wonderful health food that you make it bad for you. And if you are going to be successful in controlling this species of mindless eating, you should apply the same choco-logic to all of your foods.

There will be times—at breakfast, lunch, or dinner—when you have eaten enough of your meal to become satisfied, but there's still food left on your plate. That's when the clean-your-plate problem pops up and you magically turn into a goldfish—"Oh look, food." And then you eat that food because your mouth wants it.

This problem is driving your overconsumption of not just chocolate but also all of your foods! So, do with your meals exactly what you're doing with your chocolate. And if you can break that psychological reflex to eat chocolate just because it's sitting in front of you (and you absolutely can!), then you can break the very same reflex that causes the clean-your-plate problem to transform you into a mindlessly overeating, overplump goldfish.

Every day for at least 2 weeks, here's what you do: Leave a couple of yummy morsels of whatever you're eating (salmon, a pork chop, chili . . . whatever) on your plate. Hang out there for a while. Finish your wine or water or tea, or just sit and talk with the people around you. After at least 5 minutes, put that food in a container, in the trash, or back in the pan.

Make yourself do this at each meal by leaving "the throwbacks" on your plate. Just as it was with your chocolate, it may seem difficult at first as you consciously take ownership over your internal psychological reflexes. They are engrained and don't want to be broken. But over the next several meals, you need to think about how that difficulty changes. Soon you'll begin to notice that the urgency eases even though it once welled up inside you to the point where you had to mentally, manually, say no to yourself. At this point, you will have applied your chocolate-eating lesson to all of your foods and started to free yourself from the mental urgency that was fueling your weight and health struggles all along.

SUCCESS STORY
Tom McFalls

AGE: 56

POUNDS LOST: 36

CHOCOLATE TIP: *"I have a bag of chocolate in my freezer at all times. I love it frozen. When it's cold, it lasts longer and I enjoy it more."*

"I was overweight and felt like I didn't have any energy. I tried a couple of different things, and nothing seemed to work for me," Tom McFalls explains.

When his physician said his blood sugar and cholesterol levels were too high, Tom knew he had to make a change. He began to search for a program that still allowed him to eat his favorite foods and discovered the Eat Chocolate, Lose Weight plan.

"I was so surprised to learn that it's okay to eat chocolate and lose weight. I love chocolate! I would eat chocolate candy bars at least a few times a week," he confesses. "It was my favorite dessert. I would choose it over anything else—except chocolate cake. So, when I found out I could have chocolate every day, I was in."

According to Tom, years of overeating and unbalanced portions contributed most to his weight struggles. "I shoved the food down my throat; I was inhaling my food and not even enjoying it. I thought I was, but I really wasn't. I learned that you need to slow down, enjoy your food, and actually taste it," Tom says—and that's exactly what he learned to do. "It was much, much easier than I expected by far. It made so much sense."

He also quickly learned how to control his portion sizes. "About 3 weeks into the program, I was sitting at the dinner table one night, and I realized I was the only one with a small plate. And I didn't feel deprived at all," he reveals.

In addition, Tom noticed a significant change in his eating habits with chocolate. "Before the program, dark chocolate tasted sour to me—it had no flavor. Halfway through, it tasted great; it tasted sweet. Now, when I eat a regular milk chocolate bar, it doesn't taste like chocolate to me," he says. "When you pull your sweet tooth, foods begin to taste better. When you have too much sugar in your diet, you do not taste how good your food is. You're missing out on the flavors."

Tom lost 10 pounds in the first 2 weeks and another 10 pounds by Week 8. Since then, he's lost another 16 pounds and has gone from a size 40 to 36. "It's amazing! I pinch myself because I can't believe I lost this much weight. People see me now and ask, 'What happened to you?' and I tell them that I started this program."

The plan has had such a positive effect on Tom that he's convinced his family and friends to try it, too. "When I told my golf partner about this program, he embraced it and lost 15 pounds in the first 3 weeks. He and his kids still eat that way."

Tom's advice for anyone thinking about trying the Eat Chocolate, Lose Weight program? Start today! "What are you waiting for? Just do it, because the longer you wait, the longer it's going to take to lose the weight," he exclaims. "You're the one who's empowered. You make your own decisions, and that's why it works."

How Much Is Too Much?

Lose Your Sweet Tooth with Chocolate

Answer this question: Do you want to manage your weight? Really? If the answer is yes, then cut the sugar from your diet. Look at the ingredients of the food products you normally purchase to identify additive sugar. Find it. Cut it out. Need a rule? *Lose the sugar, lose the weight.*

So where does that leave chocolate? Many people falsely think of chocolate as a sweet or a candy. Of course it's true that chocolate can be oversweetened, so adulterated with additives that the name "candy" certainly applies. But solid dark chocolate itself is no more a candy than cocoa-licious crispy cereals are an important part of a balanced breakfast.

When I say that you need to lose the sugar to lose the weight, that has absolutely nothing to do with solid dark chocolate. And it has everything to do with the sodas and the additive sugars in our food products.

But back to my first question. If you don't really care about controlling your weight, well then, no worries. Break out the chocolate-flavored sugar that we call candy and wash that back with a diet soda because you think it "cancels out" somewhere in your gastric netherworld. However, if you actually do want to manage your weight, then you'll identify the additive sugars in all of your food products and then cut them out. As for your chocolate, that means you should go dark.

Why You Should
Eat Dark **CHOCOLATE**

There's a very obvious reason why you should eat high-cocoa chocolate. The healthy stuff in the dark chocolate comes from the cocoa itself, and that does about a billion healthy things for you: It protects your heart, acts as an antibiotic and an antiplatelet (preventing platelets from sticking together and potentially clogging your artery wall), raises your good cholesterol, lowers your bad cholesterol, can prevent the DNA damage that can lead to tumors, can help prevent the proliferation of tumors, and can even help control blood sugar for diabetics. So eat the chocolate. You need this every day.

But there is an even more important reason why you should eat high-cocoa dark chocolate. That's because the more cocoa your chocolate has, the less sugar it will have. And the first step toward losing the weight is to lose the sugar.

I looked at one particular brand of chocolate (Lindt) to see how the calories, fat, and sugars varied for 90% cocoa, 70% cocoa, and 50% cocoa. Here is the overall change in nutrient content in Lindt chocolates (units for fat and sugars are in grams).

	90% COCOA	70% COCOA	50% COCOA	RESULT?
Calories	5.3	6.0	5.3	No difference
Fat	.50	.40	.37	35% decrease
Sugars	.08	.29	.50	84% increase

In the last column, I show the percent difference in calories, fat, and sugars between the highest levels of cocoa (90%) and the lowest levels (50%). As you go from darker to sweeter, note the changes: The calories are equivalent, the grams of fat drop by 35%, but the sugar skyrockets by 84%. The increase in sugar, along with the decrease in fat, has a terrible effect on your weight, even though the calories stay the same.

This chocolate chart sums up exactly how our culture of health has led us into the weight and health problems we find ourselves in today. Check out the first row, which shows the number of calories found, per gram, in the three kinds of chocolate. The conventional wisdom of our culture of health would tell you to choose the chocolate with the lowest percent of cocoa in order to cut the fat, even though you're adding sugar, because the calories are the same.

Does this sound familiar? Remember when we were told to eat only fat-free cookies, snack cakes, yogurts, and other junk? This strategy was a terrible failure for one main reason. When manufacturers took out the fat, they still had to make the food taste good. So how did they do that? They added sugar, and lots of it. When chocolate goes from 90% to 50% cocoa, you may lose 35% of the fat, but you gain 84% more sugar. Even though the calories are the same, the added sugar drives weight problems. Here's why.

Sugar and the "Calories In, Calories Out" Model

"Calories in, calories out." This is the idea that your weight control is about no more or less than the number of calories you eat, minus the number of calories you burn. This idea is every bit as simple as it is way, way too simplistic. Food is more than just a source of fuel, and your body doesn't treat the calories it gets from fat, or sugar, or protein like generic forms of gasoline.

It's convenient for us to view our body like a machine, as if it were made by an engineer in a lab. However, it isn't and it wasn't. Our body is a miracle of dynamic biology that developed over millions of years of relationships with the things that live and grow on this planet. Thinking about it as a simple machine that someone like us would design is intellectually inane, and necessarily false. That's why the "calories in, calories out," "food is just fuel" idea cannot, in fact, work. And actually, this notion is worse than misleading, as it also results in the drastic overconsumption that you see around you.

Why is that? Calories that come from sugar cause a different digestive reaction than the calories that come in the form of fat. In other words, even though the caloric "fuel" may be identical, the two kinds of calories swing your body in two drastically different directions.

Calories from sugar are rapidly absorbed into your bloodstream. It's as if your body senses that you need those calories right away—to get a quick energy boost so you can save yourself from the lion that surely must be chasing you across the savanna. So the sugar is pushed quickly into your system to help you in your hasty lifesaving venture. Good luck.

Thus, your body makes the assumption that you will be expending those calories right away. That's why a spike in blood sugar is met with a spike in insulin from your pancreas. Insulin is the molecule that escorts all that sugar from your secret candy stash into your muscles and organs, where—so your body thinks—you'll be using it for some snatched-from-the-jaws-of-death escape maneuver.

However, most of us aren't routinely saving ourselves from actual wild animals. Not each and every day, anyway. So on the days that your blood sugar spike results simply from your poking back Day-Glo-colored, bunny-shaped marshmallow candies at your desk, all that sugar still goes from your blood into your organs and tissues. But it's not going to get used up, because you're simply reclined in your chair, watching cute kitten videos on YouTube. Watching cute kitten videos on YouTube is an exercise in *something,* but not an exercise per se.

Because of this, that very same sugar will get stored as fat. This is how a 100% fat-free item (sugar) turns into 100% fat. It gets worse, though. Yes, sugar is stored as fat, but it causes an even more perverse action in your body. It makes you tired and hungry, so that you feel like a slug and just want to hole up on the couch with a pint of Cherry Garcia and a spoon and binge-watch *Lost* episodes on Netflix. Suddenly, you're moving less, eating more.

With a sharp rise in blood sugar in your system, your body responds by making a rush of insulin. In these cases, insulin is often overproduced to create a condition known as "reactive hyperglycemia." In other words, it's as if your body sees how much sugar is coming into your blood, estimates (based on this rapid rise) how much insulin it will need, and overcompensates.

Remember, insulin is what takes sugar out of your bloodstream. So if you overproduce insulin, you clear out too much blood sugar, and then you have nothing left in there for later. Welcome to hypoglycemia.

If you've ever had what's commonly known as the "sugar blues," which is the crash you get after eating sugary foods, you know this feeling all too well. You are shaky, feel fatigued, and may have blurry vision. You notice that you're light-headed, irritable, flushed, maybe a bit down, craving sweets (again), and just hungry. That's the outcome of eating high-sugar foods. Nice, huh?

So do the math. When you eat foods filled with sugar, those calories end up making you tired. And they end up making you hungry. If you were to line up all the strategies for weight loss and put them in order of effectiveness, this would not be in the top five. It would be closer to the big fat bottom of the list. In fact, if you want to gain weight, this might be a solution for you—if it weren't so nutritionally vacuous.

By contrast, foods with fat and fiber are metabolized more slowly, and any sugars they do have in them will arrive in your bloodstream gradually, as if delivered in a timed-release manner. No sharp sugar spike. No corresponding insulin spike. No overcompensation. No midafternoon-feel-like-you-have-to-gnaw-your-way-through-the-breakroom spike.

Not only that, but foods with natural fats in them (such as the cocoa oils found in dark chocolate) help slow the rate that the stomach empties into the small intestine. So these calories are not only metabolized more slowly, but they also take more time making their way into the small intestine, where they're ultimately absorbed into the bloodstream at a slower pace.

Eating rich, wonderful dark chocolate may cause embarrassingly audible groaning, but its cocoa butter also stimulates the production of hormones that turn off hunger (cholecystokinin, for example).[1] I know it sounds weird that chocolate—the food that some cannot seem to *stop* eating—could itself be the very solution to out-of-control consumption, but it's true. It's a funny world.

It's interesting, too, how chocolate changes eating behavior. For example, I had the opportunity to speak with a wonderful gentleman, Dr. Claudio Ferri, director of the Department of Internal Medicine and Public Health at the University of L'Aquila in Coppito, Italy. I wanted to have this conversation with him because his research compares white and dark chocolate to see which is better at improving insulin sensitivity.[2] His research team was able to show that it's not the chocolate, per se, but rather the cocoa that helps to improve your body's ability to process insulin and sugar by approximately 40%.

This supports other research showing that adults who eat dark chocolate cut between-meal cravings by 17% more than those who consume white chocolate.[3] In fact, if you take into account the calories of both dark and light chocolate, the net difference comes to 8% *less* when you eat the higher-cocoa versions. In other words, darker chocolate resulted in a decrease in calorie consumption by decreasing cravings. This may be due to the increased control over blood sugar that higher-cocoa chocolate produces.

But in our conversation, I knew that Dr. Ferri's subjects had been eating either dark or white chocolate, so I wanted to know if he'd noticed anything different between these two subgroups regarding their hunger and cravings between meals. He replied, "Believe me when I tell you this, that many people came up to me and said, 'Dr. Ferri, I am just not so hungry in the afternoons!'"

Dr. Ferri is convinced that the improvements he saw were due to the cocoa itself. In fact, the chocolate he used in his research came from the oldest chocolate factory (Bonajuto) in Modeca, Sicily. He informed me that the kings in this region of Italy were brought over from Spain and insisted that their chocolate bars be made in a very particular way. That is, the chocolate had to be made according to the original Aztec tradition. Modeca's chocolatiers even went so far as to avoid heat in the preparation, avoided Dutching, and used a mortar and pestle to grind the beans into the chocolate liquor. As a result, these chocolates had significantly more polyphenols than any other chocolate. If there is an effect of dark chocolate on the control of insulin (or hunger and cravings between meals), you'll certainly find it with those chocolates.

In any case, you get the picture here. The closer your chocolate is to its original form, the better it is for you. The fewer additives and sugars it has, the less likely it is to destabilize your sugar-insulin balance. Purer chocolate leaves you less tired, less hungry.

The Bottom Line for Your Bottom Line

Whatever the biological mechanism turns out to be, I work with thousands of participants who use dark chocolate to help control cravings between meals, so I know it works. (For more on our data with corporate groups and testimonials, see pages 84–88.) But you might be thinking that, in your case, you crave more chocolate, not less. And why would that be if people are using it to control cravings? Well, there are a couple of reasons. One could be that the chocolate you're eating is way too sweet. You're not getting the cocoa or the cocoa butter, which are very beneficial for helping you to control your consumption. Instead, what you're getting is no more than a vehicle for delivering sugar to your bloodstream. If this is the case, you are essentially dialing up the hunger knob in your brain to create cravings that may not have been there before you ate those candies. If you want to fix that problem, here is your rule: Go dark. And remember: Whenever you can, don't go Dutch.

To Go Dark,
First Train Your Brain

You may read the line above and think, "If I have to 'go dark,' I might as well give up now and drown my sorrows in a Wonderbread-and-Fluffernutter sandwich, because I don't even like dark chocolate." If that's you, then my coaching is for you to put the marshmallow jar down, put the soup spoon away, and step back from the counter. Literally thousands of people have done this in our programs, so I *know* you can, too.

Just because you don't like dark chocolate now doesn't mean that you can't get there. Likewise, just because you currently like the sweeter, less healthy chocolates, that doesn't mean you have to stay there. This chapter's chocolate challenge coaches you to teach your tastes to like the healthier options—like dark chocolate!

In neuroscience, this is called "gustatory habituation," and you've probably been through this very same thing before if you've ever switched from drinking whole milk to skim milk. If you have, you know that you can't go straight back to whole milk again, because it tastes like cream. It's gross.

But that milk did not change. The milk did not go from great to gross. It was your sense of taste that changed (meaning your brain's interpretation of the taste receptors on your tongue modified over time). In other words, the tolerance for sweet that you now have can change in any direction you wish. There is a quite a bit of leeway for you there. Now think about your current level of craving for sweeter chocolates and how great it would be if you could actually want the darker weight-loss chocolate instead of the lighter weight-gain kinds.

You can get there by taking your own brain by the lobes and by using the principles of gustatory habituation to move its preferences in the direction you want (toward darker chocolate). Once that happens, your tastes will be sculpted so that you won't even want your former faves, and your infamous "sweet tooth" will be pulled out in the process! But even better is the fact that you're going to use chocolate to get your tastes from where they are now to where you want them to be—a total win-win.

When you learn this particular chocolate-eating lesson, you won't crave high levels of sugar anymore. You will become more satisfied as the quality of your chocolate increases. Yes, size matters, but in this case, eating a smaller quantity of higher-quality chocolate allows you to enjoy the most sensual, sumptuous food on the planet and still lose weight in the process.

How Your Tastes Work

Let me tell you a story about an interesting experiment. When I was in college, my genetics professor passed around little strips of paper. Everyone got the same strips. Then he told us we were going to taste only one of four possible tastes: sweet, sour, bitter, or salty. Each person in the class would say which of the four he or she happened to taste, and the professor would tally the responses in four columns on the board.

Before we started, he said, "I predict that this classroom will have some people in every category—sweet, salty, sour, bitter—but that the ratio between them will be 9 to 3 to 3 to 1." In other words, the people who thought the strip tasted sweet would number three times more than those who thought it tasted salty or sour, and nine times more than those who thought it tasted bitter.

He made this prediction and, one by one, all the students said what they tasted. The tally emerged on the board, and it ended up exactly as he had predicted: 9:3:3:1. The reason he turned out to be Nostradamus the genetics professor wasn't because he could see the future, but because the most basic ability to taste different flavors is determined by our genes, and therefore predicted by the way dominant and recessive genes are known to segregate. That's why the percentage of those who taste these strips as sweet, salty, sour, or bitter will apply to any population of people.

That said, even though your tastes are originally hardwired by your genes, there's another element that is 100% determined by your experience. The final result that sits in your mouth is a total mixture of nature and nurture. For example, when you were born, some preferred tastes were already in place like hardware (set in stone biologically, in the same way that every group on planet Earth tastes that little strip of paper at the 9:3:3:1 ratio), while other flavor faves are like software (malleable biologically, like the ability to learn to discriminate between new flavors).

So, as you might expect, you started life with flavor preferences, just like every other human. The genetically preset taste that you sought out as a child was the sweet taste. The genetically preset taste that you rejected as a child was the taste for bitter foods.[4] This is a great built-in survival strategy, actually, as many toxic plants are bitter.

As you grow up, though, nature gives way to nurture, and flavor preferences are no longer determined exclusively by your genes. A broad eating experience begins making room for other flavors as well. Of course, because adult flavor preferences (like having a colossal sweet tooth) are created based on experience—say, if you grew up in a family that ate sweetened cereal for breakfast, fruit roll-ups and a muffin with soda for lunch, followed by Sugar Daddys and Yoo-Hoos throughout the afternoon—then your brain had little chance to develop other tastes.

In this case, your sweet tooth is likely to be monster huge, worn into a solid rut by overuse since you were a child. I love you, but I have to say that sweet is for children. Sweet is cartoons; it's Halloween; it's a Superman lunchbox. You wanted sweet when you were a child because you didn't know anything different. You want sweet as an adult because you didn't learn anything different.

Like children who look for short-term gratification, the adult preference for the sweet flavor is precisely the same. There is an immediacy to the flavor that is blunt, coarse, and without discrimination. It's a child's way—the easy way. Adults continue this behavior when they smother coffee with syrup and caramel because they still favor sweet over all. And although the bitter flavors of the coffee are actually rich and complex, they will never be revealed because they're buried in sweetness.

In the same way, the normal bitterness of chocolate consists of a broad array of wonderful flavors that are typically bludgeoned to death by cloying sweetness. Listen, I want our tastes to grow up now. Sweet was what we did when we were 5 years old. We're not 5 anymore, and we'll never learn those flavors if we don't graduate from our grade school taste: sweet.

The Secret Bitter Bonus

Secrets make things cooler. They just do. And in addition to the luscious wonderfulness of cocoa, and in addition to the fact that it's good for your heart, your head, and even your blood sugar, there's an additional bonus that no one really talks about: the fact that cocoa is bitter.

Sounds weird, doesn't it? The bitter flavor of chocolate isn't typically something that anyone dances in the street about. However, this aspect of dark chocolate can actually help you control how much you eat. And this can occur through gastrointestinal hunger hormones after you eat—or even smell!—dark chocolate.[5]

In research from the Netherlands, subjects either set 30 grams of chocolate containing 85% cocoa on their tongue to melt and swallow, or they simply smelled the chocolate. Researchers found that both those who ate the very dark chocolate and those who smelled it reported decreased levels of appetite—by as much as one-third to one-half. This appetite reduction correlated with an increase in the antihunger hormone ghrelin, indicating a potential biochemical pathway through which chocolate ingestion could decrease hunger. The reason why may have to do with the fact that the hunger hormone ghrelin also decreased at the same time. Ghrelin is a neurohormone made in your stomach, and when there's a lot of it, you're hungrier. When its levels are low, you're less hungry. The idea, then, is that very dark chocolate could crank down your appetite by turning down the circulating levels of ghrelin.

And that's not all: The bitter flavor of darker chocolates appears to have this same bonus effect (turning down your hunger cravings) for another reason. If you stimulate the taste receptors for bitter flavor in experimental animals, they show a 4-hour decrease in consumption after a meal.[6] That's 4 hours of "Nah, I'm good, thanks."

Why would that be? It may have something to do with the fact that bitter flavors, like those found in cocoa (and particularly un-Dutched cocoa) can also slow the rate that your stomach empties by 30% for 45 minutes after a meal.[7] A slowed rate of digestion can lead to a slowed rate of sugar absorption into your bloodstream, which can also help prevent the insulin overproduction that gives you the hypoglycemic "sugar blues" just 1½ hours later. You stay fuller longer, so don't need to chronically nosh your way through the afternoon every day. More energy equals more calories out, and fewer calories in due to hunger cravings.

So, to sum up: Cocoa itself has a one-two knockout punch for cravings. First, the natural vegetable oils found in very dark chocolate cut cravings by creating satiety hormones, which drift up to your brain to tell you that you're full. And they also slow the rate that your stomach empties, so you keep that signal longer. Second, the taste receptors for bitter flavors may help trigger a long-term reduction of hunger.

Good **CHOCOLATE** Gone Bad

What does overt sugar do to flavor? It makes flavor sweeter, sure. But sugar also dumbs it down so it's simpler, with fewer complex flavors, and all you taste is a swamp of sweet. The effect is that all other flavors are lost beneath the swamp. And, fair enough, many people want sweets with the sensual immediacy and complexity of a sugar pill. Got it. But super-sweetened chocolate not only works against your own weight and health, it also completely obliterates the best flavors of the cocoa.

The very same thing happens to chocolate's first cousin, coffee. Have you ever seen someone in a coffee shop order a huge pail of coffee with caramel or a flavored syrup and piles of whipped cream oozing out the plastic top? That, my friends, is no longer a coffee. It has lost the right to be called coffee. It no longer inhabits coffee-ville when a normally 5-calorie beverage mushroom-clouds into 700 calories. And while I'm ranting, don't think that the "coffee" part somehow cancels out the "iced peppermint white chocolate mocha" part or that if you just make it "skinny" (by using low-fat milk), the remaining 7 billion calories actually evaporate into the dietary ether. Let me tell you something: That coffee beverage is just as much a coffee as "cheese food" is a cheese or a choco-licious breakfast cereal is a chocolate.

And this is a real problem in our culture of health, because we know coffee is a health food, and healthy cultures eat cheese and even chocolate. But we also know that bizarre products masquerading as coffee and cheese and chocolates just aren't what they claim to be. People who consume those products can't understand why in the world they're eating these "healthy" foods yet aren't making progress on their weight and health goals.

They start to doubt themselves, thinking that maybe there's something else wrong: their metabolism, their blood type, their carbs; maybe they need more peanut butter or cabbage soup, or maybe just a brand-new pair of genes.

The way out of this trap is for our tastes to grow up. They need to expand beyond sugar and develop an understanding of, and even a desire for, more than just sweet flavors. Chocolate, for example, includes a huge spectrum of bitter flavors that you've probably avoided because you thought bitter was bad, or you just gravitate toward sweeter things. Growing our tastes is something that we can control, and we should do if we want to use chocolate to lose weight.

About That Sweet Tooth

"We have developed a colossal sweet tooth," I say to thousands of people every year, and everyone nods their head in immediate assent. "Yes, we

Eat Chocolate, Lose Weight

have," they intone. But I don't think people actually realize the breadth and depth of this problem.

We consume, on average, approximately 140 pounds of sugar per person each year. Just for a second, I want you to visualize a 1-pound bag of sugar on your counter. Got that? Now, expand that out to five 1-pound bags of sugar. Now picture 10 bags. Now start piling up those sugar bags on bags on bags, row after row on top of each other with 10 more pounds, and then 50 pounds of sugar. By this time you're running out of counter space as you get to 100 pounds of sugar. Finally, picture in your head *140 pounds of sugar!*

Again, that's how much is consumed, on average, by one single person in one single year. Now, I don't eat a lot of sugar, so someone's eating mine! From the standpoint of our weight and health problems, this is the elephant in the room that few are talking about. They'd rather discuss your fat or carb or dairy intake or points or proteins or blood type or how often you eat your little mini-meals. But maybe—and I'm just throwing this out there—maybe our ponderous poundage could be addressed by not eating 140 pounds of sugar!

Need a rule? Lose the sugar, lose the weight. In fact, much of the reason chocolate consumption can become bad for you has exactly zero to do with the cocoa and everything to do with the sugar added to it. The problem is that, at least partially, our thinking is completely wrong. For example, people approach me and say, "Dr. Clower, I eat sweets because I crave sweets." They say this as if they have no control, as if they are a victim of their taste preferences. But this is exactly upside down. They crave sweets because they eat sweets, which just makes the flavor preference for sugar grow deeper and deeper.

That's why most people feel that they're something of a slave to their urgent desire for yet another super-sweetened soda. But I'm here to tell you that those cravings are completely within your control. You can *own* your own cravings, and chocolate provides the perfect food for retaking control of this facet of your health. How can you use chocolate to curb cravings? You have to train your tastes to prefer the higher-cocoa chocolates.

TAKE THE
Chocolate Challenge

Here's your challenge: Change your tastes. You can do this, and it will take 2 to 4 weeks. Your end goal is to change your own flavor faves so that you actually come to like darker chocolates. We'll do this in a simple two-step process.

WHAT DO I DO?

First, you have to use chocolate to determine where your sweet tooth is right now. The procedure for finding this out calls for choosing a brand of solid chocolate that you like and that sells bars with a range of cocoa percentages to sample: from 30% to 40% to 50%, or 60% to 70% to 80%, for example. Once you identify the brand of chocolate that offers selections with a range of cocoa percentages, you will purchase two bars. The first bar will contain the cocoa percentage that you normally consume. (If you're unsure of what percentage your typical chocolate contains, you'll have to make an educated guess.) The second will contain the cocoa percentage that has the next highest level of cocoa—this will become your testing chocolate.

To identify the starting point of your "sweet tooth," taste your normal chocolate and write down how sweet you judge it to be on a scale of 1 to 10 (you can use the journal in Chapter 11). This is a totally subjective appreciation of sweetness, but that's okay. This upper-limit, enjoyable chocolate will serve as your daily chocolate, the one that you have with your meals and during your day, as we prescribe in later chapters.

Once you've established (a) the percentage of cocoa that is your current threshold and (b) how sweet you judge that percentage to be, you are ready for the Sweet Tooth Test itself.

For this, you'll need a piece of the chocolate you've chosen as your daily chocolate and also a piece with the next highest cocoa percentage. For example, if your daily chocolate has 50% cocoa, you'll use that and the chocolate with the next highest cocoa percentage (let's say 55% cocoa, for example). You'll need both of these to help train your brain, improve your tastes, and lose your sweet tooth for good.

HOW DO I DO THIS?

You can do this test for the first time as soon as you determine the cocoa percentages of both your current preferred chocolate and your testing chocolate. Make sure to test your sweet tooth at least once—but no more than twice—a week.

The procedure for doing this involves tasting one small square (one thumb-size piece; see Chapter 2) of the darker of the two chocolates. Remember, this will be the chocolate that seems a bit too dark for your tastes at this point. Take your time, letting it melt and linger in your mouth as long as possible. When you're done, move straight to the sweeter of the two, which is currently your daily chocolate. Let one thumb-size square of that linger on your tongue. Take a deliciously long time on this.

How long is "a deliciously long time"? Basically, simply let the chocolate melt passively on your tongue. You don't need to help it out by chewing it or even sucking on it. The temperature difference between your normal body heat (98.6°F) and the melting point of the chocolate (about 90°F) will determine the melting rate. The only caveat is that cheap chocolate, which is laced with substitute oils instead of straight cocoa butter, will not melt as easily. It will also have a waxier feel in your mouth. So there is no absolute time that you need to keep the chocolate in your mouth. Just taste and keep tasting for as long as you can make the piece last.

As your daily chocolate is melting, think about how sweet it is on a scale of 1 to 10. Write that down in your journal (see Chapter 11) and compare it with the number you wrote down when you ranked that very same chocolate the last time (unless this is your first time completing the Sweet Tooth Test). For example, in your last tasting, you might have estimated that 50% chocolate had a sweetness level of 5. What does the sweetness level seem like now? After doing this test over time, you will find that your sweet tooth is becoming more and more sensitive. Soon, the same 50% cocoa chocolate might taste like a 7, and later a 9, or even a 10.

Once you judge and write down your perceived sweetness of your daily chocolate, move back to the darker chocolate. Your job now is to determine whether the flavors of that darker chocolate still seem too bitter or taste okay. This is totally subjective. If you feel that you couldn't possibly enjoy the chocolate because it's too dark, then stay at your current cocoa percentage. However, if you feel like you could get used to this level, or perhaps that you are more excited by the flavor of the richer chocolate than you are put off by the bitterness, then you are ready to move up.

If you can move up to a higher cocoa percentage, that becomes your daily chocolate. Then, at your next Sweet Tooth Test (see "What Can I Expect When I Do This?" on the opposite page for frequency of testing), you'll compare your current daily chocolate with one that has a cocoa percentage that's just a little higher. (If you decide that you can move up to the 55% cocoa, say, then you might bring in some 65% cocoa chocolate to test next.)

Here's a summary of the process:

1. Determine your baseline daily chocolate by tasting chocolates with a range of cocoa percentages.

2. Test your sweet tooth:
   a. Taste the chocolate with the percentage of cocoa that is just a bit high for you (your testing chocolate).
   b. Taste your daily chocolate and rank its sweetness on a scale of 1 to 10.
   c. Taste the testing chocolate again, and this time rank its sweetness on a scale of 1 to 10.
   d. Determine whether your tastes have changed enough so that you can move the cocoa percentage of your daily chocolate up a bit. That determination is totally up to you and about which chocolate you can enjoy eating.

WHAT CAN I EXPECT WHEN I DO THIS?

Week after week, that very same piece of chocolate—which was originally your upper limit—will begin to taste sweeter and sweeter. This will happen for a couple of reasons. First, the act of becoming a conscious eater and tasting for the sweetness in your foods will expand your palate so you can tolerate richer, less sweet chocolates. The act of tasting darker chocolate, by itself, will drive down your sweet tooth.

Other Sources of Sugar

If you actually want to "pull" your sweet tooth, you have to find these versions of sugar in all of your food products and avoid them:

- Acesulfame potassium or acesulfame-K—marketed as Sunett or Sweet One
- Agave and agave nectar
- Aspartame—marketed as NutraSweet
- Barley malt extract
- Brown rice syrup
- Brown sugar
- Corn sugar
- Corn sweetener
- Corn syrup or corn syrup solids
- Crystalline fructose
- Dehydrated cane juice
- Dextrin
- Dextrose
- Evaporated cane juice
- Evaporated cane syrup
- Fructose
- Fruit juice concentrate
- Glucose
- High-fructose corn syrup
- Honey
- Invert sugar (golden syrup)
- Lactose
- Malt syrup
- Maltodextrin
- Maltose
- Mannitol
- Maple syrup
- Molasses
- Neotame
- Raw sugar
- Rice syrup
- Saccharin
- Saccharose
- Sorbitol
- Sorghum syrup
- Sucralose—marketed as Splenda
- Sucrose
- Sugar
- Syrup
- Treacle
- Turbinado sugar
- Xylose

However, you are also going to notice the overt sugar that is put into all of your food products. As you move away from them, your taste preferences will move along with your chocolate preferences so that you crave sugar less and less.

And this is the coolest part. As your own sensitivity for sweetness gets higher and higher, something fundamental and phenomenal occurs: You change your own nervous system in a healthy direction! You train your own brain. It's hard to overestimate how transformative this can be, as you create the freedom to finally take control over the urges that have been frustrating your efforts for your entire life.

How long will this take? Everyone's sweet tooth is different, and the total time will partly depend on how often you do the Sweet Tooth Test. I recommend doing it once or twice per week, just to see how you're progressing. Doing the test more frequently won't help you pull your sweet tooth out, but it will help you see the changes as they happen.

But the biggest factor in determining how long it takes to pull out your sweet tooth is just person-to-person variability. Some people have a sweet tooth that is innately larger, or more "impacted," so to speak, and it will take longer to remove. By contrast, others have a sweet tooth that can be "pulled out" more easily. As if that wasn't enough variability, everyone has taste receptors that adapt at their own rate—some faster and some slower. All that said, there are ways we can help ourselves and game the system in our favor.

HOW DO I HELP MYSELF?

You can dramatically speed up the process by making sure that the other foods you eat don't have added sugars in them. To pull your sweet tooth and train your tastes to appreciate higher cocoa content—leading to better heart health, a cranking metabolism, and smaller pants (all the while enjoying makes-you-moan-out-loud chocolate)—you have to find the other sugars in your life and cut them out. This includes the obvious candies along with the additive sugars that are put into most of our food products.

If you don't cut the sugar out of your food, the adaptation of your taste receptors will be much, much slower—if it happens at all.

Finally, keep in mind that this process is completely synergistic. Cutting out additive sugars in food products will help you put your cravings for sweeter chocolates to bed. But it works in the other direction, too. Eating darker and darker chocolates, with less and less sugar, helps you pull your sweet cravings for all the foods you eat. This means that you will start craving not only healthier chocolates, but also healthier foods overall.

HOW CHOCOLATE SAVES YOUR DIET

To eat chocolate and lose weight doing it, you have to, have to, *have to* pull your sweet tooth and retrain your tastes. And even if you train your tastes up from sweet to solid dark chocolate, you still won't be able to fully tame your sweet tooth using chocolate alone—try as you might!

To yank out your sweet tooth for good, use chocolate to help lead you out of your dietary mess. Just as you've done with your chocolate and the faux foods we discussed in Chapter 1, go through your pantry, find the

(continued on page 70)

THE COCOA Q&A

Q: If I want to "pull" my sweet tooth, shouldn't I eat zero-calorie "diet" sweeteners?

A: The first answer is "no," followed by "absolutely not." Artificial sweeteners are hyper-sweetened, and even though they have no calories, they can actually *increase* your sweet tooth and make you crave foods that are loaded with sugar.

In fact, if you want to increase your sweet tooth cravings, a good solution for you would be to consume zero-calorie sweeteners, because they'll do just that for you and thereby undermine your efforts. This is just one reason why the consumption of artificially sweetened beverages is associated with weight gain. And recent research from Purdue University has shown that these synthetic sweeteners are also associated with increased risk of diabetes, metabolic syndrome, and even cardiovascular disease.[8]

The best way to pull your sweet tooth is to train your tastes away from high-sugar consumption, which is exactly what you will do when you take this chapter's chocolate challenge. And that is a healthy approach that will last a lifetime.

SUCCESS STORY
Mary Reid

AGE: 36

POUNDS LOST: 36

CHOCOLATE TIP: *"Always have little chocolate chips on hand (the mini kind). That way when you have a craving, you can feel like you are eating a lot more than you actually are."*

AFTER

Two years after the birth of her daughter, Mary Reid and her husband decided to have another baby. "I had gained 55 pounds with my daughter," she says. "We were trying, but nothing was happening. My doctors said I would have an easier time if I lost some weight."

That's when Mary decided to try the Eat Chocolate, Lose Weight plan. And it didn't take long before she noticed a change in her cravings. "I'm a dessert person, and when I had to pull my sweet tooth, it was a little difficult for me at first. But once I did it, I used sugar less and less in my food," she explains. "Now I can drink black coffee without sugar in it. I don't even use artificial sweeteners anymore. (I used to use two in my coffee.) I'm now more aware of how much sugar is in food. I learned how sweet food really is."

Mary had always loved dark chocolate, and she especially enjoyed being able to try different kinds of chocolate on this program. "I tried different chocolates, and that was fun because I was like, 'Oh, let me see how dark I can go before it tastes bitter.' But I have always leaned more toward dark chocolate than milk chocolate," she says.

BEFORE

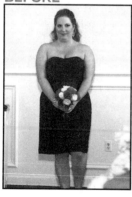

Mary had tried other programs before, but none of them worked for her in the long run. "I did other programs and lost some weight, but after that, I just went back to old habits. It just never worked. I always put the weight back on. But this plan is something that just changed the way I think about food. I'm not using it as a crutch; it's just something I learned and applied."

By the third week, she realized she could go a longer time without eating. "Normally, my brain would say, 'Okay, you ate an hour ago, so now you're hungry.' But by that point, I could hold over from lunch until dinner, and each week, the time in between my meals would get longer."

Mary decided to remain on the program after the initial 8 weeks were over and ultimately lost 36 pounds and dropped from a size 16 to a size 8. "I never wear shorts—ever. And this past summer was the first time I ever bought shorts. It was great," she exclaims. "It was very fulfilling and I felt good about it. A lot of my weight was around my waist and hips—and that's where I lost most of it."

But as good as it felt for Mary to buy a pair of summer shorts, the most rewarding part of the program was finally becoming pregnant with her son. "The week I hit the 30-pound mark (my weight-loss goal) was the week I found out I was pregnant. I really think if I hadn't lost the weight, I wouldn't be pregnant. I owe that to the program," she says.

During her first pregnancy, Mary had a lot of health issues, including water retention, high blood pressure, and preeclampsia, but she says this pregnancy has been completely different. "The entire pregnancy has been great. This time, my blood pressure was low because I was in a healthier state and eating better. I even stopped taking a daily vitamin because I was getting everything I needed from my food."

Mary experienced additional health benefits. Before starting the program, she went to a biometric screening at work, where she had her cholesterol, BMI, blood sugar, and blood pressure measured. "When I took the same screening after the program, all my numbers went down," she states.

The plan ultimately helped Mary get her life back on track. "It didn't feel like a diet because it was easy. It felt like I should have been doing it all along for my body. It's more about how I feel, how healthy I am, and how I fit into my clothes," she reveals. "What I took away was realizing what this could do for my life—not having to worry about how I have to eat certain things every day. Now, I can focus on my husband and my children."

When people ask Mary how she lost the weight, she tells them the highlights of the plan. "The great thing about it is that it's really not difficult to follow," she says. These days, Mary notes that she is both happier and healthier. "I learned to love my food again, and that's something I can pass on to my children."

products that contain sugar in all its forms, and toss them out. If you are serious about losing weight, you have to do this pantry purge.

If you don't, it's going to be really hard for you to change your cravings and to keep that sugar from creating even more weight problems than you started with. You may be able to teach your tastes to like darker and darker chocolates that contain less sugar without ridding your pantry of other sugary foods, but, honestly, you'll just be making it harder on yourself.

Chocolate can lead you out of the mess you're in and get you into some smaller pants, but you've got to help it out by purging your food products of the 140 pounds of sugar you're consuming annually. If you can manage to do this, it becomes easier and easier to sculpt your own tastes and cravings for darker chocolate.

Finally, as you retrain your tastes and get the sugar out of your life, the very same thing that is happening with your taste for chocolate (you'll *like* darker chocolate better, dislike sweeter chocolates more, and therefore choose healthier options long after you've finished reading this book) will happen with your taste for all other foods. Those super-syrupy drinks won't taste good anymore. The wicked-sweet candies will seem gross. And the bottom line for your bottom is that you'll seek out healthier foods that contain much less sugar—resulting in a lower number on that scale. Remember the rule: Lose the sugar, lose the weight. And let chocolate lead the way.

Chapter 4

The "How" of Eating Chocolate

How you eat your chocolate can determine the amount of it you eat. And the amount of chocolate you eat can determine whether this book should be called *Eat Chocolate, Lose Weight* or *Eat Chocolate, Gain Weight*. So the importance of the "how" of eating can't be overstated. And now is a perfect time to address this, because Chapter 1 covered what constitutes a good chocolate, Chapter 2 showed the first level of control at the bite and the plate, and Chapter 3 gave you the tools to pull your sweet tooth so your body mechanisms don't create cravings for more. Now we're ready to move from physiology to behavior with the "how" of eating.

The phrase "the how of eating" sounds much like "the Tao of eating," and they actually share some basic similarities. Taoists stress the process of living, rather than the adherence to reams and reams of rules and more rules. Similarly, the process of eating—the "how" of it—can help you control the amount you consume far better than some arbitrary set of strictures based on accounting for the number of carbs or fats or proteins. As mentioned in the last section, the volume of food you eat will determine whether that food is helping you gain, maintain, or lose weight. Thus, the "how" of eating turns out to be critical for ongoing chocolate weight loss and averting a very delicious dietary disaster.

For example, when I tell people I'm writing a book on chocolate and weight control, they have two reactions, one right after the other. The first reaction is to light up, eyes widening, mouth slowly opening . . . like that. The second reaction, once they reenter the atmosphere, is to ask, "Hey, how much can I have?"

And by that they mean, "I'm going to eat, and keep eating until you tell me what the absolute upper limit is, and then I will reluctantly slow down while snagging just one or two or maybe three more oh-so-small pieces for later," or something equally lame.

My response is to say, "Yes, you can eat all you want. You can have *all* the chocolate you want. All. Of. It. I want you to eat and keep eating until you are done. Then stop." When I say such things, their heads tilt sideways as their necks lose the basic ability to keep their skulls upright. Cognitive dissonance will do that.

The only reason it seems weird to say that you can eat all you want and still lose weight is because of how we've been trained by our culture to think about the phrase "all you can eat." Instead of assuming that you normally eat all you want—until you're satisfied—and then stop, we've linked the phrase "all you can eat" to wretched excess. Eating all you want is now synonymous with eating until you hate yourself and have to roll away from the couch to watch college football for 2 hours just to recover.

But that's what our culture has taught us, along with how to have a disordered relationship with food. Think about it. No healthy culture specifies how much chocolate can be eaten or micromanages the carbs and calories and points and proteins that can be consumed. No one (but us) measures out a "racquetball size" portion of vegetables or specifies a "deck of cards" size portion of meat in order to keep people from eating so much that they hurt themselves. And no healthy culture measures out allotments of chocolate and says, "Well, that's all I can have."

Healthy people in healthy cultures enjoy the chocolate they eat, until they're done with it. They eat all they want. Then they stop. They just want less because the amount they eat is kept in check by *how* they eat it. With your chocolate, this is your goal.

Don't Eat **CHOCOLATE** Like I Say

What a curious confluence of history that two of the most influential souls ever produced by our species lived more than $2^1/_2$ millennia before us, at the very same time. Confucius and Lao-tzu founded the philosophies of Confucianism and Taoism, respectively, and are even said to have met each other. But they weren't buddies. In fact, their viewpoints were just as opposite as yin and yang.

Both men faced a country scarred by political corruption and personal suffering. It was a complete mess, and they advised opposite ways to clean it up. The same could be said of the weight and health problems that we face today. Our dysfunctional culture of health has contributed to global obesity, diabetes, and all the suffering that goes along with them. It's a complete mess now, too.

Confucius, who had held the position of minister of crime, was overt and heavy-handed. He wanted to make rules for all behavior in order to institute civic obedience. So he made a slew of "Confucius says" rules. Lots of them. You had to memorize them and do exactly what they told you to do. By analogy, our traditional diets create a calculus for you to derive which poly- or monounsaturated, low-glycemic-load, protein-equivalent molecules you should eat, and precisely what ratio of this to that to the other you should have in your mashed potatoes as a function of a 2,000-calorie-per-day multimeal, multigrain diet. And if that's not enough, don't forget exactly what time of day you should eat those meals and the exact food combinations each dish should contain.

Lao-tzu took a step back. Instead of trying to regulate the specifics of every single behavior, he suggested that one should work from general principles. "Tao" actually means the "way of nature," and literally, "the path." Look around you for the principles given to us in this world. Follow those guides and the exact molecular minutia becomes academic. What's right in principle will become right in practice. How could it be otherwise?

For our diet, weight, and health, we have been directed down the long Confucian road of drastically overregulating our foods and behaviors. And while the Confucian goal of perfection by prescription is certainly possible, it's exhausting. Our adaptation of this standard approach to diet strategy could work, but who can do that every day? That's why you can stay on these diets for a good solid 3 weeks (if you're lucky) before you fall off them again. Rules chafe. Lives are complicated and chaotic.

The opposite approach is to step away from dietary micromanagement and apply the Taoist way to your diet. Eat all you want, just want less. I spoke to Dr. Yoko Arisaka, a former philosophy professor at the University of San Francisco who is now a lecturer at the University of Hildesheim in Germany, about this, and she penned an explanation much more elegant than I possibly could:

> We are originally and naturally designed to know how to nourish ourselves—that is in the Tao already, so we just need to let go of our "junk knowledge" along with junk food and junk nutrition advice and junk diet, and return to our original nature. We all have the power in us to recover that, as it is already there. We just have to trust ourselves. This is Taoist empowerment.

This strikes true. In our bog of confusing minutia, we've been coached to wring our hands for the past 50 years about the importance of calorie counting, molecule micromanagement, and outsmarting the body into weight loss. The problem is that rules are static. You are not. The world is not.

If you adopt a more Taoist approach with your chocolate, the thing that makes it bad for you—you overeating it—becomes self-limiting. You have all you need inside you (inside your original nature) to hear your body tell you when you are satisfied and when you need to stop. Once you know how to listen to your body, you can eat all you want—because you will be wanting less. And when wanting less becomes second nature, it will change your life.

How to Eat All You Want—
Just Want Less

So how do you translate a philosophy into a practical guide to eating chocolate without bingeing? First, choose the right strategy of eating. Basically, there are two choices, and each extends from a type of knowledge:

1. **Confucian strategy:** Rely on your head (which is cerebral knowledge).
2. **Taoist strategy:** Rely on your body (which is internal, somatic knowledge).

By cerebral knowledge, I mean the intellect necessary to (a) learn all the rules of behavior and (b) keep up with how many macromolecules you need in your daily allotment. Again, welcome to our Confucian world that tells you to count how many carbs and fats and points and proteins fit into an actuarial table of allotted values. It's exhausting, and you've probably already done this. You've added up your carbs, you've added up your fat grams, you've micromanaged points, and so on. How's that working out for you?

Applied to chocolate, the cerebral strategy will tell you to just have a certain quota each day (in ounces, grams, teaspoons, or drams). But this is equally weak, because everyone's body is different. Every single physiology needs a different amount of calories and nutrients based on genetics, metabolism, exercise habits, thyroid activity, daily exercise levels, and daily diet. Given this raucous chaos of person-to-person variability, what are the chances that any one-size-fits-all accounting scheme is going to be what you happen to need for your body? Zero-ish. The one-size-fits-all solution fits almost no one.

That's one problem with using the cerebral model to control your chocolate consumption. The tougher problem with this strategy, though, is that the *stop eating* signal must be cerebral as well. How much you eat must be prespecified in a tome of rules that you must remember and then adhere to. In other words, you must have enough willpower to stop when you reach your allotted amount. And you may be able to do that once, or even twice. But how long will that last—especially when you're trying to control chocolate consumption using willpower alone?

You know how Rock beats Scissors, Scissors beats Paper, and Paper beats Rock? Well, Chocolate beats Willpower almost every time. You know yourself well enough to understand how slippery that slope can be when you just have a bit and a bite, and another bit and another bite, until you've eaten way too much. If chocolate's chocolaty wonderfulness is the gas pedal that causes you to eat more of it, your willpower is a terrible brake pedal.

The second method of controlling your chocolate consumption is more Taoist and relies on body knowledge. Some people refer to this as mindful eating. This body (or somatic) knowledge adds "sensual eating" into the mix. When you taste your food, and take your time with it, and notice what you're eating and how you feel around it, you are able to hear the internal cues that let you know you have gone far enough. In this case, the stop signal is internal, not external.

This can be scary for people because they have to give up overt, cerebral control. They have to let go. Stop white-knuckling the wheel. What I have observed in thousands of participants in this approach is that the volume of food they desire becomes self-limiting. Using this Taoist, "inside-out" method, they eat all they want, but just want less.

This is a much better approach because it gets around the impossibility of having to become some kind of dietary actuary, accounting for molecules all the time, and the control of portions is expressed internally through your new eating behaviors (not externally through arbitrary rules upon rules upon rules). Learned habits, if they're good ones, work on autopilot.

Your Hunger Level Is a Moving Target

There's another reason that sensual eating through a Taoist approach is a better strategy for controlling how much chocolate you eat. The amount of food you feel the need to eat is completely changeable. Someone might prescribe a specific amount for you, but that could be more or less than you happen to need. However, if you listen to your body, it will tell you the exact amount that you should eat based on your specific needs, and not on some arbitrary value someone else has dictated. If you know anyone who has any weight to lose, then the amount of food they desire is greater than the amount they need. Those who want to lose weight, of all people, need to turn down the hunger meter so that the "want" falls in line with the "need." And you can do just that by becoming a sensual eater.

This applies just as much to all foods as it does to chocolate. For example, if you now eat your chocolate with a serving spoon, ladle, or other large kitchen utensil, that's because you're hungry for a bizarre and unhealthy amount. However, that volume can be changed so that you're hungry for a smaller pile—an amount that's actually good for you.

By the way, this adaptation process can happen in reverse, too. People who've had gastric bypass surgery (the Roux-en-Y procedure) will be left with a stomach the size of a golf ball that is able to hold about 2 tablespoons of food. However, their stomachs will stretch back out if they eat poorly—not because of the quality of food choices but because of the quantity.[1]

Think about that. You can alter the physical capacity of the stomach itself. That is the very most basic level at which you change the volume you are hungry for. The good news is that you can increase your cravings or decrease them as you wish. So if you're a little freaked out by the thought of eating chocolate, because you normally eat too much of it, just bear in mind that you are going to change that amount by dialing down your cravings.

Of course, as with everything, you cannot start at the end. If right now, for example, you eat way more than you should, you won't be able to dial that all the way down to the perfect level for your body all at once. You'll have to move your body in a healthy direction in increments. This is a process of changing some very basic elements of your physiology.

So, how do you change the amount of chocolate your body is hungry for? You do this by training it to expect a more appropriate amount over time. That means you mustn't think about the precise quantity of chocolate (or any food, for that matter) as being too much or too little. The amount you are hungry for, right now, just is what it is. We just need to move that baseline amount in a healthy direction.

The Change Begins in Your Brain

This may be surprising news, but the cravings you have for chocolate don't come from your stomach. They're actually driven by the sputtering neurons inside your brain.[2] So the key to controlling how much chocolate you're hungry for is to know how to reach into your own brain and turn down the chocolate-noshing knob.

As weird as it sounds, a large part of your brain training happens with your teeth and tongue. When you put chocolate into your mouth, never, *ever* chew it. If you do, this wonderful food will spend more time in your gullet than on your tongue, which directly impacts your brain's ability to control cravings. (There is an exception to this principle, actually, which I'll touch on in Chapter 5.) If you leave the chocolate on your palate as long as possible and just let it melt there, the sensory neural response undergoes something called "habituation," which dials down the cravings for that very thing—in this case, chocolate.

In fact, a research group at Northwestern University had subjects undergo brain scans while letting pieces of their favorite chocolate (either dark chocolate or milk chocolate) slowly melt on their tongues, just as we have you do for your starter and ender (which I will discuss shortly).[3] The researchers found that over time, "subjects commonly reported that the chocolate still tasted pleasant, but that they did not want to eat any more." This effect is called "sensory-specific satiety," which means that one particular sense (taste) becomes saturated, and therefore satisfied, with one particular food (chocolate).

In this study, over a period of seven scans, the subjects' desire for more chocolate dropped from "I really want another piece" to "I do not want to eat any more" to even "Eating more would make me sick." This growing aversion to chocolate mirrored specific changes in brain activity in the region involved in judging the value of incoming stimuli. Either this change in brain activity was causing the satiety effect, or it was reflecting it. Either way, to get your brain to move from the first pattern to the second, you must ensure that the chocolate spends more time on your palate and less time in your gullet!

Try this experiment on yourself. Get a piece of solid dark chocolate that's the size of the end joint of your thumb—no larger. Place that piece on your tongue. You can move your tongue around in your mouth, but do not chew the chocolate, and make sure it stays on your taste buds.

Now, good chocolate melts at around 90°F. Because our body temperature averages 98.6°F, the temperature difference between your mouth and the melting point of the chocolate means that it slowly melts in there and releases its flavors. And that thumb-size piece of chocolate that might look absurdly small to you at first will actually give you 2 to 3 minutes of nonstop chocolate wonderfulness.

It is the constant contact of the chocolate with your very, very happy taste buds that allows the sensory-specific satiety to kick in. People tell me all the time that this eating practice allows them to be able to control the amount of chocolate they consume. They changed how they ate it—tasting it more, chewing it less, and finally feeling that they have at least some measure of control in getting their brain to turn on the "satisfied" signal.

The total time the chocolate spends on your palate is the key factor. It's almost as if your brain wants to taste a certain amount of chocolate in order to be satisfied. So if you chew-swallow, chew-swallow, chew-swallow, then you never actually taste the chocolate. If you never actually taste it,

SUCCESS STORY
Jake A.*

AGE: 38
POUNDS LOST: 50
CHOCOLATE TIP: *"I add peanut butter to my dark chocolate meal ender, and this makes me more satisfied throughout the night."*

A former football player, Jake had trouble controlling his weight after his college days ended. And once he became a father of three and began a career that required him to sit behind a desk all day, Jake didn't know how to change his eating habits to fit his new lifestyle. "You eat a certain way as an athlete and continue to eat this way even though your amount of training decreases as you get older," he explains. "You never learn how to control it. I knew how to diet appropriately for weight lifting and other athletic activities—you either cut out all carbs or you cut out all fats. I could easily lose weight on those types of plans but could never sustain it."

This all changed when Jake attended Dr. Clower's presentation where the audience sampled the dark chocolate included in the Eat Chocolate, Lose Weight plan. This was a revolutionary moment for Jake, who loved indulging in candy.

"I have three kids, so there's frequently candy in the house, and I would eat the milk chocolate," he says. "But ever since I started eating the dark chocolate, I have no desire to eat milk chocolate anymore. It's not as satisfying. Now, I eat my dark chocolate after dinner to prevent late-night snacking."

Jake also made other changes to improve his health. "I began eating real food three times a day as opposed to the six meals I was consuming before I began the plan. It simplified my life. In addition, I made an effort to eat slowly to prevent snacking later. With this program, I learned to read the signs of my body and how much food it needs."

And Jake's changes paid off in just a few months. "Once I changed my eating style while continuing my exercise regimen, I was able to eat less and feel fuller. After about 3 months, my pants actually fit and my belly wasn't hanging over my belt. By 6 months, I was buying new clothes."

Today, Jake is 50 pounds lighter, 7 inches thinner, and more energetic than ever. He smiles and says, "It's been over a year, and I've been able to maintain my weight loss. I tend to be very reserved and laid back, but at the same time, it's really nice to hear all the compliments I receive. And it's great to be able to teach my kids how to ride their bikes and be able to run along with them and not lose my breath." On top of these benefits, Jake is still able to enjoy the food he loves. "I enjoy a lot of foods that are looked down upon in the fitness industry, like cheese, pasta, and olive oil," he says, "but this plan enables you to enjoy food the way it was intended to taste."

Name has been changed.

you have to eat a ton more of it before you sense the satiety signals from your brain. However, if a single piece melts onto your grateful taste buds, you enjoy all the flavor present in that thumb-sized morsel. That's when the sensory satiety kicks in and your brain switches on the "satisfied" signal. In other words, tasting it more causes you to eat it less; gaining flavor and losing weight in the process (another win-win).

And actually, just watch the behaviors of those who overeat and therefore have trouble with their weight. They eat very quickly, without tasting their food. It's as if they want to get it over with, or perhaps the thing they crave is not food at all but rather the act of consumption. Take a clear and honest look at yourself. Do you really love chocolate—or just the act of consuming it? You have a chance, right here, right now, to change that so you no longer confuse love with consumption.

The bottom line is that if you want to control consumption with chocolate, you have to eat like healthy people eat—slowly, in control. You want to spend as much time as possible with the chocolate on your taste buds. That's your principle.

Pace Controls Portion

Portion distortion is a primary driver of our ever-expanding, Spanx-splitting weight problems. And if you lose the portion distortion battle with chocolate, it works against you even more. To fix this problem, so you can have your weight loss and eat your chocolate, too, you have to slow down.

How much you're hungry for is only partly a function of the amount of "gas in your tank." Your hunger is also driven by how fast you eat your food. The old saying that it takes about 20 minutes for your brain to register that you're full is roughly true. The neuroscience explanation for that comes down to the satiety signals that tell your brain to turn off your hunger.[4] These signals originate from many places: your stomach, your small intestine, and even your middle intestine.

Once your food stimulates the release of all these neurohormones, they drift back up to about seven different satiety centers across the brain. These have to sum up to the feeling of fullness. However, by the time the food gets down into your gastric netherworld and triggers the satiety signals, which must then find their way back up to your brain, it's been a while. Thus, you can be absolutely full—stuffed, even—though you just haven't felt it yet because you haven't given your body a chance to hear the signals.

Need a dietary principle? What we find with our participants is that the faster you eat, the hungrier you are. The slower you eat (to a point), the less hungry you are. There is some research support for this observation as well. Women in one study, by doing nothing more than eating a meal in 30 minutes and setting the fork down between bites rather than eating a meal in 10 minutes with no breaks in consumption, decreased their calories by more than 10 percent.[5] Decreasing how much you are hungry for by 10 percent at every meal—simply by spending more time tasting it!—is one of the most useful and delicious dietary habits I can think of.

I've already talked about why this reduced hunger at the level of your tongue is true—because the sensory-specific satiety can't kick in to slow you down if you mindlessly chew-swallow, chew-swallow, chew-swallow. However, it's just as true at the level of your digestive system. If you eat quickly, without listening to your own internal cues, you're more likely to overeat while you're waiting for your body to send its satiety stop signals. Pace, then, is critical for both levels of control over the amount of chocolate you consume. Learning this lesson allows your body to register satiety so that you stop before you overdo it.

So, allow your chocolate to spend plenty of time in your mouth. Your goal with this is not to finish as quickly as possible but rather to get as much pleasure out of the chocolate as you can. When you do, your body's natural mechanisms turn off cravings: in your mouth through sensory-specific satiety and in your gut through the hormones that cause your brain to sense satisfaction. (If you are looking for a physiological substrate that explains how our Taoist approach works by listening to the natural mechanisms that are already present in your body, this would be it.) In other words, taking more time with the chocolate leaves you needing, and wanting, less of it. Exactly how long should you leave it on your tongue? *Puh-lease.* I'm just not going to specify the minutia for you. Leave the chocolate on your palate until it melts and is gone. That's how long.

When to Eat Your **CHOCOLATE**

Isn't it deliciously ironic that one item on planet Earth that the most people have the most trouble consuming the least of is chocolate, and yet chocolate is the very substance that can help them control consumption in the first place—and therefore control calories and ultimately weight. In other words, the item we most fear as a driver of our weight problem can be its solution.

Before Your Meals

You can use chocolate to control consumption before you even begin a meal. As we discussed, eating dark chocolate before a meal makes you consume significantly fewer calories during that meal (17% fewer calories) than eating sweeter milk chocolate.[6] In Chapter 3, we also showed that darker chocolate may have more fat and less sugar than lighter, sweeter chocolate, but equivalent calories. Thus, if you eat dark chocolate before a meal, the additional chocolaty calories can be offset by a reduction in the calories you consume at the plate. Why would that be?

The cocoa butter in chocolate can slow the rate of digestion, so you absorb food more slowly. This prevents the rapid spike of blood sugar from triggering the insulin that removes energy from your blood, leaving you tired and hungry. And we now know that chocolate also triggers the release of satiety signals from your gut that turn off hunger. Combine this with the fact that chocolate left to linger lovingly on the palate creates sensory-specific satiety—and all of this happens before you ever sit down for dinner!

By using chocolate to help prevent cravings before you start eating, you're more likely to be in control when eating other foods, and you won't overconsume them in a way that makes them become bad for you. In other words, instead of chocolate being the food you are the most afraid of because it causes your calorie intake to spin out of control, you actually need to embrace it precisely because it can help you rein in those meal-time calories in the first place. Chocolate is not your problem; it's your solution. So a solution for chocolate weight loss is for you to add chocolate as a regular starter to your meals.

That's the good news. The caution is that in the study cited above, subjects ate 100 grams of chocolate 2 hours prior to a meal. A whole 100 grams! That's equal to 3.5 ounces of chocolate, or one of those large bars. I'm not going to advise you to eat that much chocolate before a single meal. How much then? If you're using dark chocolate, one thumb-size piece is all you need before lunch, and another before dinner.

After Your Meals

In my wellness programs, I coach people all over the world to incorporate something called "the ender" into their daily dietary habits. The ender is what you eat after your meal is over. Think of it as a rich, wonderful, audible-groaning punctuation mark at the end of your meal.

In Mediterranean countries such as France, Italy, and Spain, you might get something like cheese after your lunch or dinner. Not cheese food, aerosol spray cheese, or that neon nacho cheese plastic, but the full-fat stuff. That's what thin, healthy people eat every day.

When we apply the ender technique in our programs, participants typically reduce between-meal snacking because they're just not hungry anymore. Figure 1 is taken from a post-program survey of more than 1,300 participants who were asked, "Have you decreased your between-meal snacking?" The answer: Fully 68.7% said yes, 12.7% said no, and 18.6% said that between-meal snacking was never really an issue for them.

Figure 1

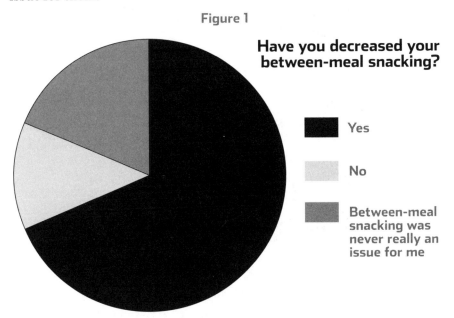

Have you decreased your between-meal snacking?

■ Yes

☐ No

▨ Between-meal snacking was never really an issue for me

These participants were also asked to indicate the number of between-meal snacks they typically had before, and then after using the ender technique of our program. The average number of between-meal snacks that this population had prior to adding the ender to their lives was 2.92 (see Figure 2 on page 86). Think about that for just a minute. What if you were having three meals per day, plus about three snacks in between meals on top of that? You'd be eating all the time!

However, after practicing the ender technique, the average number of snacks people were hungry for dropped from almost 3 to only 1.37. More than half of their daily snacking calories disappeared after they added an ender to both their lunch and their dinner. It's important to note that participants did not control chronic consumption because they micromanaged molecules (the Confucian approach). The control was not from an external set of rules on top of more rules. They succeeded because they were not as hungry and responded to internal cues from their body.

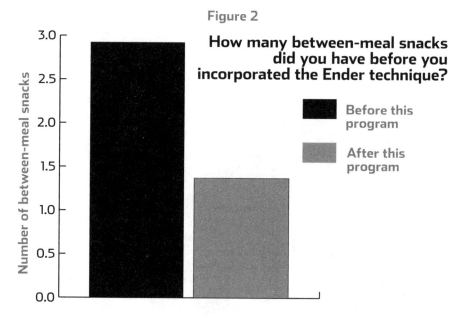

Figure 2

How many between-meal snacks did you have before you incorporated the Ender technique?

Before this program

After this program

Number of between-meal snacks

A thoughtful person may ask, "What does the reduction of between-meal snacking have to do with the amount of food eaten at the meal itself?" After all, a current fad diet that coaches people to eat every 3 hours suggests that eating fewer between-meal snacks will lead to eating more at the following meal itself. So let's test that little theory.

After 8 weeks of cutting between-meal snacking by more than half and substantially returning to a three-meals-per-day pattern (by the way, this is the same three-meals-per-day pattern we used about 50 years ago when we were healthier and thinner than we are today), here's what we found.

Participants did not in fact increase the amount of food consumed at meals. In fact, an amazing 85.1% of them reported actually *decreasing the amount* they consumed at mealtimes (see Figure 3). Only 3.3% reported increasing the amount they ate at mealtimes and 11.5% reported that they didn't need to control their portions. Furthermore, of those who reduced portions at the plate:

- Fully 51.8% reduced them by one-quarter.

- Another 23.6% reduced them by one-third.

Eat Chocolate, Lose Weight

- Another 9.9% reduced them by one-half.

- A total of 1.5% reduced them by more than one-half.

- And 13.2% found they didn't actually need to reduce them.

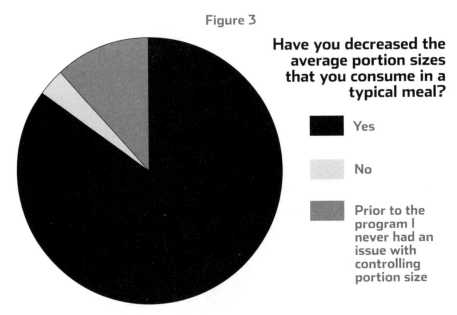

Figure 3

Have you decreased the average portion sizes that you consume in a typical meal?

Yes

No

Prior to the program I never had an issue with controlling portion size

So, while you're having your chocolate, just do the math. It's not tough math, and you won't need a calculator, a slide rule, or even an abacus. Less consumption at the plate plus less consumption between meals should equal reduced calories, and that should equal less weight, right? It's simple arithmetic.

This idea, of course, also disagrees with the eat-every-3-hours scheme. According to this idea, if you do not eat every 3 hours, your metabolism will shut down, driving your body into the so-called starvation mode, in which your body holds on to its fat. This, we are told, prevents you from losing weight.

We can test this little dietary whopper as well, to see the effect that cutting between-meal snacking has on weight itself. As it turns out, this is not just a dietary whopper. It's a whopper with cheese. Despite adding the wonderful rich, delicious, decadent, audible-groaning ender to their lunches and dinners, despite eating small at the plate and cutting between-meal snacking by more than half, participants did in fact lose weight. Duh. This is a total victory for common sense.

Of the 1,300-plus participants, 59.8% indicated that they had lost weight (see Figure 4). Another 20.9% said that they didn't lose weight, and 19.3% said they didn't need to lose weight (many people join the program just to learn how they or their children can eat better). Average weight loss after 8 weeks of postmeal enders and reduced between-meal consumption was 7.1 pounds.

Figure 4

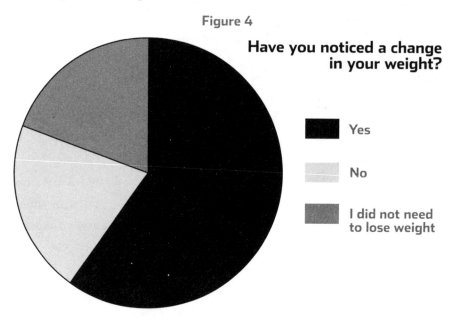

Have you noticed a change in your weight?

Yes

No

I did not need to lose weight

So yes, these data just reiterate that you can add chocolate to your life and lose weight by doing it. You really can stop eating all the time and still lose weight. So eat chocolate in control and in association with your meals. When you do, expect to see the results in yourself that I see with my clients globally. You will, on average, be better able to control volume at the meal. Plus, you'll be less likely to have to snack between meals. You'll eat all you want at the plate, but just be hungry for less. It's honestly no surprise that you'll lose weight. After all, when you're not eating your way through the afternoon, because you're just not as hungry, those extra pounds will disappear. In Chapter 7, I'm going to talk about another element—increased activity—which also helps you along this route. Moreover, it turns out that chocolate can help you with that as well.

TAKE THE
Chocolate Challenge

Here's a definite challenge for you: Eat all you want—just want less. To do that, you will need to become a conscious eater and increase your awareness of the natural mechanisms within your body. Learning the internal cues of satiety and satisfaction allows you to discard the standard dietary strategy of overt molecule micromanagement.

WHAT DO I DO?

First of all, even though you will use chocolate to control consumption, don't think about it in a mechanistic or reductionist way, abstracted from your eating habits. It's not some medicinal "one-a-day" for you to take like some silly vitamin pill. It's not a pill, and it's certainly not a weight-loss drug. It's an amazing food that needs to complement your daily routines, such as regular meals.

So include your daily chocolate as a wraparound to your meal, as both the starter and ender to your lunches and your dinners. The key, of course, is to follow the guidelines laid out in prior chapters. That is, to make sure your daily chocolate is as solid and as dark as your sweet tooth currently allows. Chocolate's satiating properties will affect the amount you consume at meals. Just do not overconsume your chocolate.

HOW DO I DO THIS?

Reserve one or two thumb-size pieces of your daily chocolate as the starter to your lunch and another one or two as the starter to your dinner.

Do the same for your ender: Reserve one or two thumb-size pieces as the ender to your lunch and another one or two to follow your dinner.

For your starter, it will take about 30 minutes to an hour for the satiety-producing effects of the chocolate to kick in. So between 30 and 45 minutes before your meal, have your starter piece and make it last as long as possible.

For both the starter and the ender, use the "how" of eating described in this chapter. Leave the very small piece on your palate and let it slowly melt onto your grateful tongue. Taste the rich, nutty, tannic flavors in your chocolate. "Love on" your chocolate.

WHAT CAN I EXPECT WHEN I DO THIS?

Here's what you're looking for: Your starter chocolate will have an impact on the amount of food you are hungry for at the meal. For this to work, though, you have to pay attention to the level of satisfaction you experience while you're eating. As you move through your meal, check in with your body to judge whether you're satisfied yet. Once you reach that point, stop.

THE COCOA Q&A

Q: If I have more chocolate as my starter and ender, will I be able to better control my portions and snacking?

A: Nope, sorry. More is not better, no matter how much you want it to be.

The beneficial impact of chocolate to control portion distortion and between-meal munchies will not improve by adding more. The optimal amount for every person will be different, but it is safe to say that you should stick to one thumb-size piece (two tops) of high-cocoa chocolate as a starter and an ender.

The key, of course, is that the increased calories of the high-cocoa chocolate should be more than made up for by the effects of the chocolate: increased metabolism + increased energy + decreased consumption at meals + decreased consumption between meals.

Expect the amount of food you'll be hungry for at the meal to lessen, because of the chocolate. How much it decreases is totally variable and depends on your current level of overconsumption. Just how much your current consumptive "wants" exceed your current consumptive "needs" will impact the degree of this decrease.

Tune in. Note how your hunger and cravings change over time. Note how it feels to listen for, and actually hear, your body's internal stop signal. Expect that the amount your body actually needs is smaller than you've been coached to believe (hence the weight concerns, right?). Be at peace with, and trust the mechanisms of, your physiology when it tells you it's satisfied.

For the ender, wait 5 to 15 minutes after your meal and have your thumb-size piece. You'll then eat it just as you did the starter, by leaving it on your palate, taking your time, and focusing on flavor and taste.

Here's what to expect. As I've shown above, the addition of the ender makes the food you ate more likely to stick with you over time. In other words, you'll be less likely to get the munchies between meals. To begin with, I want you to simply take note of how the ender lengthens the time between the end of your meal and the next time you become hungry. It increases that time by allowing you to better utilize the food you do have on board.

If you normally get hungry in the afternoons around a certain time, say 2:30 p.m., see if the ender extends that to 3:00 or 3:30, or even all the way through the afternoon. Write down the new time to keep track of it. Likewise, if you typically get hungry later in the evenings, notice how the ender reduces that craving. Again, when that occurs, write it down to give yourself a record of how your cravings are coming under control over time.

Finally, expect to get better at hearing the signals from your body as you practice. At first, it may be tough to sense satiety and satisfaction because you have so little experience doing it. But becoming self-aware is a skill. You have to practice it and train it like a muscle. The more you attend to the ways of your body, its path, its Tao, the easier you'll be able to hear and respond to it. Don't be discouraged by this. Just continue to attend to the signals your body is sending you.

HOW DO I HELP MYSELF?

One of the best things you can do to help your body align how much it wants with how much it actually needs for weight control is to sleep well. Do not skimp on this! In fact, for the next 8 weeks, I want you to be very rigorous about getting in bed at an early hour and making sure you get plenty of sleep.

The reason this is so important is that lack of sleep can be taken by your body as an internal stressor, which can create cravings. Notice what happens the day after you've had an awful night's sleep. You find that you are noshy through the day! That hunger is probably not because you're "out of fuel" but because of how your body interprets the stressful nature of sleep deprivation. So, if you want to help yourself out, get some serious shut-eye during the next 8 weeks.

HOW CHOCOLATE SAVES YOUR DIET

Chocolate is brilliant. I get that. But as wonderful as it is, you cannot expect chocolate to overcome the other bad habits that are working against it. If you want your chocolate to help you succeed—and let me tell you, you want your chocolate to help you succeed—then you have to apply these chocolate-eating lessons across the board, to all of your eating behaviors.

How do you do that? In the immortal words of Inigo Montoya, "*Let me 'splain. No, there is too much. Let me sum up.*"

Start with good-quality chocolate, which simply means that it's normal and not altered with synthetic ingredients. Now, apply that principle to all of your foods—eat normal foods, not faux-food weirdness. When

Eat Chocolate, Lose Weight

you do this, you will automatically eat more natural fats, fiber, and protein, along with less overt sugar. All of this helps your chocolate control cravings between meals. See? It's like you guys are a team!

Finally, you're eating your chocolate slowly, and that lusciously slow pace helps you control how much you eat at any one time. Likewise, the amount of food you're hungry for, at the plate, is also a function of how fast you eat it. If you take your time with your lunch and with your dinner, and don't gobble it all down in 2 minutes, you will be hungry for an amount that better lines up with your "needs" than with your "wants."

So eat your food just like you eat your chocolate. Take your time with high-quality food, and you will be rewarded with low-quantity consumption both during and between meals. Ever wonder how healthy cultures can eat the richest, most wonderful foods on earth and still be thin and healthy? This is how they do it, and you can do it, too, by letting chocolate be your guide.

SUCCESS STORY
Julie Smink

AGE: 50

POUNDS LOST: 24

CHOCOLATE TIP: *"Don't chew your chocolate. Let it melt in your mouth. It will taste richer, it will last longer, and you'll eat less of it and still be satisfied."*

AFTER

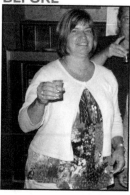

"I met my husband later in life. We got married when I was 39, and within 3 months, I was pregnant," Julie Smink explains. "Between being busy with a new marriage, a new baby, and a new house, I thought that would help me lose the baby weight, but that's not what happened."

Up until that point in her life, Julie always had her weight under control. "I had been a cheerleading coach for 27 years, so this was the first time in my entire life that I was carrying too much weight. I didn't know what to do about it because I'd never had a weight problem before," she says. "For a while, I was okay with it, but eventually the doctor started questioning why I wasn't dropping the weight. 'You're technically obese,' he told me. I was dumbfounded."

Julie wanted to get her weight under control while still being able to indulge in her lifelong love of chocolate. "Because my grandmother worked at Reese's, she would bring home fresh peanut butter cups off the line. I grew up eating that stuff constantly. Growing up so close to Hershey, Pennsylvania, even the air smelled like chocolate after it rained. Chocolate has been a part of my life forever, and because I never had a weight problem, I never thought of it as an issue," she shares.

BEFORE

So, when she found out about *Eat Chocolate, Lose Weight,* Julie knew she had found the plan for her. "Over the years, my tastes have changed, and I developed a taste for darker chocolate. I've always kept it in my desk drawer, and my grandmother's candy dish still sits in my living room full of Hershey's Kisses," she says. "I once thought dark chocolate was too bitter, but I've transitioned over the years. I still like milk chocolate but prefer dark chocolate now."

The most important thing Julie learned from the program was how to eat properly. "Learning to make my chocolate last 10 minutes—not 10 seconds—changed my life and my eating habits. Now, I cannot eat a piece of chocolate in the same old way. If I try to chew a piece of chocolate, it tastes like wax. The flavor of dark chocolate is so much richer and intense if you savor it," she says.

She also learned how to balance her portions. "I finally understand what real food is, and I learned tricks to control my portions, like asking for half of the food in a to-go box and using more time to eat the meal. That way, I not only stop when I'm full, but I also have food for tomorrow," she says.

In addition, *Eat Chocolate, Lose Weight* helped Julie learn to manage her stress. "Sometimes my job is stressful because I have to protect our company's data, and I found I tended to be a stress eater. Now I keep packs of almonds or some dark chocolate in my desk drawer, and I take a 'chocolate break': I take it out, bite a small piece, close my eyes, breathe deeply, and let the chocolate melt. By the time I get through the whole piece, I've taken about 10 minutes for myself and gotten over my stress, and then I get back to work."

Julie initially knew the plan was working within the first few weeks. "I was running late, and I ran downstairs to get a pair of jeans out of the laundry basket. I put them on and buttoned them up and ran to the top of the stairs. And when my husband saw me, he said they looked really good on me. And that's when it hit me that I didn't have to struggle to put them on," she explains. "I have two pairs of pants that were my 'fat clothes.' I don't get rid of them because every time I put them on, they're a reminder of the fact that I don't want to go back there."

After losing 24 pounds and dropping three sizes, Julie feels better than she has in a long time. "I'm lighter now than I have been in more than 10 years. I sleep better. I don't struggle with menopausal night sweats or indigestion. The hot flashes are almost completely gone, and I no longer need to see a chiropractor," she says. "I feel more confident now. I've always been a pretty outgoing person, but I didn't realize how those extra pounds made me feel about myself."

Julie says the plan isn't just about losing weight—it's about making a lifestyle change. "This isn't a diet because the word 'diet' has such a negative connotation to it. It's just guidance and making better choices, and everyone can do that. It's not about what you have to give up—it's about everything in moderation."

Chapter 5

Sensual Eating with Chocolate

I was giving a "Sensual Eating" seminar at a conference of administrators who get totally geeked out over rules, procedures, and policy positions. Nice, huh? About 150 stuffy people, sitting in a stuffy conference room, as stuffy presenters drone on and on about worksite OSHA benefit structure allocation, blah, blah, blah. So for those who hadn't already lapsed into a policy platform–induced coma, I think the words "sensual" and "eating" definitely caught their attention.

During my presentation, I had them compare fresh strawberries versus fresh-from-the-plastic-bag strawberry-flavored rope candy. The first part of this test is to lightly rub the outside of the berry with your fingers and take in the aroma. This stimulates saliva, which is basically just your mouth yelling to your brain, "Me too, me too, me too!" Then, with the smell still lingering deeply in their collective nostrils and their eyes closed, I had them bite slowly through the tartly sweet flesh and lightly open the berry with their teeth and tongue to release the sweetly tart flavors. Postures suddenly went limp in a room now filled with the random audible groans of some happy, happy administrators.

Next, I had them smell the chemically flavored, Day-Glo strawberry candy. This didn't go so well. After coming off that prior experience of simultaneous strawberry mouth-gasms, the synthetic, fresh-from-the-chem-lab smell was noxious by comparison. You should have seen their faces. It was like an ad for the TV show *Fear Factor*.

They were supposed to taste it, but over half the people in this room didn't go past the smell test. These people, whose job it is to research, create, and enforce "procedures," were going totally rogue on me! They wouldn't follow through because the comparison between real versus fake, friend versus faux, turned the candy from a great little afternoon snack into a repulsive, disgusting, no-good, awful oral calamity.

Of those who actually went through with it and put the candy into their mouths, approximately half looked up and actually—I kid you not—spit it out into their napkins. The interesting thing about this little experiment wasn't just that you could get that much reaction out of a room full of otherwise somnolescent professionals, but that many of them came up to me afterward to say that they normally liked those candies. However, now I've ruined their lives by showing them how nasty they are. Now they can't go back, and they're going to miss their candy! Bummer. I guess I'm just a bad human being.

This perfectly illustrates why sensual eating is so important to your overall health. Not because I'm such an awful person, but because when you taste—really taste—your food, it turns out to be really, really hard to make poor eating choices. Honestly, the only way fast-food nastiness and junk-food junk are tolerable is if you have zero to compare it with (so you don't know any different), or if you slam it back so fast that it spends more time in your gullet than on your palate. Either way, sensual eating is the solution. And just try to name one food that's better than chocolate to use for sensual eating practice. There just isn't one.

Learn to Love Your
CHOCOLATE. Really.

You may be thinking that, sure, the phrase "sensual eating" and chocolate are perfect for each other—got it. But the problem comes when you love your chocolate so much that you can't stop eating it. The problem comes when you look back at the pile of wrappers surrounding you on the couch, or the sheer volume of chocolate just eaten after a bout of choco-love. Isn't it a problem to love your chocolate too much?

The answer is no, absolutely not. The problem is not about love at all but about the sense we have learned that love is equivalent to consumption. This misconception about love and food is exactly what leads to overconsumption, which leads to consuming more calories, which leads to the weight gain that ultimately leads to the larger pants.

I was on the phone with the health editor for one of the largest-circulation newspapers in the United States today. She asked me how Mediterranean people could eat so much amazing food and still be thinner and healthier than us. I blathered about data for a while before she stopped me and said, "Will. Will, Will! Whoa, there. It's a short article. All I need is a bullet point."

I laughed and said, "Okay. They can do what they do because they *love* their food." She paused for a long time. Finally, she said, "No, that's not right. *Our* problem is that we *love* our food too much."

Her conclusion reflects one of the most persistent problems we have with our food: this confusion between love and consumption. And we've been taught that equation from Day 1. Think about the classic Cookie Monster character on the very popular children's show *Sesame Street*. He's depicted as funny when he's gobbling down a million cookies, with his gravelly voice saying how much he loves them and a spray of cookie shrapnel going everywhere.

Our children learn from this that if you love cookies, you gobble them up. And you should do so as fast as you possibly can. This is how our culture of health defines love as consumption. I'm not picking on this kids' show per se, because it's not the cause, but a reflection of something we all believe so implicitly. And that implicit belief is so engrained in us that it comes out in our behavior—even when we're all grown up.

For example, as adults we're told to eat at the seafood restaurant because of the "endless shrimp" deal (not because of the flavor of the shrimp); you go to the Chinese restaurant for the "bottomless buffet" (not because of the quality of the Hunan); and for a mere 39 cents more you can get a bucket of french fries with your burger at your local fast-food chain. I want you to watch commercials and ads through this filter and notice how they depict someone who is enjoying their food. Mouths are poised open for a monster-size chocolate bar, or burger, or drink, or steak.

What you see in advertisements is a reflection of ourselves. It's like looking into a mirror, because marketers will find out exactly what we want to hear and then tell us exactly that. These are our own biases and beliefs, affixed to their company logo. Therefore, what has become our most basic bias around eating? Quantity *is* quality and volume *is* value. Worse, we have turned love into consumption.

I don't care what relationship you're in—with your spouse, your job, your hobby, your pet, your food—when love becomes consumption, you're in a disordered relationship. And unfortunately that's the relationship we have developed with our food today, which has led to weight gain, obesity, and the raft of health issues that trail in its oversized wake. Everyone says that they love their chocolate, but what does that mean? Is it love they're talking about, or is it just the consumption of it?

Now ask yourself this question: When you say you love your chocolate, what do you mean? Are you only satisfied with your chocolate after you've eaten a lot of it? Or are you able to eat a smaller amount of higher-quality chocolate and no more? Be honest with yourself. Now is the moment. If, for you, love is consumption, we have to correct this disordered relationship.

This chapter retrains us to really love our chocolate. And it's not done by eating a bucketful of it or by inhaling it like you see done in commercials, but by actually focusing on its sensual aspects: the flavor, the savor, and the aroma. Being sensual with your chocolate will improve your relationship with it, but it will also improve your relationship with all of your food. And when your relationship with food is improved, the quality of that food goes up, the quantity comes down, and you get all the health benefits it offers without eating so much of it that you make it bad for your health.

Sensual Eating
with **CHOCOLATE**

If you're not taking the time to notice the different tastes within your food, you're like a canine that cannot see color. You have no idea what you're missing—or that you're even missing anything, for that matter. You're just living in a gray-flavored world. If you want to color your senses, all you have to do is open your mind to the sensuality of the food you're eating.

Do you remember how, as we discussed in the previous chapter, the solution to controlling portions started in your brain? Well, now it is your brain that stands between you and sensual eating. More to the point, what keeps us from being sensual with our chocolate is the overintellectualization of every single thing we do.

Case in point: The overintellectualization of our lives. After all, humans are incredibly smart. We just are. But being really high on intellect can create a deficit in the other important aspects of ourselves, like the sensual dimension.

This is exactly what we do with our chocolate and all of our food, by dissecting the minutia of a meal to parse out just how much of this or that molecule we should be eating (2,000 calories per day as the baseline, with 30% of that composition coming from fats, 40% from carbohydrates, and 40% from proteins).

The alternative to this mental rabbit hole is to be sensual. In other words, to pay attention to your senses. Of course, we're always sensual in some base, unconscious way because we have to see and feel and hear and taste and smell just to navigate through the world. But throughout most of your day, those sensations are on autopilot. You're not consciously aware of them. Sure, you can choose to focus on the things you smell, or taste, or feel, or see if you want to, but most of the time they're just quietly working away in the background.

When you choose to focus on your sensations though, you become conscious of them, awake to them. And this makes you aware of the flavor and aroma and texture in ways you have never been before. As I'll explain in the next few paragraphs, this also creates the physiological conditions that help you improve the quality of the chocolate you're eating and decrease the quantity you're putting away. Thus—and here's the take-home message—being a sensual eater with your chocolate increases the quality of your eating while decreasing the quantity in the long term. Sensual eating is the antidote to overeating.

In fact, researchers set out to understand the factors that cause cravings to decrease over time.[1] For example, it could be that you eat, fill up, and stop eating simply because you have ingested enough calories; this is the standard "food is fuel" idea. Alternatively, it could be that the Off switch of eating happens when you "wear out" on a flavor or taste. To test this, these researchers conducted a study comparing two dietary conditions: one high-calorie and the other low-calorie. In each case, they had subjects taste a small amount of a food and rate their desire for more than 10 repetitions. The time between each repetition was 2 minutes. They found that the decreasing drive to consume after "repeated presentations of the same food stimulus is affected by the sensory characteristics of the food rather than the caloric content."

So, do the math here. If "the sensory characteristics of the food" is a factor in helping you prevent overconsumption, and you are gulping your food so fast as you're stopped at the red light that you don't even notice how it tastes, then you will never even notice the sensory characteristics—and therefore, you will overconsume. The good news is that if you take your time and attend to these sensory characteristics, you'll be more likely to keep your caloric load to a level that supports a lower number on your scale.

In other words, sensual eating is a solution for all of your foods, not just chocolate. But if you're going to harness sensual eating to help you control consumption, and therefore calories, and weight, and your pants size, there's no better food on planet Earth to start with than chocolate. But to break out of your current behavioral biases, you're going to have to practice. This isn't hard practice, and the only thing it takes from you is the consistency needed to just stick with it.

Overcoming Your Main Obstacle: You

You have to want to change. I had a friend named Roberta, who worked with me in the lab at Syracuse University. This was during my first year back after returning from doing research work in France. She was thin, but nevertheless kept a bag of little mini candy bars in her desk drawer. It was funny, too, because when I was a kid, this particular brand of candy bar was my favorite, *favorite* candy of choice. At one point during some journal review, she offered one to me. Remembering my childhood fondness for them, I peeled back the plastic and popped it in my mouth. Ewww. It was totally gross, wickedly sweet, waxy chocolate.

After the meeting, I went straight back to my desk. I had brought back from France some Côte d'Or chocolate, which is a Belgian variety I like to call "from God" (a.k.a. amazingly awesome). After rinsing out my mouth with Borax and a Brillo pad, I approached Roberta to ask her if she would like to try some of my chocolate. I was so excited to give her this wonderful deliciousness to replace those things she was putting in her mouth.

She said to me, "Will, I'm not going to do it. I don't want your chocolate, thanks."

I was stunned. Why would she not? Hell, I suffered through her schlocky candy bar and she won't even try my chocolate? So I replied, "Why? It's really good, I promise!"

Then she explained, "I know it's good. In fact, I know exactly how wonderful that chocolate is. That's why I won't eat it. It's so good that if I have it, I won't want my candy bars anymore! And I don't want to not like them."

Now there's some honesty and self-awareness! Most of my friends

Eat Chocolate, Lose Weight

relent and start eating decent food after I harangue them enough, but I never turned Roberta from the dark reaches of that candy bar. She just didn't want it.

For you, when you're ready to start training your tastes for chocolate in a healthy direction, just be prepared that you may be turning your own tastes against a favorite comfort food. You'll replace it with a better one, but you need to be willing from the outset to let those former faves go. And to do that, let's start by thinking about the aspects of chocolate that you perhaps haven't paid too much attention to once you've opened its wrapper.

Visual Appearance

Chocolate is more than just brown. "Brown" is a nothing description. I mean, yes, chocolate is brown. But if you took a minute to compare different chocolates in different ways, you'd see that chocolates vary from light to dark, depending on the bean they are made from or because of the additives applied. Once you know to look for these variations, you'll see that "chocolate brown" can be anything from ruddy violet to rustic red to charcoal brown.

Why is this important? Because we don't eat just with our mouths; we eat with our eyes, as well. And the visual appreciation of the thing you're about to eat can preset your expectations. As a principle of neuropsychology, those preset expectations can color (pun entirely intended) your expectation of the flavor.

When you open up the wrapper, your chocolate should appear dark and shiny, and if you break it, you should hear a nice crisp snap. However, sometimes you may see a little whitish discoloration that makes it appear as though it may have gone bad. This discoloration is most likely a common "bloom" in one of two varieties: a sugar bloom or a fat bloom.

In a sugar bloom, the chocolate may have simply come into contact with moisture of some kind. It doesn't happen just when something wet gets spilled on it. Sugar blooms can also happen if there are rapid swings in temperature that produce condensation on the surface of the chocolate. For example, if your chocolate is stored in the refrigerator and then warmed quickly, the condensation can cause a sugar bloom. But even if you happen to live in an area of high humidity, you can also get this kind of bloom.

In a fat bloom, the grayish mottled discoloration is composed of crystals from the cocoa butter itself. When the chocolate is produced, six types of these crystals are formed as the chocolate hardens. A process called "tempering" is used to make sure that only stable crystals are formed. However, if this is not done well, over time the nature of the crystals can change and you will get the fat bloom.

How do you know whether you have a fat bloom or a sugar bloom? If it's a sugar bloom (caused by moisture), and you put some moisture on there, the ashy appearance will go away. Just lick your finger and touch the chocolate to see. In either case, whether it's a fat bloom or a sugar bloom, the chocolate is certainly edible and its flavor isn't affected a great deal. In the case of the fat bloom, you may notice a textural difference in your mouth.

Aroma

Smell is a basic sense. It's hardware. It's part of the standard package (typically) that we all just get. However, this sense can be learned and improved on: There's a software element to it as well, which can be programmed to detect more aromas, better, over time. And all you have to do to detect these aromas is, very simply, to practice taking notice of what you smell.

You can treat smell as nothing more than one of your five senses, or you can treat it as a gift that informs your tastes with many variations and notes of aromas in your food and drink. And if you are going to develop this aspect of your life, there is no better food to use than chocolate to train your senses. In fact, there are many flavor components to chocolate—including more than 600 different aromas.

That said, the nutty, sensual aroma of chocolate can easily be lost. You can pound it out by adding too much sugar. You can hide it completely by eating the chocolate cold. And there won't be much to smell if you eat chocolate that's been cheapened by replacing its cocoa butter with some species of vegetable oil.

So let's discuss a couple of rules on smelling your chocolate. First, it must be at room temperature, much like cheese or wine, in order to liberate the aromas. Next, you can warm it further by taking a small piece and rubbing it gently between your fingers. Bring that close to your nose, close your eyes, and take in the smell. Here's what to think about as you smell the chocolate: Try to discern whether the aromas are fruity, nutty, floral, or even earthy.

If you don't detect those aromas at first, that's okay. Honestly, it's difficult to pick them up if you haven't compared one type of chocolate with another. It's the comparison and contrast of multiple kinds of aromas that informs you of the varieties of nutty, fruity, floral, or earthy aromas. By trying multiple kinds of chocolate and by doing this smell test each time, you'll become better at picking out the differences over time. Think of it as acquiring a skill: The more you practice, the better you become.

Sensual Flavors

Smelling your chocolate is actually a wonderful prelude to tasting your chocolate. That's because when you smell your chocolate, it goes into the olfactory region of your brain, which then informs your consciousness about the upcoming flavor of the chocolate within the taste region. So when you smell your chocolate before you eat it and notice how it enhances the flavor, you have basically just juiced your brain to be better able to taste the chocolate before it even hits your palate.

When first tasting chocolate, most people assume that it has a single flavor. At the most basic level you hear, "Oh, this tastes like chocolate." But "chocolate" has many layers of flavors—and an estimated 1,500 flavor components. These flavor variants arise from the specific species of bean used to make the chocolate (Criollo, Trinitario, Forastero, or some combination of those). Each of these types of beans has a totally unique flavor, just like the Cabernet, Pinot, and Shiraz grapes produce completely different flavors of wine.

Also, chocolate's final flavor, like wine's, doesn't come just from the bean itself but also from the earth in which it grew. The Criollo, Trinitario, and Forastero beans will produce a chocolate that tastes different depending on the growing region.[2] Here are the flavors you should think about when you're tasting your chocolate:

The Fourth Dimension of Sensual Eating

You don't have to be an Einstein to know that the fourth dimension is time. What does this have to do with chocolate? The flavors that come from your chocolate change over time. Like Willy Wonka's Everlasting Gobstoppers, the early flavors come, then go, and finally give way to the middle and then the late flavors. Thus, if you're an Einstein yourself, you'll have the patience to taste these time-traveling flavors as they come and go.

By the way, you may have heard that Albert Einstein was eating chocolate when he came upon the theory of relativity and that early in his career, while he was working at the patent office, he approved the patent for Toblerone chocolate. However, regardless of just how much I want these little choco-facts to be true, they just aren't. Sorry.

EARLY FLAVORS

When you first place a piece of chocolate in your mouth, the taste receptors on your tongue register flavors in your brain, in combination with the smell of the food you're eating. The first flavor you'll be aware of when you taste your chocolate will be the sweetness. If there is a lot of overt sugar in the chocolate, it will be noticeable at the very beginning.

MIDDLE FLAVORS

After a few minutes, the middle tastes will move away from blunt sweetness to reveal more of the actual underlying flavors. For example, you may begin to taste a floral component, like a light orange flower note. Other subtly sweet sensations will give way to a more fruity taste, like plum or raisin.

- **Nuttiness:** think roasted chestnuts or hazelnuts
- **Fruit:** think plums or raisins
- **Floral:** think orange or rose
- **Spices:** think vanilla or cinnamon

If you can't pick out these flavors at first, don't worry or think that it's you. It may simply be that you have cheap chocolate, and there's really nothing there to smell or taste. But even if you do have chocolate with

As simplistic sweetness fades into flavored sweetness, the fruit flavor may then fade into a slightly tart or acidic element. Just as when you eat a piece of fruit and notice the sweetness before the tartness, the same is true when you eat chocolate. At this point in the progression of middle flavors, the tartness will start to carry tannic notes. Some describe these as "earthy" or "leathery." This may seem weird to you, because you've probably never tasted earth or leather. But you recall the smell of the loamy earth of a forest floor or the soft hide of rubbed leather. So, if you think of these aromas while you're tasting the middle portion of your chocolate, you'll see the similarities and realize how your chocolate tastes like these smells smell.

LATE FLAVORS

The last flavors to reveal themselves are the bitter flavors. The bitter receptor is the most sensitive of all taste receptors on your tongue, possibly because bitter flavors are often associated with plants that are toxic, and it's beneficial to be able to detect these even at minute levels.[3] And in fact, your brain can detect bitterness more acutely than any other flavor. That said, many bitter foods are excellent for your health as well, such as coffee, cocoa, hops, olives, bitter greens, etc.

The bitter flavors in chocolate are like the sweet and sour flavors in that they also carry associated flavors with them. These are the flavors that will linger on your palate after the chocolate has melted and been swallowed. You will note these as the smokier flavors.

Just realizing that there are early, middle, and late flavors that are all totally unique will help you taste them. Tasting for those evolving flavors will ultimately lead you to choose the better chocolates that are also healthier for you. And this new understanding will help you avoid those schlocky chocolates that have no more flavor than the waxy oils from which they're made.

decent flavors on board, it actually takes practice to be able to pick out even a few of the notes. Again, it's just like practicing tasting wine, and over time becoming able to distinguish the different flavors.

Unlocking the Flavors

As we've discussed, the first key is to make sure that your chocolate opens onto your palate and stays there as long as possible. Don't rush this. You can use your teeth if you want, but the point is not to chew up your chocolate in order to swallow it down (so that you can go back and get more to chew and swallow). If I were writing a book on how to eat chocolate and *gain* weight, that would be my prescription.

When you're tasting chocolate, the point of using your teeth is simply to open up the inside of the chocolate onto your awaiting, grateful, gleeful, newly happy taste buds. Lightly break the chocolate open and then leave it alone to liberate the deliciousness between your tongue and the roof of your mouth. Your teeth have done all they need to do.

Texture

While you're tasting your chocolate for the immediate, medium, and late flavors, you should also think about its texture. Another term for texture is the "mouthfeel" that your chocolate gives you.

The procedure for doing this is to take the chocolate into your mouth and to lightly press it against the roof of your mouth with your tongue. Then gently move your tongue over the bottom of the chocolate from the front of your tongue to the back. Note the feel of it: Is it smooth and creamy or powdery and gritty? If there is an inert waxiness to your chocolate, this is when you'll pick up that for sure.

Tasting for texture is even more important if you want to lose weight, because this can help you stop eating nasty chocolate that just isn't as good for you. Cheap chocolates substitute cheaper oils for the cocoa butter, which is the source of the fatty acids that are good for your heart, among many other things. Thus, once you start noticing the texture of your chocolates and selecting those with smoother finishes, you'll be less likely to choose unhealthy versions. And now that you know the basics of what to look (and taste) for in your chocolate, let's talk about a few guidelines to keep in mind as you learn to become sensual with your chocolate.

Before Each Tasting

Before tasting your chocolate, it's important to cleanse your palate. I was speaking at a gathering of French people, talking about diet and food, when I was cornered by this man who was probably 4-feet-nothing tall, but who was all up in my face about the importance of having the salad *after* the main course. "Nehver before, do you hear! Nehver! Zee salahd must have dressing of vinagre to cleanse your palate before zee dezzert, you know. It is zee simple chemistry of acids. Zey clean your mouth, zen you can taste zee dezzert!"

As animated and adamant as this gentleman was, he was absolutely right. If you want to be able to better taste your chocolate, clean your mouth first. Water is average for this; a very small piece of bread is better; but best would be something slightly acidic with no sugar (such as vinegar in a salad dressing or a chilly tart sorbet).

Cleansing your mouth before you taste your chocolate is a great idea, because otherwise the flavors of your wonderful chocolate will be masked. Then, when you have another piece, your brain won't get the message and neither will you. How sad would that be?

The Procedure for Tasting

Let your chocolate come to room temperature. This, by the way, is what you should do with a lot of things. When your beer is ice cold, you cannot taste it as well. There are many reasons why an ice-cold beer is good, but flavor isn't actually one of them. The same thing is true with cheese. If you eat cheese right out of the fridge, you won't be able to taste the flavors as much as you will when it has had a chance to come up to room temperature (around 70°F).

Likewise, unless you live in some Sahara-type locale without air-conditioning, where you're afraid your chocolate is going to turn into a molten puddle that you'll have to lap up from the wrapper, just leave your chocolate in the cupboard and grab your pieces when you're ready to eat them.

How Much Can I Have?

To answer this question, we need to break it up into three separate questions: (1) How much can I have at each bite? (2) How much can I have at each tasting event? And (3) How many times can I have these tasting events each week?

Let's start with the bite. From the standpoint of sensual eating, you can diminish your ability to taste your food by trying to do too much at one time. Take the long view. Know that you've got a while. This is a process. Relax into it. Breathe.

In other words, when you taste your chocolates, the size that you put in your mouth shouldn't be nearly as large as the state of Wisconsin. You shouldn't have to unhinge your jaws just to get it in there. A larger chocolate wad in your cheek does not provide larger flavor or appreciation, and it certainly doesn't help you fit into smaller pants.

So, when you taste your chocolate, use our rule of thumb and take just one thumb-size bite. If you look at the size of this chocolate and think that it's way too small, then you're thinking about it in the wrong way. You're thinking about it in terms of consumption rather than flavor. Your tongue can detect chocolate flavors at molecular levels. And the number of molecules in your thumb-size piece of chocolate is enormous. Thus, that square has all the flavor you will ever need, without the high volume that turns your chocolate into a liability for your weight and your health.

Now, when you are doing a sensual eating comparison, how much should you have at each event? When you select the chocolates that you will compare, have no more than four thumb-size pieces at a time. After about four pieces, your taste sensations will lose discrimination. They won't be able to pick out the differences as well. You want to get all the flavor your chocolate has to offer and to become good at tasting it. And to get good at tasting it, you'll need to plan for this process to take years, not days. All that means is that you have to practice eating your chocolate longer. Bummer, right?

Finally, how often should you do these tastings during a given week? Only do these tastings on the weekends. You'll have your daily chocolates that you consume in association with your meals (the starter and the ender) each day in order to help control consumption (during the meal and after the meal, respectively). However, this is a great activity to do on a Saturday or Sunday with friends, when you have more time on your hands and you're not juggling a million things at the same time.

Write It Down

I've had wine that has totally taken me by surprise. It was so shockingly delicious that I tried to peel off the label so I wouldn't forget what vintage it was. A better idea when you're tasting chocolate is to keep a journal so that you can write down not only the specific brand of chocolate but also the flavors as you notice them.

There's no right or wrong way to do this, so feel free to create your own rating system. But the simplest version would be to rank each chocolate in two ways: First, rank how much you love the flavor, aroma, and texture on a scale from 1 to 5. Second, note any special flavors you detect, such as nutty, fruity, floral, leathery, earthy, or tannic. And the best scenario for your tasting practice is to do it together with a number of people. In this case, do the taste testing in two rounds. During the first round, have everyone write down what they notice as specified above. While you're cleansing your palate between tastes, have everyone read their tasting notes. Then retaste the same chocolate, keeping in mind the flavors that were noticed by the others. When you retaste, you'll be more likely to pick up on the additional tastes that went unnoticed the first time around.

More Friendly with Two

Sensual eating, it turns out, is much more friendly with two—flavors, that is. Pairing chocolate with sympathetic flavors just makes your mouth that much happier, as you can uncover tastes in the chocolate that you couldn't have noticed by eating the very same chocolate on its own. Think about complementary flavors that you can add, such as cheese or wine or any red fruit. Just as with your chocolate tasting, there are no right or wrong pairings, but below are a couple of tried-and-true combinations to get you started.

Strawberries. Take just a moment to think about chocolate-covered strawberries. Think about the rich, dark chocolate lingering over the red tartness of the berry. This pairing is especially good when the chocolate is as dark and creamy as the berries are fresh and perky. Once it's in your mouth, the flavor parade begins with sweet, followed by tart, and then the deeper tannins finish the show.

Peanut butter. Peanut butter is like type O blood: It goes with everything. And chocolate is a perfect example. However, unlike the taste coupling of a chocolate-enrobed strawberry, the marriage of peanut butter and chocolate offers a different contrast. In this case, there is no sweet sharpness of berry to bite against the richness of chocolate's cocoa.

Because of this, pairing good peanut butter with good chocolate makes the bitter tannins jump out even more. Strawberries are so overwhelmingly tart that they swamp those more subtle flavors in the chocolate. But with peanut butter, the tannins are released from the background of flavor into the foreground of your awareness.

Wine. The bad news: There are so many complex flavors inside *both* the wine and the chocolate that you're not able to fully taste just how they interact with each other without a lot of practice. The good news: There are so many complex flavors inside *both* the wine and the chocolate that you're not able to fully taste just how they interact with each other without a lot of practice.

When you want to taste wine and chocolate together, there are some basic commonsense rules. Ready? Lighter wines go with lighter chocolates, while darker wines go with darker chocolates. Darker chocolates pair well with heavy tannin zinfandels and cabernets. On the other hand, a pinot noir or a lighter merlot are best for the more subtle flavors of lighter chocolates. Finally, if you have a number of wine-chocolate combinations to taste, always start with the lighter ones and move to the darker ones, because starting out with strong flavors on your palate can make it harder to pick out the more subtle flavors tasted afterward.

Bear in mind, too, that the order of the tasting matters. Start with your chocolate, and do not add the wine until the chocolate flavors have started to open up. If it takes a minute for them to develop, that's okay; wait on the addition of the wine.

TAKE THE
Chocolate Challenge

Change your tastes. There. That's your chocolate challenge. Because if you change what you have a taste for, you'll choose healthier foods. And even better, you'll choose healthier foods not because you're following some dumb dietary prescription that you can stick with for a good solid 2 weeks before you're off it again. You'll choose healthier foods because you happen to like them better. At that point, you're not micromanaging molecules—you're just living your life. That's your goal, and this chocolate challenge will help you get there.

WHAT DO I DO?

In Chapter 3, you learned to pull your sweet tooth with a vertical tasting. In other words, you tasted the same kind of chocolate but with different levels of sugar in it. For this chocolate challenge, you will do a "horizontal" tasting.

However, do not start this horizontal chocolate challenge until you have completed the vertical challenge in Chapter 3. How do you "complete" the Sweet Tooth Test? It's completed when the daily chocolate for which you have conditioned your tastes is 70% cocoa or greater (any amount darker than this is actually better). Once your tastes have adapted to that cocoa threshold, you'll then be able to taste the unique flavors found in high-quality chocolates. On the other hand, if your taste buds are still being bludgeoned by the sugar in your milk chocolates, you won't be able to detect all that your chocolate has to offer.

So just wait until you've gotten your tastes beyond the 70% threshold before moving on to this more advanced chocolate challenge. Once you're "there," it is time to take up this horizontal chocolate challenge. But what do I mean by "horizontal"?

A horizontal tasting is typically done with wine, and this involves tasting a couple of wines that are from exactly the same grape and the same year, but from different vineyards. For chocolate, though, you'll taste versions that contain the same percentage of cocoa, but from two different producers or from two different kinds of cocoa beans.

This horizontal challenge is much more difficult than the vertical challenge that helps pull your sweet tooth, because sugar is such a blunt, obvious taste. This horizontal challenge requires another level of awareness for the flavors in your chocolate. However, just as the learning is more difficult, the reward is that much better, too.

Once you complete this challenge and have changed your tastes in a healthy direction, I want you to see how far you've come. To do that, you'll do a probe tasting of a former chocolate that you perhaps once enjoyed (something like the candy bar I used to love). To see how much your tastes have improved, compare your new chocolates with the former faves you once craved.

HOW DO I DO THIS?

To do the horizontal tasting, you'll have to find chocolates that have the same cocoa percentage but that come from different locations or manufacturers. If your local chocolate shop doesn't carry enough variety to provide this comparison, it's easy enough to order them online.

Mainstream, off-the-shelf, everyday chocolates will give you the greatest contrast to train your tastes because some will be made with cocoa butter and others with substitute oils. You'll notice the waxy difference between them right away. Move on from here though, and compare old-world chocolates versus new-world ones (in other words, comparing chocolates made with South American cocoa beans versus African cocoa beans). Other delicious horizontal tastings are nationalistic: Swiss chocolate versus Belgian, for example.

Once you have identified the pairings for your horizontal tasting, use the techniques in this chapter to taste them side by side. The challenge will be conducted in stages. First, taste one of your chocolates, think about the flavors you notice, and write down your impressions. Next, cleanse your palate, and then move on to the second chocolate. During your tasting of the second version, you need to note two things: the flavors you perceive and also the difference between that chocolate and the first one. Again, write this down in your journal to keep track of your progress.

After the first comparison, rinse your palate and repeat with the same pairing. This time, when you compare the two chocolates, you'll have a better idea of what to expect. Thus, the second tasting will bring out even more of the contrast between them.

For the Probe

After you have practiced your horizontal tastings for 2 weeks, find a cheap chocolate—preferably one that you used to like before you started changing your own tastes. Bear in mind that you actually liked that chocolate at one point in your life. Note: Do not do the probe trial more often than once every 2 weeks, as you need to allow your tastes time to acclimate to the better flavors.

Treat this probe trial no different than any other horizontal tasting you do. First, taste the higher-quality chocolate that you have been eating. Then rinse your mouth and taste the former fave; rinse and repeat. Note the differences between them. However, in this case, also take note of how much you have changed your own tastes. Write down how much your tastes have changed and, more important, what this means for your weight and health.

WHAT CAN I EXPECT WHEN I DO THIS?

First of all, expect that you can do this. You may be thinking that chocolate tasting sounds like wine tasting, which can be viewed as some kind of purist pursuit of pinky-extending, hint-of-oak-smelling, highbrow snoots. Because of this, you might think that such a tasting just isn't your game.

I'm going to tell you that you can not only do this, but you can also become good at it. The only thing that stands in your way is practice. Repetition. That's all. If you start the horizontal test and think you can't tell the difference between the two types of chocolate, don't worry, because you will absolutely get better at it the more you do it. Think about it like a muscle: It's totally a flavor appreciation muscle that you can tone up or let wither. And again, the only thing required for this kind of "taste toning" is repetition. Oh, bummer, that means you have to taste more.

Also, if you do this chocolate challenge with other people, you may taste something completely different than they did. That doesn't mean you "missed" something, or that they're making something up because you didn't taste it in your piece. It just means that there's no right or wrong taste because everyone's neurosensory taste system is different. In fact, no two people perceive the very same flavor in the very same way. So if someone else is picking up that hint of oak, and you're not, well, that's just them. You'll taste other flavors.

For all these reasons, don't shuffle between different kinds of chocolates too quickly. For example, let's say you've compared a Belgian 70% chocolate to a Swiss 70%. Even if you've detected clear differences between them from the beginning, the differences you notice will change as you get better at detecting the different flavors contained in chocolate.

However, the most life-changing difference will come from the probe trial. You'll notice that the flavor you once loved, and perhaps went way out of your way to get, now tastes nasty and gross. The amount of time it takes to get to this point will vary from person to person. But I promise you that your first probe trial will shock you. The second probe will reinforce it. And if you make it to a third probe trial, I'll be surprised. By this point, most people simply cannot go back to the bad chocolate—ever again.

Expect to have your eyes opened in a couple of ways. First, you'll realize how poorly you ate and wonder how you could have possibly eaten that schlocky chocolate. More important, though, you'll realize the empowerment and freedom that come from taking ownership of your health. You made a change so fundamental that it altered the physiology of your own brain, creating new cravings that now make unhealthy food taste bad to you. You did that, and that is nothing short of absolutely amazing.

HOW DO I HELP MYSELF?

Don't treat your chocolate like a pill that you pop into your mouth just because you were told to. It's important to create routines around eating your chocolate in association with meals, for both your vertical Sweet Tooth Test and your horizontal sensual tasting. Why? Well, one study showed that the appreciation of the flavors in your food increases when it is eaten in a regular or ritual way.[4] ("Ritual" in this context doesn't mean you have to go as far as including candles or chanting or gongs, but just doing things in a predictable way. When I was a kid, we set the table, said a prayer, and then ate. That's a perfect example of a routine or ritual that precedes eating.)

For this study, people ate chocolate by unwrapping one portion, eating, waiting a bit, and then unwrapping a second portion, eating, then waiting a bit longer. This routine not only caused subjects to actually like the chocolate more (15% more compared to the "random eating" condition), but it also extended the length of time they spent eating the chocolate.

As we now know, enjoying your food and taking your time with it also help you control consumption by giving your brain a chance to hear the signals that you're full before you overrun them by eating too quickly. And from the standpoint of your brain, patterning routines around eating creates an operant link between the behavior and the upcoming flavor (the food). Thus, the next time you prepare food or chocolate for consumption, your brain will know that something delicious is coming, and this will enhance your appreciation of it.

How else can you help yourself? Return to the family table. Eat with the people you love in your life—in a pattern that is predictable. If that means eating together, do that. If it means having an appetizer before the main meal, do that. If it means we all sit down and contribute something

THE COCOA Q&A

Q: How long will it take to change my taste preferences?

A: Every physiology is different, so there will be a lot of variability from person to person. You can start to notice changes in what you have a preference for in as little as 1 week, but this process will continue for years. For others, it may take up to 4 weeks to notice a change.

This is such an important question, though, because if your tastes have not changed in that time, there may be other behaviors that are standing in the way. If this happens, you need to step back, take an inventory of the foods you're eating, and make sure that everything is real food.

The reason this process can take so long comes down to just how fundamental this change is. You are making a transformational change of your cravings, moving the baseline of taste preference in a healthy direction. When this happens, you make healthier choices just because that's what you enjoy more.

So be patient with yourself—until you've been doing this for about 4 weeks. You should notice a difference in your taste preferences by then. And if you don't, it's time to take a look at the foods you're eating to make sure you're not somehow standing in your own way.

Eat Chocolate, Lose Weight

about our day, well, that's just perfect. In the end, these rituals around eating are as good for your body as they are for your soul. Oh, and by the way, you parents get to find out who your kids are in the process. Bonus.

HOW CHOCOLATE SAVES YOUR DIET

Now think of how you can apply the change you learned through this chocolate challenge to your entire diet. You changed your taste preferences for bad chocolate to good chocolate, and you can make this shift with all of your foods.

What if you craved fruit instead of plasticized fruit sheets? What if you craved vegetables instead of prepackaged packets of oversalted, oversugared food products? If that is who you have become, then you will exchange high-quality for high-quantity consumption by doing nothing more than eating what you love.

You can get from here to there. You can change your own physiology—your own brain—for the better. Just apply the lessons from this chocolate challenge across the board. In other words, practice tasting for flavors in your sauces, breads, fish, and veggies. The more you do it, the better you'll get. And just like with this chocolate challenge, the only thing standing between you and this level of freedom is repetition. Taste, and you begin the process of sculpting a healthy flavor appreciation.

By the way, people ask me all the time how they can help their kids eat healthier. You can tell them all the rules of what to eat, for sure. But the Confucian, top-down, cerebral strategy (see Chapter 4), in which they have to (a) remember what their parents said and (b) *care* to remember what their parents said, is useless. It will never stick for long. The solution for our children is to get them to taste, and to talk about what they're tasting. If you can get them to discriminate between good foods and bad foods, then you will have created an internal guide for them that will work when they've forgotten all your reams and reams of rules and more rules. Inside out, that's your solution. And that's a beautiful thing.

SUCCESS STORY
Rose Batiste

AGE: 52

POUNDS LOST: 30

CHOCOLATE TIP: *"Really savor your chocolate ender. Think of it as your reward at the end of your meals."*

"My grandmother loved dark chocolate, and that's what she always gave me as a treat as a little girl," Rose Batiste shares. "So I've always loved dark chocolate. I ate chocolate every day. Before this program, chocolate wasn't an 'ender'; it was a beginning, a meal, and an ender."

But it wasn't *what* Rose ate that caused her weight problems; it was *how* she ate. "I was working long hours and just grabbing food whenever I could. My time was limited, and I wasn't mindful about what I was eating. I ate mostly fast food and processed food. I wasn't active at all," she says, noting that she tried countless times to lose the weight, but nothing worked. "I'd tried every diet, every pill, every gimmick, but they were just too hard and required too much thought and planning."

Tired of struggling with her weight, Rose knew she needed to find a weight-loss plan that gave her the freedom to eat more of the food she enjoyed. "I was tired of buying bigger clothes all the time. I kept buying larger and larger sizes instead of fitting into what I had. I knew it was time to try something new."

So when she heard how simple and unrestrictive the Eat Chocolate, Lose Weight plan was, she decided to give it a try. After starting the plan, Rose quickly learned the importance of the chocolate ender. "It's like the period at the end of the sentence. Now I look forward to it, and it's about savoring that moment."

And once she learned that, the program became even easier and she noticed even more results. "I knew the program was working when I realized I could get through the day without sugar. I didn't need to have sugar in my coffee or to have cookies or doughnuts for breakfast. Once I was off sugar and ate something sweet again, it tasted too sweet—too concentrated."

Rose ultimately lost 30 pounds. She also dropped several clothing sizes, going from a 12 to an 8, all without ever feeling unsatisfied. "You never feel deprived when you have the piece of chocolate at the end of your meals. It's all about savoring." For Rose, sensual eating was the key to her success. "You can eat anything you enjoy, but you have to take your time and not just shove it down your throat. All you have to do is be aware of what you're eating and enjoy it."

Chapter 6

Chocolate on the Brain

I received my doctorate in neuroscience about a thousand years ago from Emory University. What I understand from all that training is how your brain controls behavior, and how your behavior impacts your brain. It's a circle. But today, instead of teaching primates to play video games for juice and Craisins, I teach adults the healthy behavioral habits that lead to controlled consumption, conscious eating, and smaller pants.

In fact, I provide "Chocolate Eating Lessons" for corporations to teach their employees how to eat healthfully. And as much as monkeys love their juice, humans are even more motivated by chocolate. I have to admit, though, that to say employees love those Chocolate Eating Lessons may be a true statement, but it's also totally misleading. Think this through: I give seminars in which people get chocolate, and then I ask them how they liked the presentation. I don't care what job you have, if you host a meeting and throw chocolate at people, your evaluations go *way* up. It's not even fair. It's almost like cheating.

Nevertheless, participants leave understanding the importance of high-quality versus high-quantity eating. They also learn why chocolate is a health food and what constitutes healthy chocolate and what doesn't. Finally, they learn the "how" of eating chocolate, which controls overconsumption, as we discussed in Chapter 4. Best of all, these Chocolate Eating Lessons apply to all daily dietary decisions, and thus become the perfect example for how you should eat all of your food at all times.

One of the reasons I love providing the Chocolate Eating Lessons is that I can see the unique role that chocolate plays across both the body and the brain of each participant. For example, all the lovely, warm and fuzzy things you feel about chocolate actually take root in your neurons, branch out into your emotions, and then end in your behaviors. And there's no better food to connect the dots between mind and body than the deliciously emotional, palpably physical response we all have to eating pure chocolate.

By the way, if you're looking for a "missing piece" in dietary advice, it's precisely this connection between the mental and the physical spheres that has been largely avoided in our search for that magic diet that will solve (or dissolve) our weight problems. However, to gain any kind of control over the drives that drive our eating behaviors, we have to address the complete picture. And chocolate is perfect in this respect, because it sits at the connection between emotional and physical worlds. Using brain-imaging scans, scientists from Northwestern University, in Chicago, found that eating even one square of chocolate and allowing it to melt on your tongue activates pleasure areas of the brain, such as the orbital frontal cortex.[1] This is also associated with the release of feel-good chemicals in your brain, which can lead to lower stress hormones, and thus impact your metabolism and therefore your weight.[2] But getting from here to there, from larger pleasure to smaller pants, requires an understanding of every level in the cascade from brain to body.

I have to say, though, as someone who coaches thousands of people on how to use chocolate to eat well, lose weight, and love their food again, that the problem with chocolate is not the actual chocolate. In other words, the problem with chocolate is not the physical properties of chocolate (which are massively healthy), but instead our mental baggage about this food. We think of it as a candy or a vice.

This attitude is completely counterproductive, and it's time we rethink our beliefs about this wonderful food, our overall health, and, yes, even chocolate weight loss. It's only once you remove the sense of denial and self-loathing you were coached into applying to your chocolate eating that you can reduce your internal stress and make it easier to achieve your weight-loss goals. But you have to stop gripping the handlebars so tightly. Ease off a bit. Relax around your food. And chocolate can help you do that.

Stressing Stress Inside Your Brain

Weight loss is tough. It just is. And one of the reasons it can be so hard comes down to the fact that there are many other factors besides food and feeding that impact your weight. Stress, for example, creates hormones, such as cortisol, in your blood and brain that are associated with increased obesity (one study found that obese women have twice the cortisol of women of normal weight),[3] abdominal fat,[4] adrenal exhaustion, and even diabetes. Therefore, trying to maintain a 100% fat-free, carb-free, calorie-free lifestyle can increase your stress levels and totally frustrate your attempts to keep that scale under control. And it just so happens that the very same chocolate that can help get your weight under control can also produce long-term improvements in your level of stress.

The idea that chocolate can "bring the happy" strikes us as true. We've all heard the stories of people who swear that they feel better when eating chocolate, that they crave it, and that it's just plain better than sex. Be that as it may, this chocolate euphoria does have a neuroscientific basis that comes from the psychoactive chemicals naturally found in chocolate and the brain reactions they produce, which can help you control stress and anxiety in the process.

As you might guess, your brain's pleasure centers love chocolate as much as you do. And a major reason is because chocolate stimulates your brain's pleasure receptors with one of its chemicals, known as anandamide. By the way, the word *anandamide* originates from the Sanskrit word *ananda*, meaning "bliss" and "joy." Tell me that doesn't sound just about right! Also, when you leave chocolate on your palate for an extended amount of time, this very same anandamide molecule goes one step further: It enhances your appreciation of chocolate's sweetness![5] This is amazingly cool because darker chocolates not only have more of these anandamides than milk chocolate, but they also have less sugar. And even though there's less sugar, your appreciation for the smaller amount of remaining sugar is amplified because of the additional anandamide. Doing the choco-math here, there's less sugar to drive your weight problems but a heightened appreciation of it to satisfy your sweet tooth. That's a win-win if I've ever heard one!

After tickling your brain's pleasure receptors with anandamide, chocolate also spikes your endorphin levels to activate entire pleasure regions of your brain, creating very happy brain cells. These chocolate-induced warm fuzzies are bolstered by another drug found naturally in cocoa, phenylethylamine, or PEA. PEA is known as the "love drug" because it also happens to be released in your brain when you fall in love. Downstream of anandamide, the endorphin party floats along with the love drug itself, leading to the production of serotonin, which (surprise, surprise!) stimulates more positive feelings in the new pleasure-palooza you have going on in the brain. It's one big biochemical Kumbayah.

All these biochemical brain reactions explain why people feel better when they eat chocolate. Unfortunately, they may also be why patients with higher clinical depression scores eat more chocolate at a sitting than those who aren't depressed.[6] Basically, they self-medicate to make themselves feel better by increasing these positive neurochemicals.

And it's fine to make yourself feel better. When you're hungry, you eat and immediately feel better. When you're sluggish, you get up and move to feel better. But in the case of chocolate, the problem is that the benefits attained from this form of self-stimulation can rise, fall, and go away, leaving an aftereffect of "unhappy." And because the original happy effect is short-lived, a person would have to dose up, then dose up again, then again and again until that entire bag of chocolate is empty.

Eat Chocolate, Lose Weight

That's really what everyone's worried about: eating chocolate until the eating of it becomes a problem. There is no Stop signal—there is no Off switch. When this happens, the person doesn't respond to hunger and satiety cues that should curtail consumption, because the eating is not about nutrition or hunger or fullness. These emotional eaters consume for reasons that have nothing to do with food. For them, food is not the end; it's a means to some other end. It fills a void, and the trouble is, the void they're trying to fill cannot be filled by chocolate—or any other food for that matter.

Is this kind of uncontrolled consumption driven by emotion? Habit? A search for comfort? Self-medication? The answer is yes, to all of the above—but in different proportions for different people at different times under different conditions. And there's nothing approaching anything in the vicinity of a one-size-fits-all solution for that chaos of variability.

One more degree of freedom—as if there just weren't enough before—is that even though chocolate can be the object of a disordered relationship with food, it can also be very stabilizing for emotions, stress, and even anxiety . . . in some cases, but not in others. Clear as mud?

The good news is that there's a principle that cuts the clutter and gives us a very simple guideline for eating chocolate to help manage emotions: *Prevention is good. Treatment is bad.*

Prevention, Not Treatment

In health care, there is an axiom: Prevention is cheaper than treatment. Doing what you can to prevent problems on the front end will always cost less than treating them after the problem has arisen. This approach is just as effective on a personal level, as the following examples demonstrate.

Costs: Buying smoking-cessation gum is cheaper than treating lung cancer; healthy eating is cheaper than a quadruple bypass; clicking on your seat belt is cheaper than digging glass out of your skull in the emergency room.

Health: Getting a colonoscopy is less inconvenient than wearing an external bag on your abdomen; eating well is less inconvenient than losing a foot to diabetes; walking around the block once a day is less of a pain than having your face paralyzed for the rest of your life from a stroke.

The same axiom is true for the linkage between chocolate and stress. Chocolate can improve your emotional state when it's used in a preventative way. But it can be totally counterproductive if you turn to chocolate as a solution to your stress—as a treatment for your daily stress load. By eating chocolate in response to a bad day or bad feelings (or boredom, or anything else), you not only take it out of the "health food" category, but you also quickly turn it into an "unhealthy food." Your brain's short-lived feel-good effects slide down the slippery slope of empty cravings that can ultimately feed the problem of obsessive consumption. The distinction to remember is that the impact of chocolate on your emotional state hinges on when and how you take it: whether it is proactive or reactive.

THE COCOA Q&A

Q: How do I keep myself from eating too much chocolate, especially when I'm stressed?

A: The key is to leave your small piece of chocolate on your tongue for as long as possible. This does two important things, both of which can help reduce your stress-induced overconsumption.

First, if you don't chew it or suck on it, that chocolate piece will take a very long time to melt—how long will depend on its quality and thickness. This added time you spend slowly tasting your chocolate is time you're not popping more into your mouth.

Even better, leaving chocolate on your palate will induce sensory-specific satiety. Basically, you just wear out on the taste. It's as if your brain interprets that you're eating the entire time.

All of that said, if you think you have compulsive eating patterns, it will take you a while to retrain your brain so that you don't fall into compulsive eating with your chocolate. To do this, give yourself 2 weeks in which you bring a set amount ꞓcolate to work (like two thumb-size pieces). And if you eat your chocolate ꞓre, just make sure to use the techniques we've discussed. Allowing yourself to ꞓlate, but in a controlled amount, will be the key to your success.

Reactive Chocolate:
A Short-Term Mood Massage

It's important to separate the psychological impact of eating chocolate from the physiological. The psychological side is like software, and represents the mental association between the behavior of eating chocolate and pleasure. This association can be formed and broken and reformed again. The pleasure you perceive from this association is as short-lived as the release and breakdown of the neurochemicals bouncing around in your brain.

The short-term emotional impact of chocolate is commonly seen in those who crave chocolate, the so-called chocolate addicts.[7] In a study published in the *British Journal of Clinical Psychology,* 40 women—20 self-identified chocolate addicts and 20 who did not have this emotional attachment (the control group)—were instructed to eat chocolate every day for 7 days, and their feelings of depression and guilt were rated through a standardized process. It's interesting that, even though chocolate addicts might go on for days about how they "love" their chocolate, it was this group that felt guilty about their behavior, and were noted as more depressed than the control group.

This is amazing in one way, because these are people who were in a study. They agreed to the rules of the study, which included eating chocolate every day for just 7 days. They had a ready-made excuse for their behavior! It wasn't as if they were off breaking some arbitrary rule about chocolate eating that they'd set for themselves. They weren't sneaking chocolate from their kids' Halloween stash or fantasizing about being Augustus Gloop in Willy Wonka land. They were in a research study and were instructed to do what they did.

Despite this, after the short-term improvement of mood had passed, the chocolate lovers still felt guilty. They still felt depressed. And eating chocolate did not help them. It was just a little mood massage that lasted only a little while. One research group actually timed it, to find out how long this brain blip lasts. They discovered that the little mood massage lasts about 3 minutes. Then it's gone.[8]

When I spoke with Beatrice Golomb, professor of medicine at the University of California in San Diego, about the link she discovered between consistent chocolate consumption and weight loss, she also pointed out that chocolate can lead to an increase in serotonin in the short term, which then affects mood. However, for those who are already depressed, chocolate consumption can act like a tipping point to swing them into depression. In her observations, such changes in mood associated with chocolate consumption occurred in about 2 minutes.

Still, she wisely cautioned against making sweeping generalizations about chocolate and short-term mood changes, because every physiology is unique. For example, some coffee drinkers are fast metabolizers and others are not; so while some need more to get going in the morning, others are so sensitive that they can only have decaf.

The same is true regarding the effect of cocoa on emotional health. Some people will experience a stronger effect than others—a higher boost or a deeper depression that could last just a little while or for much longer. You cannot know beforehand which physiology you have. So when you read that the time of the short-term mood enhancement is about 2 to 3 minutes, just keep in mind that your body is different from everyone else's, and chocolate could have a longer or shorter, greater or lesser effect.

Even though chocolate's short-term mood massage may vary in specific time or extent, it does appear and disappear for everyone. The high can be followed by a low, particularly in those who have a tendency toward depressed moods, making eating chocolate a terrible solution for those looking for something to make themselves feel better.

As a matter of fact, one research group found that emotional eaters who used chocolate as a way to treat a bad mood were actually more likely to have those bad feelings persist than those who didn't use it as such a treatment. In other words, when used to treat *existing* anxiety or stress, chocolate made the problem persist even longer.[9]

And think about how this condition can very quickly slip out of control. If a person continues this strategy (eating chocolate to fix his or her

Eat Chocolate, Lose Weight

emotional state), the person's mood, as shown by research, doesn't actually improve. This, of course, makes it more likely that anxiety and/or depression will persist, which increases the odds that he or she will turn to chocolate later. And this process will only continue. At that point, you're sliding down a slippery chocolate slope straight into a bog of emotional awfulness.

Chocolate Prevention

So let's set the record straight in zero uncertain terms: Eating chocolate is not going to take away the fact that your report is late or that your kids have raging hormones and attitude. It's not going to shield you from crazy drivers. And if you are using chocolate to basically self-medicate, you can certainly do that, but your very best-case scenario is that you'd just be treating symptoms. At worst, you are just making the problem worse.

A better solution is to use chocolate to reduce the risk that the problem will happen in the first place. As I said, chocolate will not be able to prevent others from driving you crazy. Nothing and no one can do that. What it can do is help you keep the outside stressors on the outside and prevent them from getting under your skin and into your heart and mind, where they will do the most harm.

For example, if you're a person who is stressed on a chronic basis, eating 40 grams of chocolate (about eight thumb-size pieces, or 1 ounce) every day for 2 weeks can help lower your stress levels, according to a 2009 study.[10] How? Consuming this amount of chocolate for this long actually decreases the stress hormones that flood your blood.

Moreover, the cortisol stress hormones that chocolate puts to bed are the same hormones that can trigger fatty deposits, adrenal exhaustion, and even muscle wasting.[11] So, keep in mind that while you're getting all calm and happy with your daily dose of wonderfulness, you're also coaxing your bodily biochemistry to give you an even better shot at sustaining weight loss in the process.

But does the statistical decrease in cortisol in the blood actually make you feel less crappy? Less stressed? Less anxious? It's one thing to measure a hormone in the context of some research study and show that its level in the bloodstream moves up or down. But the real question is whether eating chocolate results in improved feelings in the long term.

As the continual bearer of good news, let me just tell you that the answer is a big, chocolaty yes. A 2010 study published in the *Journal of Psychopharmacology* reported on 72 subjects who ate cocoa polyphenols daily, and then ranked how they felt on a validated psychological survey to see whether their measures of anxiety changed as a result of the daily consumption. The study showed that after 30 days, the subjects' anxiety had decreased by 10 percent, while their measures of calmness had increased by another 10 percent. In addition, the subjects reported feeling better and even experiencing less depression.[12]

A key to this important study is that it was done with (relatively) normal people who had never been diagnosed with clinical depression. It's not like the subjects came in with anxiety, and someone said, "Oh, you have anxiety. Let's throw some chocolate at you and see what happens." These were ordinary people with ordinary levels of anxiety and depression who found an improvement in their emotional state when they had a little chocolate every day. The improvement in emotional stability came only after sustained exposure to chocolate: 2 weeks of it. But keep in mind that the total volume they ate each day is *not* the issue. In other words, don't think you can short-circuit the issue by having *all* of your 2 weeks' worth of chocolate in one session. You can't "pull an all-nighter" or "cram" to get it all in at once. Think of it exactly as if you had a regimented prescription from a physician who directed you to take one pill every day for 2 weeks. If you think you can go ahead and get this little chore out of the way by downing all 14 of them at once, you're going to end up hurting yourself.

Eat Chocolate, Lose Weight

CHOCOLATE's Long-Term Emotional Benefit

By contrast, if you have a little high-cocoa chocolate every day, positive mood states like sense of satisfaction and self-rated scores on "calmness" and "contentedness" will improve. As research has shown, these improvements happen when the chocolate is taken over 30 days. However, there's no short-term effect. In other words, the cocoa polyphenols don't immediately boost mood, satisfaction, calmness, or contentedness. This happens only when chocolate is eaten slowly and steadily.

This result, however, may seem totally counterintuitive based on your own personal experience. For example, if you put chocolate in your mouth and let it slowly melt, you basically have a delivery device for wonderfulness—right on your palate. So the idea that it takes a full 30 days to get from your current emotional state to satisfaction, calmness, and contentedness sounds like a divorced-from-reality research flub. After all, you know that it doesn't take 30 days before you start groaning audibly after eating your chocolate—it takes about 30 seconds after it melts in your mouth. But this is exactly the difference I've been emphasizing in this chapter, between short-term psychological blips and long-term physiological changes. To be clear, both kinds of feelings of satisfaction and wonderfulness are very real. They're just different functions in your brain.

These different functions are hinted at by the source of the positive emotions. The short-term happy dance in your brain may come from neurostimulation through some combination of anandamide, PEA, serotonin, and/or endorphins. Other studies indicate that the long-term reduction in anxiety may also require one other factor: the polyphenols found specifically in cocoa. Because of this, emotional eaters could get their short-term mood massage from any species of chocolate, whether good for you, bad for you, or indifferent. But the long-term reduction in anxiety, stress, and even depression requires cocoa's polyphenols (and therefore, high-cocoa chocolate).

For example, in a 2010 study, researchers looked at the impact of cocoa polyphenols on chronic fatigue syndrome in two groups of people over an 8-week period.[13] They gave one group 85% cocoa chocolate and the second group something that tasted just the same as that chocolate and even had the same number of calories. Basically, this second group ate the same product but without the polyphenols. Each group consumed 15 grams of their respective foods, three times per day. (And if you're wondering how eating the equivalent of nine thumb-size pieces of 85% cocoa chocolate daily impacted their weight, there was no weight gain at all after 8 weeks of eating this amount. None.)

So what was the difference identified between these two groups after 8 weeks? Those eating the 85% cocoa chocolate with elevated polyphenols reported a 35% reduction in fatigue, a 37% reduction in anxiety, and a 45% reduction in depression. By comparison, those who ate the very same product but without the polyphenols reported slight increases in every one of those emotional measures, compared with their pre-study baselines.

To get this kind of improvement in 8 weeks is impressive, for sure. But even more impressive is the fact that the subjects in the study had all been diagnosed with chronic fatigue syndrome. These aren't simply people who are run-down at the end of a day. They are individuals with a chronic condition. And the solution was a slow and steady approach of applying a little high-cocoa chocolate consistently over 8 weeks.

It's funny how fads come and go, with all kinds of crazy pills and powders and products proffered as solutions. But the more we look at what it takes to be healthy, the more we always return to common sense. The golden mean of moderation and consistency will save your life. It's not sexy. You can't pack it into a pill or sell it at health food stores. But the golden mean of moderation and consistency will save your life.

One More Thing to Remember

We've established that the short-term effect of eating chocolate is a kind of mental mood massage that lasts just long enough for you to reach for another candy from the sack. On the other hand, concrete emotional benefits take between 2 to 8 weeks to develop, and they require consistent tasting.

I understand how oh so sad you must be to learn that you should have a little chocolate each day in order for it to benefit your emotional state. But let me benefit your emotional state a bit more by letting you know that this same strategy—long-term, controlled consumption of high-cocoa chocolate—has other benefits that you're going to want to remember.

I spoke again with Dr. Claudio Ferri at Italy's University of L'Aquila about his work with elderly people who had been shown to have mild cognitive impairments. (What does "mild cognitive impairment" mean? Basically, it's like when your grandparents can't recall your name until they cycle through the names of all of your siblings first, and the cousins, and the cat, and your neighbor from first grade.) Dr. Ferri found that, in this grandparental group, their cognitive performance improved after 8 weeks of consistently consuming cocoa polyphenols. Even better, the higher the level of polyphenols consumed, the more improvements that were seen.[14] But you don't have to wait until you're elderly and diagnosed with mild cognitive impairment to get this benefit. You should start before you get to that stage, because by that time, you'll be more likely to forget to remember that you need it!

We all slip little by little into the fog of forgetfulness as we age. And it's the small things that reveal this mental erosion. Like when you're in your house, thinking about a million things, and then go down into the basement. Once you get down there, you look around, wait, survey the inevitable mess, and wonder why in the world you went into the basement to begin with. Now you're grumpy, because you know you can remember. You strain, trying to will your brain to pull back the simple errand that was right between your ears not even 2 minutes ago. Finally, you slump, give up, and reluctantly climb back up the stairs. Then it hits you . . . socks!

Wouldn't it be wonderful to have something to help us put that experience off for just a while longer? Sure, this steady senility-creep gets you two laps out of your trip to the basement just to get your socks—and that's an extra workout added to your day. But if you don't want to travel two sets of stairs just to retrieve your clothes from the downstairs dryer, you might want to add a little high-cocoa chocolate to your life on a consistent basis for about 8 weeks.

TAKE THE
Chocolate Challenge

Use chocolate to achieve lower stress in the long term. Likewise, prevent chocolate from increasing your current stress levels.

For this chocolate challenge, it's vital to reemphasize that people eat chocolate for many reasons that have exactly zero to do with hunger, flavor, or savor. They eat it because they're bored. They eat it because they're happy. They eat it because they're sad. They eat it because they're hopeful that something will happen to make them happy. Or they eat it because they're worried that something will happen to make them sad. It's emotional quicksand.

Because of this, the challenge to use chocolate to help control stress and anxiety must be put in the right perspective, like meditation. For example, meditation can encourage your body's physiology to move from a stressful state, called the "sympathetic response" (commonly known as the "fight or flight" response), into its opposite, more relaxed state: the parasympathetic response. These two systems are your body's equivalent of yin and yang, the passive and the aggressive, the calm and the storm.

Eat Chocolate, Lose Weight

Meditation can help your body shift itself from the sympathetic stress response into the parasympathetic calm response. What meditation cannot do is make people stop driving like lunatics. It cannot make teenagers *not* act like teenagers. It cannot make the external stressors go away. It can only help your body deal with them better.

The same thing is true of chocolate. Many people use chocolate to fill holes in their lives, even though that space they are hoping to fill has no bottom. And certainly not a bottom that chocolate can fill. Can chocolate help your emotional state move in a healthy direction? Yes. Is it a magical panacea that will take away the craziness of the world and the hurt and the harm and the hurricanes in your life? Of course not.

I wish I could tell you that eating chocolate will wash away the stress, and that may be exactly what we all want to hear. In fact, we're coached by our culture to think in terms of binary, simple solutions (it's good for you or it's not; it's right or it's wrong; it's fattening or it's slimming). The tougher, more honest fact is that our lives operate in the smooth continuous analog nature of nuance.

So take this chocolate challenge. Eat your chocolate consistently as described in this process. When you do, expect to still have crazy drivers in your life, wonky teenagers with attitude, and all the other daily dilemmas you face. But also expect to be better able to find a measure of peace around them.

WHAT DO I DO?

Let's choose an amount of chocolate to have based on research. Make it 40 grams of high-cocoa chocolate (at least 70% cocoa), which you'll eat every day for 8 weeks. To give you a ballpark idea of how much chocolate is equal to 40 grams, one of those large rectangular bars is typically 100 grams, and your typical thumb-size piece weighs in at about 5 grams or approximately 0.12 ounce. Thus, your daily dose will be about eight thumb-size pieces (or about 1 ounce). Keep in mind that you cannot have that amount all at one sitting. Spread that total out during the day.

In fact, one of the advantages of this book is that the chocolate challenges you complete provide a structure for your consumption: Have one or two thumb-size pieces for your starter and the same for your ender—both for lunch and for dinner; have chocolate in order to pull your sweet tooth or to increase your energy level in association with your exercise patterns. All of these routines help you keep chocolate consumption under control so you can get the mood-boosting benefit without eating so much that it becomes bad for you.

For this particular chocolate challenge, the effect you can expect to experience will come from two factors, both of which must be present to get any emotional benefit at all: cocoa concentration and consistency.

As for the cocoa content, darker is better if you want to improve the anxiety-lowering benefits of your chocolate. In other words, 70% cocoa is good, but 80% is better. So when you're choosing your chocolate, edge toward higher concentrations, as your tastes allow.

That's the "quality" part. As for "quantity," it's not clear from the research that having more than 40 grams per day is going to help you feel even better. So for now, just keep it steady at this level. Plus, you'll likely not get the emotional benefit you're looking for unless you're consistent over time. This is every bit as important as the cocoa content. It's the steady background level of cocoa catechins that will, over time, help reduce your stress levels.

Again, and this totally bears repeating, stressful events occur on the outside. It's only when we allow them to get to us (on our insides) that they become problems in our lives. Chocolate cannot take away the crazy. What it can do is assist you in helping to keep the outside stressors on the outside. This will protect your inner calm.

Just like everything else we've talked about in this book, chocolate is not a magic pill for stress, or weight loss, or fitness. Nor can it fix anything all on its own. Your chocolate needs you to take the lead before it can become the most delicious helper you've ever had!

HOW DO I DO THIS?

No matter how many of the chocolate challenges you're taking to get your weight and health under control, don't add the 40 grams of additional chocolate on top of the other amounts you're already eating throughout the day. Just add up the sum of the high-cocoa chocolate you do eat, and be sure not to exceed the 40-gram total each day. Do you *have* to eat at least 40 grams of high-cocoa chocolate every day to get the effect? Absolutely not. If you're worried about calories, you could simply substitute cocoa powder to get the daily polyphenols you need.

By the way, if you aren't eating chocolate that is at least 70% cocoa, hold off on this challenge for now. Once you adjust your tastes so that you can enjoy 70% cocoa and higher, then begin this challenge.

WHAT CAN I EXPECT WHEN I DO THIS?

I'm afraid that this chocolate challenge, above all the others, is as important as it is squishy. With all the other chocolate challenges, I give you nice, concrete measures to look for. With the starter, you'll be hungry for smaller portions, which you'll see with your own eyes. When you're working on losing your sweet tooth, your cravings for sugar will decrease by a definite amount. With the ender, your between-meal snacking will drop by a discrete amount. It's all very scientific and quantified.

In each case, I'm giving you the ability to have real, measurable outcomes that you can set up, monitor, and review for yourself. With this challenge, you're likely to feel a change after the 2nd, 3rd, or 4th week. But what kind of change, and how can we track that? Basically, you should notice that you feel less anxious and stressed, all other things being equal—in other words, if there are no new or unexpected stressors in your life. But that's the thing. *All things are never equal!* Life is not static, and the crazy stressors of this world are sometimes greater and sometimes less depending on the month, week, day, or even hour. This variability makes it hard for you to detect the emotional improvements that you will experience with this challenge.

That said, you should see noticeable improvements in your mood. You may feel more even-tempered—less quick to react harshly and more likely to have patience. Also, notice how your general level of anxiety changes over the next 8 weeks. This may be hard to pick up on over time, because the regular high-cocoa consumption will help you be less distracted by your anxiousness—definitely a good thing.

I know that these measures are soft and qualitative and that we can't put numbers on them. But these are some of the most important improvements that chocolate can provide. In this case, listen to how you feel over time, and note the improvements you perceive. In addition, use the journal in Chapter 11 to record the changes you observe in yourself.

HOW DO I HELP MYSELF?

Chocolate needs your help. And it's so good to you in every bite that the least you can do is give a little love back. You can help your chocolate boost your long-term emotional health by setting aside 10 minutes every morning. That's all. It's simple to do and requires only a mini-meditation, during which you will observe the following procedure.

First, get into a comfortable, quiet place where you won't be disturbed for 10 minutes. Close your eyes and focus on breathing from your belly, not from your chest. It's important to get into the habit of belly breathing, because this action stimulates your body's internal relaxation response. By contrast, chest breathing stimulates the "fight or flight" nervous system response. So, to make sure you're moving your emotional state in the right direction, during this mini-meditation, place your hand on your belly to make sure it's expanding and contracting with each breath.

This mini-meditation can reduce your cortisol levels, but keep in mind that it's not just the act of closing your eyes and being quiet that causes this important internal change. It happens when you clear the mental desktop and return to a singular focus. In other words, you focus on one single thing and all the other cares and thoughts and worries are set aside for just that brief time period. But your distractible brain is prone to wandering, and you may find that daily concerns begin to find their way back into your thoughts.

The solution to this problem, so you can find your singular focus, is to speak a single word, softly, throughout the mini-meditation. This word should connote peace, ease, and relaxation. The word you softly say to yourself assists your meditation by keeping your focus on that word. If your mind happens to wander and you lose your singular focus, that's okay. Just refocus on your word and you'll get it back.

Do this mini-meditation daily for 8 weeks, and you will move your body into a relaxation response state (away from the "fight or flight" state). Even better, the combination of this mini-meditation with daily high-cocoa chocolate consumption becomes a powerful shield to help you keep outside stressors on the outside and to prevent them from getting to your insides, where they can cause damage.

HOW CHOCOLATE SAVES YOUR DIET

Again, people eat for many reasons that have nothing to do with hunger or fullness or even the food itself. This chapter encourages you to eat chocolate, but do it for the right reasons. Eating a little chocolate each day can be very healthy for both your physical and emotional heart. But if you eat it in response to emotional swings, whether positive or negative, you'll only be digging a deeper hole.

The same is true for everything. Think about it in terms of wine. If you have one to two glasses per day, it could help you live 10 extra years (10 happy years). But if you have a week's worth of wine in one sitting to "drown your sorrows," that same alcohol can destroy your life.

The principle is the same: Your chocolate, your wine, and, in fact, all of your foods should be consumed in small portions over time. When any are eaten to fill an emotional void, they only make the problem worse. When eaten for the right reasons, they are a daily blessing to be enjoyed.

SUCCESS STORY
Joe Pientka

AGE: 47

POUNDS LOST: 15

CHOCOLATE TIP: *"Try different kinds of dark chocolate. I found a kind with raspberries in it, which I love. It really satisfies me."*

"My meals had just gotten out of control. I would snack all day and eat meals at a rapid pace," Joe Pientka says. "I was trying to eat what I thought was healthy, but I was eating too much. I was having a lot of diet soda and thought that was okay because it was diet. My body was out of whack and I was hungry all the time."

Joe wanted to lose the weight, but in order to do that, he needed to know how to eat simply and how to eat better. When he heard about the Eat Chocolate, Lose Weight program, he knew he had to try it. "It made sense to me as I learned more about it," he says. "It was how I wanted to live—eating natural foods and avoiding chemicals."

Joe says his transition from milk chocolate to dark chocolate felt natural. "Before the program, I didn't have much of a sweet tooth. I would occasionally eat milk chocolate with caramel or almonds, but I crave fats more than sweets. Dark chocolate reminds me of coffee—and I really like coffee. That really satisfied me inside somehow. In the time that I've been doing this, I seem to go back to the same type of dark chocolate that I really enjoy. As long as it's a good-quality dark chocolate, I like it. It's very smooth—like a good cup of coffee."

Once he started the program, Joe realized it was easier than he expected. "Once you understand the principles, it's easy to follow. You don't have to count calories. All you have to do is eat the right foods." He also regained control over his eating habits and cravings. "The best thing I learned is how to slow down my eating at meals. The second best thing I learned was to not cave in to having a lot of snacks," Joe explains.

In 8 weeks, Joe lost 15 pounds and two pants sizes. "It felt great to complete the program. People could notice I lost weight. I had more energy and a new outlook—a spark—that went beyond the weight loss and improved my attitude," he says. And Joe is not the only one who has benefited from the program. "My family changed their eating patterns, too. We now buy better-quality foods and avoid processed food."

In addition, the plan helped Joe control his stress. "When your stress levels go up, your old habits tend to come back. Before, I would eat too quickly, but now I can keep myself in check," he says, noting his improved blood pressure and cholesterol levels. "Now, my levels have straightened out, and I attribute that to this plan."

For Joe, the Eat Chocolate, Lose Weight plan was more than just a weight-loss program—it changed his life. "Now I have more energy, I feel better, and it just changed how I go through life. It's a combination of losing the weight, not feeling sluggish, eating the right foods, and not having guilt. It all plays into my overall well-being."

Chapter 7

The Chocolate Workout

O kay, just relax. Breathe in, breathe out, because I'm going to turn your thinking on its head yet again. We know that working out in the gym is supposed to be for the type A, go-getter people who really take care of their bodies, right? Eating chocolate every day, by contrast, is said to be for the slackers who don't really care about their physique.

In fact, most people think that chocolate and exercise have a quirky kind of relationship: Exercise is what you have to do to atone for the sin of eating chocolate, and chocolate is what you get to eat as a treat for having gone through the pain of exercise: "If I want to eat that chocolate bar, I'll have to pound out 10 miles on the treadmill or else I'll gain 10 pounds!" In other words, chocolate is to exercise as pleasure is to pain, and the equation between these two must balance.

However, feeling like you have to make up for something like eating chocolate is silly. High-cocoa chocolate is not a problem you have to "work off." Actually, it's the solution you have to "work on," because it gives you more energy to exercise in the first place, it lets you stay active longer without fatigue, and it even helps your muscles repair themselves after you exercise. Chocolate also reduces muscle fatigue, making it great for those athletic types who like running on the treadmill and competing in events such as the Ironman and the Tough Mudder. These people actually need high-cocoa chocolate in their diets on a regular basis if they want to be better competitors.

But what if you're not one of those athletes? Well, eating chocolate can benefit you as well. Let's say you just enjoy moving and being active by gardening or walking or playing on a league team for some sport, or by taking a hike or bike for an afternoon—let's call this the "active living" group. This group also gets the very same benefits—before, during, and after a workout—as the competitive athletes do from regular consumption of high-cocoa chocolate.

So, here's the summary, right up front: High-cocoa chocolate helps you start exercising, keeps you going longer during your workout, and helps your muscles recover faster from your activity. In this way, you can think of chocolate as parentheses around your workout. This chapter details the effect of chocolate, whether you want to up your athletic game or just need a little metabolic oomph in your day.

Activity versus Exercise

Before we get started talking about how chocolate helps you get fit, I have to put this chocolate-induced fitness fantasy into context by making three points:

1. We have to be clear on what chocolate can—and cannot—do.
2. We need to understand how chocolate impacts fitness versus activity.
3. We must realize why we need to change our minds about chocolate and fitness.

What Can Chocolate Do for Fitness?

First, let's just make sure you're tethered to reality. Chocolate, even the high-cocoa kind that you should be eating, will not make you fit. Sorry. You can't poke down a bar of 70% dark chocolate and be totally ripped by morning. It's just not going to happen.

Instead, it'll do for your fitness exactly what it does for your weight. High-cocoa chocolate creates the conditions inside your body that help you succeed in weight loss. It's not going to make you thin. It's not going to make you fit. It's just going to make it easier for you to make those things happen. It's your little helper, so you can get from where you are now to where you want to be—whether that goal involves weight loss or fitness.

How Chocolate Impacts Fitness versus Activity

Most of the research on cocoa and its effect on muscles, stamina, and cardiovascular parameters is done with athletes—those people who happily spend hours and hours grunting away and sweating through their clothes. I happen to love those people, because I've been that person my whole life. However, most of the dieters I work with are not athletes. They're just people—employees in companies. They don't want to "gut it out" on the elliptical machine while being yelled at by some Jillian Michaels wannabe; they just want to manage their weight and health.

Even though our culture of health tells us that we have to be athletes—and the research literature supports this idea by looking pretty much at only this group—you do *not* have to turn into a gym rat and become an athlete, unless you already are one. You cannot be who you are not. If you do happen to be an athlete, that's great. But if you're just an ordinary person who harbors no plans to dunk from the foul line or swim the English Channel, I've got good news. You don't have to have dreams of superior athletic ability to get the beneficial fitness effects of high-cocoa chocolate.

Just to be clear, you absolutely do need to be active every day. Just do things. Get outside. Move your bones. Find your way off the couch for more than trips to the fridge and back. Find ways to fit consistent movement into your daily routines, and chocolate will help you out as well.

How Chocolate Will Change
Your Mind about Fitness

Here's what we're taught: Our body is a machine, and when we eat, we're basically just putting fuel in the tank. This idea is so fundamentally flawed (as outlined in Chapter 3) that it's not only misleading, but it's also contributing to the overconsumption that actually fuels the health problems we see around us. Whoosh, over the cliff we go.

In the case of fitness, here's why it's so far off the mark. The idea leads people to believe that once they run or walk or bike or do any activity, they've used up their fuel. Hence, if they're "on empty," they have used up their gasoline and have to whip into the gas station to fill up again. Time to refuel. Go eat. Have a nutrient bar. And people will do this even though they're not hungry, because this is how we're taught to think about exercise.

That may be how an invented car works, but it's exactly nothing like how our body works. That's because—and I'm going to let you in on a little secret here—we're not actually machines invented by some guy named Otto in a lab somewhere back in the late 1800s. We're biological organisms and have developed a symbiotic relationship with the other biological organisms that exist on this planet. And that synergy has developed over the past 4.5 billion years.

Although it would be oh so convenient for our egos if our bodies turned out to work just like a machine invented 150 years ago, about 2 seconds of thought makes that perspective totally silly. And the fact that our bodies operate nothing like a machine should be our premise. Unfortunately, it is our living assumption. And that assumption is dead wrong.

For example, if your body were a machine, then exercise would use up the "fuel." When the fuel was gone, you'd be empty. So you should be prompted to eat more so you could refill the tank (in other words, you'd get hungry). However, this is exactly the opposite of what actually takes place.[1]

When you are active at a medium to high intensity, a natural shutdown of hunger occurs. In other words, you finish your exercise and then find that you're just not hungry. The phenomenon is so well known in research that it has its own name: exercise-induced anorexia.[2] By the way, for those of you who lift weights, weight-bearing exercises have an even greater exercise-induced effect on satiety than non-weight-bearing "cardio" exercises do.[3]

Of course, this doesn't mean that exercise makes you anorexic. It only means that you are less likely to crave food after you work out, even if you've expended a lot of calories. The reason your body shuts down hunger is that exertion is treated as a specific kind of biological stressor. This species of stress leads your body to reroute blood toward your lungs, brain, and muscles, where it thinks you need it. (This is a form of the "fight or flight" response of your sympathetic nervous system.) Therefore, blood is removed from your gut, where you would need it to receive, utilize, and digest your food. But if you're in an active state, you're not going to be eating, so your body reallocates its limited resources. Hence, you're just not hungry. And as a result, hunger cravings are reduced after exercise because of the way your body has adapted to dynamically respond to its changing demands for survival.

In fact, studies have linked this very same exercise-induced hunger suppression to the ability to control your chocolate consumption. Researchers looked at individuals who typically craved chocolate and determined how much they ate each day. Then the subjects were instructed to walk at a moderate intensity for 15 minutes. The exercise-induced hunger suppression decreased the likelihood that they would eat chocolate by almost half![4]

So if you crave chocolate and want to have some measure of control over those cravings, you now know what to do. Go for a "chocolate walk"; I recommend a 30-minute stroll at a moderate intensity. When you're done with that walk, judge how your previous cravings have changed.

How long will this exercise-induced hunger suppression last? Every person is different, so you'll have to be your own little lab animal. That's because each physiology will require a different amount of time to come down from its "fight or flight" mode, and into the more relaxed state where you can then digest food. The time it takes to go from one state to another accounts for the time of the hunger suppression that you experience.

How Chocolate Boosts Your Energy

Chocolate can increase your energy levels through the specific kind of antioxidants most abundant in cocoa: catechins and epicatechins. These antioxidants do two very important things to increase your muscles' ability to create more energy for you to use. First, they increase the amount of nutrients your muscles have to work with, and then they further increase the micromolecular organelles that produce the energy itself.

To nourish and power your muscles in the first place, you have to get the nutrients into the muscular fibers. This, of course, happens when the oxygenated blood in your large arteries flows out into the smaller arteries, then into the smaller arterioles, and finally inside the muscle tissue via tiny capillaries. The diameter of a capillary is about 0.0003 inch, or about the width of one single red blood cell. In other words, your red blood cells have to go through the capillaries in a single-file line.

This spidery array of branching capillaries is so small that nutrients can pass from the bloodstream into the tissue. So, if you need more energy, you'll need more nutrients, and you'll need more capillaries to infiltrate the tissue. That's the first need.

The second requirement is to be able to turn those extra nutrients into extra energy. For this, you need the mitochondria, which are tiny organelles. What's an organelle? You know how Pluto recently got demoted from a planet to a "planette," or mini-planet? Well, an organelle is basically a mini-organ—a self-enclosed structure that performs a function for your body. Organs like the liver and kidney may be bigger and doing more things that are more central to your living another day, but your organelles are just as critical—only smaller!

Eat Chocolate, Lose Weight

The mighty mitochondria organelles are the power plants that make the energy that makes you move. Without them, you don't move. And, if you are feeling lethargic and don't want to do anything but veg out on the couch, you can blame your mitochondria. It won't do you any good, and it's not their fault anyway, but it will certainly make you feel better to blame something that you can't see or touch, and most people don't even know what they are.

"Hey, what are you doing?"

"Just being a slug on the couch. It's my mitochondria."

"Oh, that sounds awful. What is it?"

"Mitochondrial malaise, you know, a medical condition with tons of syllables."

You'll be so impressive, right up until the moment your friends discover Google.

Chocolate may be what you turn to during your attack of mitochondrial malaise, but it also happens to be a solution for that very same affliction. Not chocolate per se, but the cocoa in chocolate, which has the highest levels of epicatechins. That's because sustained cocoa consumption produces a happy downstream effect on top of the increased capillary formation in your muscles: new mitochondria formation.[5]

In other words, the epicatechins you get when you eat high-cocoa chocolate do both things that you need in order to increase your energy. This is definitely good news for athletes, as well as for anyone who wants to eat chocolate, and lose weight doing it.

But here's a mistake you cannot make. Yes, high-cocoa chocolate can create energy for you at the cellular level. Yes, this can give you the energy to get off the couch in the first place. It can also give you more energy to take whatever activity you are doing to the next level. However, chocolate is not going to save you. It can't hoist you off the couch. It can't run you down the street or get you to move. It is no more and no less than your most delicious activity support system ever. If used as a support system for your activity, it can help you help yourself.

Here's another question you may be asking. Do I have to *do* anything to get the benefits of these crazy epicatechins? In other words, does the added energy from chocolate *require* activity? If you just eat high-cocoa chocolate and don't exercise, do you still get the increase in capillaries to your muscles? Do you still get the increase in the mitochondria that increase your energy? The answer is yes. You still get them both.

And it pains me to say that. I wanted to research the science and discover that you get the benefits of high-cocoa chocolate consumption only when you also exercise. I just don't want people using this knowledge nugget to justify their inactivity. I don't want them to think, "I'll just launch into a choco-chow-down until I get the energy surge I need to do something more. But until then, my activity is basically eating chocolate, and walking to the cupboard to get more chocolate."

So, yes, you do in fact get the benefits by just eating the chocolate. However, you actually get more of a boost when you combine activity with high-cocoa chocolate consumption. The number of capillaries to your muscles increases (including your heart muscle, by the way), and the number of new mitochondria increases when those muscles are activated.

By the way, the reverse is also true. I just told you that high-cocoa chocolate can increase capillary and mitochondria growth all on its own. The same is true of exercise. On its own, exercise will increase the number of capillaries to your muscles. Likewise, exercise alone will increase the number of mitochondria generated in them. Again, though, the combination of activity plus high-cocoa chocolate provides even more of these benefits to both your skeletal and cardiac muscles.

How many more? According to one study, cocoa epicatechins alone produce a 30% increase in fatigue resistance and a 30% increase in new blood supply. However, the increase in energy that you get from combining cocoa epicatechins with exercise amounts to a boost of 50%![6] In layman's terms, that's a huge increase in your ability to complete your exercises and to go through a normal day with increased energy.

The outcome of this is simple: fatigue resistance. And think about what this would mean for you in the context of your normal day. How much would a little fatigue resistance be worth to you? For example, if someone had a pill that could reduce fatigue without also killing your liver, causing you to break out into boils, or sending you into convulsions ("Don't take it if you're pregnant or are thinking about becoming pregnant; ask your doctor if convulsions are right for you"), you'd buy that. This side effect–free fatigue resistance comes from the combination of high-cocoa chocolate and moderate activity.

How long will it take for these changes to occur? It took 2 weeks for experimental animals to see a 30% increase in fatigue resistance.[7] In a separate study, it took 4 weeks to see increased capillaries and mitochondria.[8] And subjects with type 2 diabetes who were administered 100 milligrams of epicatechins per day for 3 months showed a significant increase in mitochondria.[9] In fact, before taking the epicatechins, their energy-producing mitochondria had all but withered away. It was only with the addition of the high-cocoa chocolate that their mitochondria were restored.

Does that mean you have to have chocolate every day for 3 months before you see improvements in your energy levels? (Okay, worse things could happen.) No, you don't have to wait 3 months. You'll see an increase in energy within those first few weeks, because the increased capillaries and mitochondria are progressive and develop over time.

It turns out, too, that as you get older, chocolate's improvement on your capillaries and energy level is even more evident. As you age, you notice yourself running out of energy more often. Where do you think that energy went? Those little mitochondria organelles, and the nutrients carried in with the capillaries, erode over time.[10] And you become lethargic.

Because of that, there are fewer of the organelles in your muscles to begin with. And as a result, the improvement older individuals realize with increased high-cocoa chocolate consumption is actually greater than that of younger people. There are so very few perks to growing older. Perhaps this is one!

One more question that will absolutely come up: Do I have to eat chocolate all the time to make sure I keep the benefits? The answer to that question is no, not at all. Think about the change you're causing, which is essentially that you're adding "hardware" to your musculature. You're adding physical capillaries and physical organelles. Once in place, they won't poof out of existence in the very nanosecond you stop being active and eating high-cocoa chocolate. It will take a period of inactivity for them to resorb and pull back out of the muscles you're apparently not using anymore.

The result is that even after you're done training, your endurance gains linger because they're in place as new hardware. In fact, researchers have found that the cocoa-induced improvements are sustained for up to 14 days after you stop exercising and taking the catechins.[11]

Before You're Active?
CHOCOLATE.

When you exercise, your bones knock against each other, tendons pull, and muscles break down. Your body typically responds to this physical wear and tear with some degree of oxidative stress. Cocoa is a massive antioxidant that contains flavonols that are also anti-inflammatory.[12] I know people who take anti-inflammatory pills, even though those meds have well-known side effects like nausea, vomiting, diarrhea, constipation, dizziness, fluid retention, and also little things like kidney failure, liver failure, and prolonged bleeding after an injury.

You might predict that the anti-inflammatory impact of regular consumption of high-cocoa dark chocolate would help reduce the damaging effects of prolonged oxidative stress that occurs when you exercise. And you'd be right. In fact, in exercise cyclists who rode for an amazing $2^1/_2$ hours, one group ate 100 grams (about 3.5 ounces) of 70% dark chocolate 2 hours before cycling, a second group ate a snack containing the same macromolecules included in dark chocolate but without the cocoa, and a third group ate nothing. This design allowed researchers to see whether the cocoa lessens the anti-inflammatory markers in the blood after exercise.

They found that the cyclists who had eaten nothing and also those who had eaten the snack without cocoa had elevated levels of isoprostane in the blood (a potent inflammatory molecule that heightens the feeling of pain). Meanwhile, a full hour after exercise, the group that had eaten dark chocolate had levels of inflammatory pain-producing molecules (isoprostanes) that were no different from those before they'd even started exercising.[13] In other words, preloading with dark chocolate can help prevent post-exercise pain.

How much chocolate do you need to get this effect? Honestly, you won't have to add additional chocolate to get this benefit. Just eating it consistently, as we've discussed, is enough. The improvement has less to do with adding more chocolate and more to do with just making sure that you have a little and have it consistently.

One more question: Should you eat chocolate a certain number of minutes before exercising? No, it's not a pill or a fuel pellet that gives you instant energy for your upcoming exercise. It provides a sustained effect, which comes from sustained consumption over time. Again, you don't need high volume; you just need consistency.

After You're Active?
CHOCOLATE.

Remember the anti-inflammatory properties of cocoa that we just talked about? They are why chocolate helps your muscles recover after they have exerted themselves. To investigate this, researchers studied athletes who exercised hard twice a day—once in the morning and then again in the afternoon. In between these two exercise sessions, researchers gave one group of athletes a cocoa drink and the other group a simple carbohydrate replacement drink.

The question? Which one of these drinks is better at providing more energy after a fatiguing morning practice? In other words, which is the better recovery drink?

During the afternoon session, both groups of athletes did a shuttle run exercise until they were completely fatigued. Those who'd had the cocoa drink took a full 2 minutes longer to fatigue than those who'd had the standard carbohydrate replacement schlock—a significant amount of time when running.[14]

And the same result was found for exercise cyclists. Basically, the cyclists were put through two bouts of intensive exercise. After the first one, they had a 4-hour recovery period during which they were given a recovery drink: either chocolate milk or a standard carbohydrate replacement drink. Then they were put back on the bicycles to ride until they were totally exhausted. So, which drink leads to better performance during the next "ride to exhaustion"? It turns out that those who had consumed chocolate milk prior to their second workout were able to produce 57% more energy during their workout than those who'd had the standard carbohydrate replacement drink. And despite the fact that the chocolate milk and the carbohydrate replacement drink had the same amount of carbohydrates, the subjects who'd consumed chocolate milk were able to cycle 49% longer than the group who'd consumed the carbohydrate replacement beverage.[15] As a matter of fact, consuming chocolate provides a fivefold reduction in your perception of soreness, compared to drinking carbohydrate replacement beverages.[16] In these studies, the recovery effect of cocoa appears greatest when you have it about 30 minutes after your exercise.[17]

In most of these studies, the researchers used a drink with cocoa in it. You don't have to consume your chocolate in the form of a beverage though. A drink is just the most convenient source if you're an athlete, because you're thirsty anyway, and you don't feel like eating anything. All that said, there is a red flag regarding commercial chocolate milk products and their use as recovery drinks. You have to watch out for what manufacturers put into the milk—sugar, for example. If you're an athlete doing two killer bouts of exercise per day, you can probably afford the sugar in the chocolate milk drink. But if you're a casual exerciser, this can become a problem, and you shouldn't consume those drinks. In this case, an easier solution is to finish your activity, relax, drink some water, and nurse a couple of thumb-size bites of high-cocoa chocolate while you're catching your breath.

TAKE THE
Chocolate Challenge

Use chocolate to increase your fitness level. All the research discussed above shows how high-cocoa chocolate can increase your energy and also the amount of time before exhaustion sets in. What a great opportunity this is to make chocolate your solution to getting fit!

WHAT DO I DO?

To use chocolate as your little helper, you have to know your own level of fitness to begin with. Get your baseline (which we will discuss in the next section) so you know what, if any, effect chocolate actually has on you. Every person has a different physiology, a different history, and a different capacity for improvement. For all these reasons, chocolate has a different effect on each person. And you won't know its effect on you unless you understand where you're starting from.

After you get your baseline, you will eat high-cocoa chocolate both before and after you exercise. Continue to do the activity or exercise that you normally do, but now start to note the following:

- **Before your exercise:** Have your daily energy levels improved?

- **During your exercise:** Are you able to complete your routine faster or go longer?

- **After your exercise:** Do your muscles feel as sore as they did before you incorporated high-cocoa chocolate into your diet?

Basically, you're doing a thoughtful analysis with your own body. Like a scientist, you're finding out where you are starting from (your baseline), applying a test condition, and finally, measuring the effect of that condition on your original baseline measurements. It's smart, and lets you know exactly what works for you, in what way, and by how much.

HOW DO I DO THIS?

Get your baseline by determining two measures: one subjective and one objective. The objective measure is the duration of your activity (how long, how far, and how often you do it). If you run for 30 minutes each day, you might note how far you run in that 30 minutes, or how fast you run during that time. Use the same format for any activity you do, whether it's walking, riding a bike, gardening, etc.

How Much Chocolate Can You Have If You Exercise?

Following the instructions in this book, you will eat your chocolate in association with meals, to pull your sweet tooth, to control chronic consumption, and to help your muscles recover after you exercise. In each case, the amounts you eat will be small, but they can add up! So please, make sure you don't exceed the maximum allotment, based on the percentage of cocoa you're eating (see Chapter 2, page 36).

When you exercise, you should consume two thumb-size pieces of chocolate—one about 30 minutes before a workout and the other about 30 minutes after. Alternatively, you can have one piece before and a cocoa-based recovery drink afterward (see "The Cocoa Q&A" on page 157 for details).

The subjective measure is how you feel, on a scale that ranges from pumped, to great, to fine, to weak, to zombie. You'll take this measure before and then after you exercise. Keep in mind that the subjective measure (how you "feel") is every bit as important as the objective measure. It's just going to have more variability in it each time.

For this chocolate challenge, make sure that the exercise you're doing during the pre-chocolate period is the same as what you're doing during the post-chocolate period. That way, you'll be comparing apples to apples. Just be consistent with your activity throughout this challenge so you can see if there's a true effect.

During the control week, keep track of the objective measures in your journal—how long and how far—along with the subjective measure: how you feel after your exercise. Once you start the chocolate phase, you'll write down exactly the same measures, but note how those change over time.

WHAT CAN I EXPECT WHEN I DO THIS?

Are you a man or a mouse? The mouse data say that it takes a couple of weeks for chocolate to increase the muscle capillaries and mighty mitochondria that give you more energy throughout the day. However, the little bit of human data that exist show an increase after 3 months. My guess is that you'll be somewhere in between those two time frames, and that middle ground will depend on many different things: how much you've been exercising already, how good your diet has been to this point, your age, your gender, etc.

Even with all that crazy variability, person to person, here's what you can expect: With the objective measurement, your endurance will improve over time. With the subjective measurement, your feelings about exercise will improve as well. In other words, it will be less burdensome on you as you go along.

The rate of this progress will be specific to your body and how it responds. You're blazing your own trail here. The improvement you realize from your chocolate in increased energy, endurance, and performance will be unlike anyone else's. So trust yourself. Whether you're improving at a rapid rate or a more modest one, be at peace with that and keep moving. You'll continue to improve your fitness, and chocolate will make it easier for you to do that over time.

Plus, if you were to exercise without adding chocolate to your life, you would still increase your objective measures (how far you can go, how fast, etc.). But according to all these data, you will do that more quickly by adding just a couple of thumb-size bites of chocolate on a consistent basis. And this challenge will help you determine exactly how much your efforts have helped you improve and how much better you feel about it.

HOW DO I HELP MYSELF?

The very best way to help your workout is to cut out extraneous sugar. The additive sugars that food manufacturers put into their processed food products can sap your energy, leaving you tired and even hungry. And the last thing you want to do when you feel that way is to work out. Thus, if you want chocolate to boost your energy levels even more, be rigorous about cutting out all sugar.

This doesn't mean that you should eliminate all carbohydrates, because fruits and vegetables are wonderful for you. Moreover, the natural fiber they contain lowers the glycemic index of that food to help prevent the insulin response from happening. The same is true, but to a lesser extent, for complex carbohydrates like potatoes, rice, or bread. If you eat these foods along with some natural form of fat, fiber, or protein (pasta with olive oil, bread with peanut butter, or rice with beans), then you will lower the glycemic index of those starches so they don't sap your energy in the next 2 hours.

HOW CHOCOLATE SAVES YOUR DIET

High-cocoa chocolate does a lot of wonderful things for your muscles and vascular system. In this chapter, I've emphasized a number of times that having massive amounts of chocolate isn't the thing that's going to improve your fitness level. The benefit you want is not going to come from a high volume but rather from being consistent. Have a little chocolate every day, and you will realize the benefits over time.

The way to apply this chocolate eating lesson to your entire life is to apply the same strategy to your activity. If you're a fitness buff or an athlete of some stripe, you may feel the need to hit the gym for concentrated bouts of grunting. For everyone else, though, exercise needs to be distributed through your day, consistently.

As with your chocolate consumption, being fit is not about increasing numbers of higher-intensity bouts of exercise, but is instead about moving throughout your day and doing that consistently. In other words, if you can move, move. If you can walk, walk. If you're on the phone with someone and you walk around during the call, that counts. If you can fit movement into your daily life activities on a consistent basis, you win.

Here's the thing: You can often hear people say in a complaining voice how they "have to walk" to get something. For them, walking is an

THE COCOA Q&A

Q: Which is better as a recovery aid: solid chocolate or chocolate milk?

A: First of all, unless you make it yourself, chocolate milk is okay but not great for you. Conventional chocolate milk drinks are loaded with syrups, stabilizers, and other junk that's not at all recommended for better health. However, if you take cocoa (especially un-Dutched cocoa) and mix it into milk, that would be an exceptional recovery drink.

As for solid chocolate, it is good, but not as good as cocoa delivered in liquid form for muscle recovery. That's because your body is still in digestive lockdown after exercise. In other words, it routes blood to your muscles, lungs, and brain and away from your viscera, where digestion takes place.

So, in this case, a fluid form of cocoa (cocoa in milk, for example) is preferable to a solid form (chocolate) because you'll be better able to digest it, and therefore absorb it. Plus, the added protein in milk can help with muscle recovery after a strenuous bout of exercise.

inconvenience when they could take a car, a tram, a Segway, the escalator, the elevator, or any number of inventions we've come up with to save us from the inconvenience of putting one foot in front of the other.

However, when you're 80 years old and you can no longer get yourself from point A to B without having to be handled by your family, you're going to hate it. You're going to wish with all your heart that you had the opportunity to be inconvenienced in that way. What a joy it would be to have the independence and freedom to "have to walk" to get something. Moving is a gift and a miracle. It's a freedom that you don't appreciate until the very moment it's gone from your life and you find yourself dependent on others with no way out of that trap.

If you want to keep that freedom as you age, there is a solution. If you want to be able to move then, you need to move now. Move every chance you get, and you'll be better able to move when you get older. You don't have to be heroic or ballistic, just be consistent.

Here's the rule: Do not walk because you have to. Walk because you *can*. And when you add a little chocolate every day, you get the added energy boost you need to be active longer throughout your life.

SUCCESS STORY
Donna Hume

AGE: 48

POUNDS LOST: 65

CHOCOLATE TIP: *"Keep going. Just because you have a bad day—or two or three—where you get off track, doesn't mean you should give up. This is a process, and retraining your brain and body takes time; allow yourself that time."*

"I had always done the diet, the deprivation, and it wasn't working," says Donna Hume, who had struggled with weight loss for 20 years. "Every time I tried another diet, I lost 15 or 20 pounds and gained it back." Her desk job didn't make matters better either. "The majority of what I do is in front of the computer and on the telephone. I would come in at 8 a.m., and before I knew it, it was noon and I hadn't moved."

As a self-described picky eater and chocolate lover, Donna needed a program that was both sustainable and enjoyable. "Give me chocolate ice cream, brownies, or chocolate cake and I'm in heaven. It's not something I'm willing to give up," she exclaims. "When I heard I could have chocolate on this plan, I was like, 'I'm on board with that!'"

Shortly after starting the program, Donna noticed a change in her eating habits. "Before, I would graze and snack all day," she admits. "Now, once I've had my chocolate ender, I know my meal is over. It's really helped to control my cravings."

Donna soon began noticing other changes as well. "I would go out to lunch with coworkers once a week, and I would make better choices than before. And I started doing it automatically," she says, noting that on other programs, it was a struggle to know what to eat. "Whenever I'm on a diet, I think about it all the time: I can't have this, I can't have that. On this program, it's about what you *can* have," she says.

Donna also increased her amount of exercise while on the Eat Chocolate, Lose Weight plan. "I started exercising, and now I'm motivated to move more. I force myself to get up at least once an hour and take a little walk."

Amazingly, she lost 15 pounds in 8 weeks, which inspired her to keep going. "I think it became so ingrained that it became a habit and I just continued. It didn't feel like I finished a 'program.'" Donna not only lost weight during the holiday season on the program, but she also maintained her weight loss while recuperating from surgery. "After I went in for surgery (that's usually a 6- to 8-week recovery), I was back to work in 4 weeks," she says. "I bounced back quickly, and I even tried to walk while I was recovering. I started with 5 minutes a day. It doesn't sound like a lot, but my body just felt better." She ultimately lost 65 pounds and went from a size 22 to a size 12.

For Donna, this wasn't just another weight-loss program. It was a lifestyle change. "It's not like the other programs out there. I don't even want to call it a program. It will teach you how to eat in the real world and set you up for the future."

Take Your "Vitamin Ch": Why Chocolate Is a Superfood

I f I told you to think of a health food, you would immediately come back to me with standard foods like kale, açaí berries, or even dietary catchphrases like low-fat, low-carb, organic, farm-raised, 100% natural, and so on. But you might be surprised to know that high-cocoa chocolate has the cancer-fighting properties of broccoli, the antioxidant boost of carrot sticks, and even the heart-healthy power of a glass of wine. In fact, this amazing superfood has so many health properties that it really should be its own vitamin—vitamin Ch! This is yet another reason why I prescribe this over-the-counter vitamin Ch for your daily consumption.

What's funny is that even though it's so good for you, the thought of taking a chocolate "prescription" almost sounds frightening. Whenever you hear of research that points out ever more of the raucous health benefits you can get by eating cocoa, the commentary portion of the study always apologizes for the results. Every single time, like a prerecorded message, researchers say they'd never recommend that you eat this food that is so great for your heart, diabetes, stress reduction, arteries, stamina, and so on. But why? Why in the world wouldn't they wholeheartedly endorse something that's so effective for so many people in so many ways? What are they afraid of?

Can you imagine what would happen if all of these benefits were found not in a food but in a pill that could be sold by pharmaceutical companies? This pill would be offered to doctors to prescribe to their patients, and it would be a blockbuster! Drug companies would sell a billion of them, and doctors would prescribe them without hesitation. Too bad chocolate doesn't come in a pill.

If it were a pill, it would improve your heart health like cholesterol-lowering medications such as statins do, only without the little disclaimer voice on the commercial warning you that it might harm your liver ("Ask your doctor if liver failure is right for you"). If it were a pill, you could take it for depression, only without the possibility of it increasing the frequency of sad, troublesome thoughts ("Ask your doctor if suicidal ideation is right for you"). However, in the standard refrain, we hear that people cannot be advised to take a healthy food like chocolate every day, because they may make it bad for themselves by having too much of it. And it's strange, too, because pills can be overconsumed just like food can. And when pills aren't taken as prescribed, the side effects can (typically) become even worse. However, that stops exactly zero doctors from prescribing more and more meds for us.

The standard worry about taking too much chocolate is a complete double standard. The same hand-wringing was applied to wine, when it was first discovered that wine contains so many positive health properties. "Oh, we can't recommend that you drink wine because you might overdo it." And by the way, our medical researchers "discovered" that wine was good for you even though everyone else on planet Earth already knew that. We had to discover what was already known. And the same is true for chocolate. In healthy cultures like France, Italy, and Switzerland, people eat chocolate every day. But somehow we in the United States can't do that until we discover what everyone else already knows: Chocolate is a health food. Only then do we say, so proudly, "Hey, look what we discovered!"

So, given the fact that healthy cultures eat chocolate all the time and research has yet to show anything but confirmatory evidence about the health effects of high-cocoa chocolate, it seems logical that you should eat chocolate every day, like a delicious vitamin. Just control your daily medicinal vitamin Ch as described in the first few chapters of this book, and make sure it's high in cocoa.

Bonus Effects of **CHOCOLATE**

We've already discussed the reasons why chocolate can help you control your weight (by increasing your metabolism, increasing the amount of time you can exercise before exhaustion sets in, reducing cravings, and controlling consumption). And even better, it can be used to help pull your sweet tooth so that the foods you do crave are lower in sugar.

However, there are many bonus effects of chocolate that violate some of the most entrenched "myth-conceptions" about this wonderful health food. These remove perhaps the last few concerns you may have about adding chocolate to your daily life. We'll review these one by one, but just look at this list of bonuses you can expect from eating high-cocoa chocolate:

- Better skin
- Healthier teeth
- Reduced cancer risk
- More control for diabetics
- Improved heart health
- Controlled hypertension
- Improved sexual health

Chocolate and Your Skin

I remember my dad telling my sister that the reason she had acne was that she loved eating chocolate and that chocolate causes zits. This was the conventional wisdom at the time, but researchers still get equivocal results even after 40 years of asking the question "Does eating chocolate cause acne?" Some say yes, while others say no. In other words, the jury is definitely still out.

One explanation for this scientific waffling is that acne may be associated with chocolate consumption but not *caused* by it. Something may be carried along with the chocolate, which simply wasn't controlled for in the original experiments. For example, there's some evidence that dairy may contribute to facial blemishes, so the cases finding a positive association between acne and chocolate may actually be due to the dairy in the lighter milk chocolates.

As the rash research rages on, other results support the conclusion that chocolate is actually incredibly good for your skin and can even decrease the likelihood that you will get a sunburn. In that way, chocolate acts like a sunscreen but without also blocking vitamin D.

In a study in London, researchers gave two groups of pale-skinned volunteers chocolate to eat for 12 weeks. One group received a high-flavonol chocolate, such as the kind you might get with a high-cocoa chocolate. The second got a "low-flavonol" chocolate, such as you might get with lighter milk chocolate. After 12 weeks, they assessed the skin of these participants with UV light to see whether cocoa provided any added protection to the skin from erythema (a.k.a. sunburn).

The results were amazing. Those who ate low-flavonol chocolate had no benefit at all. In other words, the amount of UV radiation that caused a sunburn before they started eating their milky chocolate was the same as the amount that caused a sunburn after they ate it. However, those who ate the high-flavonol chocolate doubled their protection compared to the baseline.[1] Doubled. Less than 2 weeks of eating high-flavonol chocolate produced skin that was protected from burning even at twice the UV level.

One of the reasons for this protective effect may be the fact that high-cocoa chocolate can increase circulation into the skin itself. Women who consume high-flavonol chocolate drinks can get more blood from the fine capillaries into the topmost layers of the skin (those within only 1 millimeter of the surface). When this happens, you get the healthy oxygenation your skin needs to help protect itself.[2]

Think about what this can do for you over time. Let's say you get this UV protection, which will help prevent damage from the sun's rays. That's great—but you're also getting increased bloodflow to the very top surface of your skin, with more nutrients and more oxygenation. This helps produce healthier skin that looks and feels better, too.

It turns out that this is exactly what happens. After women had high-flavonol cocoa for 12 weeks, researchers discovered, their skin was more hydrated! How many people do you know who buy hydrating creams and rubs and whatnot? In this case, 12 weeks of enjoying delicious high-flavonol cocoa reduced the loss of moisture in the skin by about 25%! What cream can promise that?

For the women in this study, my guess is that they're less concerned with the scientific terminology of "micro-vascularization" and "minimal erythemal dose" and more interested in how the high-cocoa flavonols make their skin look and feel. Other researchers have discovered that the "skin surface showed a significant decrease of skin roughness and scaling," thanks to high-cocoa chocolate.[3] What all of this means is that by eating high-flavonol chocolate, your skin becomes smoother, healthier, less dried out and so less prone to wrinkling, and more resistant to the UV rays that damage your collagen fibers, leading to slackening of the skin.

This is obviously great news, although there is a caveat. In these studies, the scientists had subjects ingest an amount of flavonol equal to about 100 grams of 70% chocolate every day. That would be like eating one of those large rectangular chocolate bars every day. You're not going to want to eat that much each day for 12 weeks. Of course, if you eat chocolate with a higher cocoa content, you'll be getting more of the flavonols that are so good for your skin, even in a smaller dose.

But don't sweat the details on this. You don't have to clone their research study to get the benefits they describe. Just eat high-cocoa chocolate and be consistent about it. The higher the cocoa percentage and the more consistent you are with your consumption of it, the better the effects will be on your grateful, more supple, less-desiccated skin.

Chocolate and Your Teeth

Have you ever heard that you should not eat chocolate because it will "rot your teeth"? It turns out that this is just a case of mistaken identity. Those high-sugar confections that masquerade as "chocolates" because they've got a patina of chocolate schmear over the top can certainly contribute to dental cavities. But the chocolate in this case is just a victim of guilt by association. The sugars cause the cavities, not the cocoa component.

In fact, the news is even better than that. Not only will high-cocoa chocolate not cause cavities, but also your dentist will love you even more because it can prevent those cavities from forming in the first place! Cocoa polyphenols can decrease the formation of biofilm on your teeth and also the production of acid by the streptococcus bacteria.[4]

In a study conducted at the College of Dental Sciences and Hospital in Davangere, India, children were instructed not to practice any oral hygiene, such as brushing and flossing, for 4 solid days! On the morning of the 4th day, one group was given a "chocolate mouthwash" (actually, just a wash that contained cocoa antioxidants). The second group was given a placebo mouthwash with nothing in it. In the cocoa-mouthwash group, the bacteria decreased by 20.9%, compared with that in the placebo group—and there was a decrease of 49.6% in plaque formation.[5]

These results were replicated with white lab mice, which were fed white chocolate (with a whopping 35% sucrose). But one subgroup was given extract from cocoa powder. The researchers then looked to see which group ended up with dental cavities. They found that the addition of cocoa powder extract blocked bacteria from causing the dental cavities that normally happen under these conditions.[6] The antibacterial source of the cavity-fighting yumminess comes from the cocoa bean husk.[7] We need this in our toothpaste. (Can you imagine someone marketing a "chocolate toothpaste"? How counterintuitive would that be to our society's way of thinking about chocolate?)

Chocolate and Cancer Prevention

Your body transforms part of the food you eat into energy to keep your muscles and organs functioning, and the rest of it becomes unsanitary waste that must be eliminated from your digestive system. Once eliminated, it must then be carried away from your home, or else it can cause people to become sick.

Similarly, every one of your cells takes in nutrients, transforms them into energy, and then uses that energy to power your muscles and organs. And again, there is a leftover by-product of this normal metabolic process that is basically a form of cellular waste, which must also be removed from the cellular environment. This is known as reactive oxygen species (ROS).

In the case of your cells, the scientific research clearly shows that ROS waste products must be removed from your system or they can build, build, build and contribute to your getting sick, sometimes in the form of cancer. One way they do this is by causing damage to your DNA, which can create the mutations that start, and sustain, deadly cancers.[8] If you've heard health authorities say that you need antioxidant foods, this is why. Antioxidants act like the garbagemen of your body, coming by to remove the ROS molecules so they don't pile up into a metabolic mess.

High-cocoa chocolate is one of those antioxidant foods that can pick up and clean up the ROS molecules in your system. In fact, cells incubated with cocoa extract or its main antioxidant, epicatechin, lower the amount of ROS that is produced by your cells. And it does this in a dose-dependent manner: the more epicatechin, the lower the damaging ROS.[9] In other words, the antioxidants in cocoa can help stop the formation of the cellular waste that can lead to cancer before

Eat Chocolate, Lose Weight

it even starts. But what if you already have cells that have been exposed to so much ROS that they are damaged, mutated, and becoming cancerous? Can these antioxidants *treat,* as well as *prevent,* cancer formation at the cellular level?

It's impossible to say yes to this . . . for now. However, the evidence is very, very suggestive that cocoa antioxidants can inhibit existing breast cancer cells from proliferating out of control.[10] And there's more. Researchers treated experimental animals that developed lung cancer with another in cocoa's closet of flavonols known as proanthocyanidins. The result? The animals experienced a "significant reduction in the incidence and multiplicity of carcinomas."[11] This was not a small effect, either. In the case of colon cancer cells, cocoa polyphenols reduced their proliferation by an amazing 70%.[12] You can ask your doctor, but I'm betting that high-cocoa chocolate is the most delicious treatment there is for reducing the out-of-control growth of cancer cells.

Lung. Colon. Breast. As far as cancer goes, these are the biggies, accounting for more deaths than any other type of cancer (see the table).[13]

CANCER TYPE	DEATHS EVERY YEAR
Lung	159,480
Colon	50,830
Breast	39,620

What would it be like if the creation of cancer cells could be stopped or slowed? What would it be like if these 249,930 souls, *almost a quarter of a million people every single year,* could reduce their chance of developing cancer cells in the first place? Then, even if the cells were produced, what if you could take something that could help keep them from replicating out of control? It would be lifesaving, that's what it would be. And the available research so far indicates that cocoa polyphenols can interrupt the initiation, promotion, and proliferation of cancer.

Are you a mouse in a cancer study? No. Can you incubate your cancer cells in cocoa polyphenols in a petri dish? Of course not. And are the quantities used in these research studies similar to the amounts you could get from a chocolate bar? Sometimes yes, sometimes no. Given these limitations to the existing research, one solution would be for you to wait another 15 or 20 years before you take steps to prevent cancer in your body. You could certainly wait until all the studies have been done and redone and everyone agrees with one another in a unison of scientific harmony.

Alternatively, you could eat high-cocoa chocolate, and eat it in control. After all, even now the research does in fact indicate that there is a cellular pathway through which cocoa stops cancer cells from being produced and prevents them from taking over your breast, colon, and lungs. While you're waiting on scientists to agree on something, you might as well just eat high-cocoa chocolate, and eat it in control.

Chocolate and Diabetes

For many nutritionists, the idea that chocolate consumption should not be discouraged for diabetics—and especially that it *should* be encouraged—creates a stress response to spike their own blood sugars through the roof. But this is another example of how newer research is replacing older ways of thinking.

First of all, a principal characteristic of diabetes is uncontrolled blood sugar: It swings too high (hyperglycemia, which can lead to diabetic coma, known as ketoacidosis), or it swings too low (hypoglycemia, which can lead to seizures or unconsciousness). So, any consumption of any food that makes you lose control of your blood sugar regulation should not be encouraged—ever.

Fortunately, according to a study in the research journal *Diabetic Medicine,* high-cocoa chocolate does not cause the blood sugar of diabetics to swing out of control.[14] In this study, those with type 2 diabetes ate

45 grams (about 1.5 ounces) of high-cocoa chocolate every single day for 4 weeks. The scientists found that the subjects' blood sugar control did not suffer at all. (And guess what—neither did their weight!) How's that for good news?

Another consequence of diabetes? The downstream impact of this disease can wreak havoc on your blood vessels, leading to high blood pressure and heart disease. However, high-cocoa chocolate may actually provide relief. A German research group has shown that consistent consumption of cocoa rich in flavonol antioxidants—taken three times every day for 30 days—improved artery function by 30%![15] This suggests that the consistent consumption of cocoa with high levels of antioxidants, such as the un-Dutched variety I've advised, may actually help treat the symptoms of this disease.

But what if you are a borderline diabetic, or just want to make sure that you don't slip into full-blown diabetes? The evidence shows that high-cocoa chocolate may be able to help here as well. A 2005 study published in the *American Journal of Clinical Nutrition* showed that healthy subjects who ate 100 grams (about 3.5 ounces) of high-cocoa

THE COCOA Q&A

Q: Wouldn't it be better for me to just take megadoses of antioxidant vitamins than to get my antioxidants from chocolate?

A: No. Multivitamin megadoses can actually be very harmful and are not recommended. If you abstract one single element of a healthy food and provide it to the body in a gelatin caplet, you are giving your body doses that are not physiological. Also, you are giving your body those elements outside the context of all the other things that grow in the plant itself. Many times, it's the total combination of all the components of a health food that produce the healthy effect. That's why the health properties of the catechins in cocoa are tied up in the consumption of the bean itself, and the very best way to maximize the health benefits of chocolate is to eat it as close to its original form as possible: un-Dutched, solid, dark chocolate.

chocolate every day for 2 weeks actually had improved insulin sensitivity (the ability of your body to get sugar out of your blood and into your tissues where it is needed).[16]

Again, the science here is new and the biochemical mechanisms for exactly how this happens is just now being worked out,[17] but what is clear is that a new research trail leads directly from chocolate to cocoa to antioxidants to improved insulin sensitivity—and therefore, lower blood sugar. Whether to help stabilize the effects of this condition, or to help prevent them from developing in the first place, this cocoa trail has a very tasty beginning and a very healthful end.

Taking Chocolate to Heart

Do you ever feel like, with health advice, the rug gets pulled out from under you all the time? "Margarine is going to save your life!" Oh, yeah, sorry about that advice. Margarine is actually killing your heart. "You have got to drink *at least* eight 8-ounce glasses of water every day." Um, right, so, about that advice . . . there was never any data supporting that one, either. We've clearly established that what's bad for you today used to be good for you; what's good for you today used to be bad for you. No wonder we're so confused about what to put in our mouths.

A case in point is the evil saturated fats that are supposed to kill your heart. They're another key reason we're told to avoid eating chocolate, because chocolate contains saturated fats. How can chocolate be good for your heart and still have those saturated fats that we're told are mucking up the works? It turns out that, like many evil villains, they're just misunderstood, and all saturated fats aren't all bad for you all the time. There's a good side to them, too! That's why chocolate's theory-offending saturated fats turn out to be heart healthy. They originate from cocoa butter, with one-third of them consisting of stearic acid. Stearic acid doesn't raise your bad cholesterol at all. Moreover, it's actually good for your heart because your liver converts it into oleic acid, which is a heart-healthy, monounsaturated fat. Another one-third of them are the healthy monounsaturated fats to start with. Those fats may be one reason why chocolate's polyphenols raise your good cholesterol (HDL)[18] and lower your bad cholesterol (LDL).[19]

Of course, just because HDL and LDL move in the right direction, it doesn't necessarily mean that high-cocoa chocolate consumption actually does lead to lower rates of heart disease. After all, the theories have been plenty wrong plenty of times before. It would be more convincing if you could show that those who eat more chocolate have less heart disease. The problem with that approach is that you would need thousands of people in that study to get the statistical strength to be able to say whether the result you found was significant and not just spurious. Luckily, we have just that.

Researchers at Brigham and Women's Hospital studied the massive National Heart, Lung, and Blood Institute's Family Health Study, with a whopping 4,970 participants, ages 25 to 93 years old. After controlling for every variable under the sun (age, gender, prior familial cardiovascular risk, education, non-chocolate candy consumption, smoking, alcohol, exercise, fruit and vegetable consumption, etc.), they discovered that people who ate more chocolate did in fact have fewer incidences of heart disease.[20] One of the reasons for this may be that chocolate helps fight the chronic vascular inflammation that can lead to atherosclerosis.[21] The volume of people studied and the rigorous nature of the comparison make this a conclusion that is really hard to blow off.

Even better, the heart disease benefit was dose dependent—the higher the dose, the higher the protection. Chocolate consumption one to three times per month was good at preventing heart disease; one to four times per week was better at it; and the greatest reduction in actual incidents of heart disease occurred with those who had chocolate five or more times per week. In other words, chocolate consumption and heart disease are inversely related: When one goes up, the other goes down. By the way, those who had non-chocolate candy had a 49% *greater* prevalence of heart disease.[22]

In addition to this chocolate boost of heart health, magnetic resonance imaging (MRI) studies show that chocolate can open up blood vessel circulation, allowing more oxygen-rich blood to reach your heart muscle and also your brain. In fact, subjects who consumed high-cocoa chocolate (150 milligrams of cocoa flavonols) daily for just 5 days had greater bloodflow to the brain when they performed cognitive tasks than those who did not have the chocolate.[23] So don't forget to have your chocolate, or you may just forget to have your chocolate.

Given all this goodness, chocolate honestly should be prescribed for daily use. Can you imagine some doctor telling you to take your daily dose of vitamin Ch? Don't hold your breath. Until you get a prescription for some 70%-plus-cocoa chocolate, do your heart a favor and have some every day—in control. Get a Pez dispenser if you have to.

Chocolate and Your Blood Pressure

Think about your arteries as skin-thin pipes. Blood runs through them. And sometimes, like when you stand up, exert yourself, or exercise, the pressure inside those tubes increases. If those skin-thin membranes that hold in your blood have too much pressure on them, the weakest spot along the pipeline will split open. The blood will then spill out into your body, and everything downstream that was supposed to be irrigated with nutrition and oxygen will be deprived. That, my friend, is called a stroke.

You might think that the solution to this little problem would be to have stiffer pipes, because that would prevent the blood from breaking through. But the opposite is actually closer to the truth. You need arteries that are more flexible. That's because when the pressure increases, your

Chocolate: A Myth-Conception

It's called the "Halloween effect." You know what happens when your kids come home with their Halloween haul, groaning beneath their pillowcases of candy that your otherwise friendly neighbors gave them to pour into their veins? The kids soon thereafter bounce off the walls, and basically zing through the house in fast-forward until their batteries run out and they collapse in their beds, still a-twitchin'.

Most people assume the culprit behind the freak-out frenzy is the sugar. However, research studies have confirmed over and over that sugar itself is not causing this ballistic behavior, as we've been led to believe. Some have suggested that it's the dyes and synthetics in the candies that cause the problem. Others point to chocolate.

One reason chocolate gets a finger pointed its way is because people assumed that chocolate is loaded with caffeine. I've heard so many people say that they can't eat chocolate after lunch because they're afraid they won't be able to sleep at night. Or perhaps they get too jittery after drinking regular coffee and they assume chocolate will have the same effect. Let me help you out here.

Chocolate doesn't contain much caffeine. Let that little Whopper Junior go. It does, however, contain its second cousin, twice removed, called theobromine. They're related, both being chemicals in the methylxanthine family. However, theobromine is a couple of molecules short of caffeine—three, to be exact. Because of this, and despite the otherwise identical chemical structure, chocolate's theobromine acts much differently than its hyperactive coffee cousin caffeine (see the table).

THEOBROMINE	CAFFEINE
Mild stimulatory effect	Strong stimulatory effect
Very slow to take effect	Acts quickly
Lasts a long time	Quick effect, but quick decline
After 10 hours, 50% in bloodstream	After 5 hours, 50% in bloodstream
Increases sense of calm	Makes you more alert
Stimulates cardiovascular system	Stimulates cardiovascular system
Stimulates muscular system	Stimulates respiratory system
Not addictive	Physically addictive
Mild diuretic	Larger diuretic

All that said, if you happen to be very sensitive to caffeine, even the mild stimulatory effect that theobromine can have may be enough to keep you awake. However, this effect will depend on the person. In other words, you will never know if high-cocoa chocolate affects you specifically until you give it a shot. Test it out, with an open mind, to see just what effect it has.

vessels need to expand and contract like a balloon, so the added pressure is relieved. Your arteries need to be able to breathe with the ebb and flow of the increases and decreases of passing blood pressure so they don't break open. That's what you want for your arteries.

As you might expect, because I've already devoted so much ink to this topic, cocoa increases the flexibility of your blood vessels—what's known as "flow-mediated dilation." In other words, research has shown that when individuals drank a high-cocoa beverage consistently for 7 days, their flow-mediated dilation (and therefore blood pressure) improved more with each day of consumption. On Day 3, the flow-mediated dilation was improved by approximately 40%, on Day 5 it improved by 65%, and after 1 week, it improved by 70%![24] However, when the cocoa was withdrawn for a week, the flow-mediated dilation returned back to baseline.

In other words, consistent consumption of high-cocoa products can increase the flexibility of your arteries over time. This is the likely reason why four meta-analyses of randomized control trials found that ingesting cocoa epicatechins (about 50 grams of 70%-cocoa chocolate daily) reduces systolic blood pressure by approximately 4.6 points and diastolic by 2.1 points.[25]

I have to say, though, that the impact of eating this much high-cocoa chocolate is modest. I wish it were more robust, actually. If this research is correct, a person with a blood pressure of, say, 130 over 100 could reach a level of 125 over 98. That's not a drastic change, to be sure. It's definitely a step in the right direction, but the better effect of chocolate on your blood pressure is not from the reduction in your systolic and diastolic numbers. The more meaningful effect comes from the improved flexibility of your arteries. When they breathe easily with the changing pressure demands, that property can help protect you from a life-threatening stroke.

The Key for Your Heart

As shown in this chapter, studies confirm that anything made from cocoa beans is an amazing health food for your heart. Not only does it help lower your blood pressure, but it also acts to keep your platelets from sticking together and clogging up the inside of your artery walls. Doctors prescribe aspirin because it does exactly the same thing. But aspirin isn't brilliant with red wine, and there are no "aspirin truffles," strawberry-dipped aspirin, or flourless aspirin torte. Moreover, chocolate doesn't directly contribute to ulcers like aspirin does.

The key for your heart is the same key you'll find for your weight and everything else. The cocoa component of chocolate is the good part. And the higher the cocoa you consume in your daily dosage, the more likely you'll be to get all the downstream heart-healthy effects from it.

Chocolate, the Aphrodisiac

"Better than sex"—that's what we hear. And with all the other wonderful things that chocolate does for our health, you might expect that this is going to extend our winning streak of wonderfulness. However, while it may turn out to be true in our hopeful minds, that seems to be where the aphrodisiac effect of chocolate ends.

A research group in Italy correlated women's chocolate consumption with their sexual activity to see whether they were related in any way. The only relationship they could find was that younger people tend to eat more chocolate and are also active sexually.[26] The key variable was more tightly related to age than to chocolate consumption. Hardly a home run conclusion. Actually, a more accurate predictor of healthy sexuality was found in women who enjoyed the moderate consumption of red wine (one to two glasses per day).[27]

TAKE THE
Chocolate Challenge

Lower your own blood pressure. Lower your bad cholesterol. That's your challenge. How do you do this? Add cocoa to your life, because doing so can help you lower high blood pressure[28] and your bad cholesterol in the process.[29] If you have normal blood pressure, don't worry, though: Cocoa exerts its lowering effect only on those who have high blood pressure.

WHAT DO I DO?

Obviously, first of all, you need to add cocoa to your life because it's wicked good for your heart. Plus, if it comes packaged in a piece of chocolate, well, that's just the price we all pay for living the healthy life! One of the main points of this book, however, is that having just a tiny bit of good stuff (in this case, the cocoa) mixed in with a pile of bad stuff (like sugar, fillers, and synthetics) is ultimately bad for you. So your challenge is to add more cocoa to your life without also adding nastiness that is terrible for your weight and health.

HOW DO I DO THIS?

As we discussed in Chapter 1, you should begin by making sure that the cocoa you have isn't Dutched. In other words, it hasn't had alkali added to it. Un-Dutched cocoa works to help reduce your blood pressure and your bad cholesterol even more than Dutched cocoa.

Before you start, you will first need to get your blood pressure taken, which you can do on your own at many drugstores with a measuring device. It's a good idea, though, to get a couple of these readings and average them to make sure your "before" value is closer to your true average. As for your cholesterol, you'll need to have a checkup with your doctor to get your current values. Alternatively, you may know what your LDL and HDL cholesterol numbers are right now. If so, you can use those numbers as your "before" reading. Just schedule a visit for a checkup to get your "after" reading.

Honestly? All you have to do to meet this particular challenge is get chocolate that is approximately 80% cocoa or higher and consume perhaps 20 grams of it each day (equal to approximately five or six thumb-size pieces, or 0.7 ounce). For it to benefit your heart health, it doesn't matter whether or not you consume it in association with meals or at any particular time of the day.

The key here is consistency. Make sure you eat it religiously, like clockwork, each day. Another important element is that you need to make sure that you don't fall into a trap that our culture of health sets for us. That is, if you eat something good for you, that allows you to eat something nasty for you. This is the candy bar–diet soda rationalization (if I chase a candy bar with a diet soda, they cancel each other out down in my gastric netherworld).

In other words, if you take your high-cocoa chocolate for 2 weeks, don't think, "Great, I'm lowering my blood pressure with chocolate. That means I can chow down on ramen noodles, pork rinds, and fried mayonnaise balls!" Taking this chocolate challenge must be done while you're also eating a reasonable, non-fried-mayonnaise-ball style of diet, which includes normal fruits and veggies.

WHAT CAN I EXPECT WHEN I DO THIS?

Give it 2 weeks. A number of studies have shown that eating 100 grams of chocolate over 15 days significantly reduces both systolic and diastolic blood pressure. That said, other studies don't require that much chocolate to see the same effect. After the 2 weeks, take your blood pressure for your "after" measurement to see the change. Just like you did in the "before" measurement with the drugstore reading, take your reading on a couple of days and average those together to make sure the value is closer to your actual average pressure. When you're at your

(continued on page 180)

SUCCESS STORY
Keith Stephens

AGE: 60
POUNDS LOST: 84
CHOCOLATE TIP: *"For your ender, leave it in your mouth until it melts. It should take about 3 to 5 minutes. If you're eating it faster than that, you're not really enjoying it fully or getting all of the benefits."*

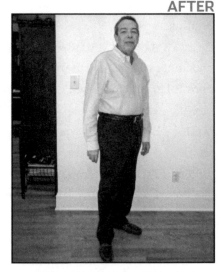

AFTER

Prior to starting the Eat Chocolate, Lose Weight plan, Keith Stephens was experiencing some health concerns. "I wasn't very active and was on a lot of blood pressure medication," he explains. "I also had osteoarthritis in both knees and had no cartilage in one of them, so I wore knee braces. In addition, I smoked for 32 years, and I was diagnosed with an aortic aneurism 17 years ago. Ironically, the day I finally decided to quit smoking was the day my aneurism tore."

Faced with a serious medical emergency, Keith immediately underwent surgery. Afterward, he was determined to turn his health around, which is when a friend suggested he try a new program. "When I came out of surgery, I signed up for the 8-week plan. At the same time, I was going through cardiac rehab, so I started working out moderately three to four times a week," he says. "The idea of eating whole foods was really appealing. That part really made sense to me, so I decided to try it."

BEFORE

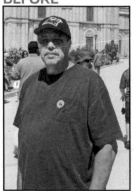

But even though his friend recommended the program and Keith understood the idea of eating "real" food, he still struggled to change the way he thought about chocolate. "I have always loved chocolate, but I was afraid to eat it in the beginning because I thought all chocolate contained a lot of calories and sugar," he shares. "But my wife gave me some dark chocolate after we discussed the program, and I started eating it every day."

And it didn't take long for Keith to notice a change in his eating habits. "I learned that you should eat whole foods and take your time eating those foods. If you take your time, your brain understands that you're full," he explains. "I also cut back on my salt and sugar intake. And I began to eat my chocolate differently. Every day after lunch, I would eat my chocolate ender. Then at home, I would have another ender after dinner—and it worked! It kept me from being hungry, and I loved the fact that I could have it every single day! In fact, I have two nutrition bars in my desk that I haven't touched in more than 2 weeks because I'm never hungry anymore."

It wasn't long before Keith started noticing even more results. He lost 16 pounds in 8 weeks, and the longer he stuck with the plan, the more confident he became. "I've dropped three shirt sizes—from XXL to large—and I've even fit into a medium lately," he says. "I'm still trying to get used to how clothes are supposed to fit. I'm so used to hiding in my clothes. When you gain weight like I did, you wear clothes to try to disguise things. Now I'm wearing clothes that are more tailored."

In fact, one of the most memorable moments Keith had while on the program happened while he was shopping for new outfits. "I was hoping to fit into size 38 pants, and the attendant said to try on a pair of pants that were even smaller—a size 36! And they fit! I started giggling and asked, 'Where are the jeans!?' My feet even went down a size!"

But Keith's new lifestyle didn't just affect his weight, it improved his overall health. In addition to no longer needing his knee brace, Keith also states that his cholesterol is the lowest it's been in years and he no longer takes vitamins. "I only just recently got my blood pressure under control (with a lot of medication help, I am sorry to say). But my cholesterol is perfect. At the last reading, my HDL was 55 and my LDL was immeasurable (0). My total cholesterol was 158."

And his energy and fitness levels couldn't be better. "I think if people saw what I could do in the last year, they'd know they could do it, too. When I first started the cardiac rehab, I could barely walk from one side of the house to the other. It's a whole different world now," he says. "I couldn't do the stretches at the beginning of my rehab, but by the end, I could do them all. I'm so much stronger now. I can walk across the parking lot without getting winded. I can now run around and play with my grandkids. It's amazing!"

When asked how he feels now, Keith states that his hard work has paid off and he has more energy than ever. "Thanks to this program, I've finally found a new way to live. I know now that food isn't my enemy; it's one of the best things in life! And it is great to take more time and actually get some enjoyment out of my food. This is not a diet and it's easy to do. And the best thing? I feel like I'm 24 again—and I was in great shape at that age!"

doctor's office to get your "after" reading on your cholesterol values, be sure to talk to your physician about what you're doing, why, and what improvements you've noticed in yourself.

HOW DO I HELP MYSELF?

The best thing you can possibly do to help chocolate improve your health is to be active, as we discussed in Chapter 7. All the positive benefits of chocolate are amplified if you are active. This doesn't mean that you have to be a superathlete, but it does mean you need to move every day, whenever you can.

Cocoa and exercise are both excellent for all the conditions covered in this chapter. And in combination with daily high-cocoa chocolate consumption, daily activity will even further enhance weight loss, decrease blood pressure, enhance cancer prevention, and boost heart health.

HOW CHOCOLATE SAVES YOUR DIET

In the end, you should see the same results in yourself as were found in the research studies. If you don't, ask yourself why that might be. It could be that your physiology is different from everyone else's. But the more likely answer is that there's something more going on: Perhaps you're still consuming too much sugar, your eating volume at the plate level is still too high, your activity level has not come up, etc. Finding that out is actually the exciting part of this entire process, as you progressively learn more about the hurdles that stand between you and a lifetime of optimal health (and chocolate)!

Chapter 9

The Eat Chocolate, Lose Weight Meal Plan

After reading this book, you may think that a meal plan goes against everything that I teach. After all, I've emphasized a more Taoist approach that provides principles over particulars. And this approach frees you to live a lifestyle of health on your own, so you don't need someone to micromanage exactly what you eat, and exactly when you eat it.

So it might seem that a meal plan, which specifies every meal of every day, is exactly the opposite of the philosophy you've read in this book. But this meal plan is structured with sample dishes and principles to follow, so you can apply it in the way that works best for you. Use it as a jumping-off point to your new life of living well on your own, every day.

You will begin this 2-week sample meal plan with the goal of learning how to apply the lessons on your own after you've completed it. And to help you pull it all together, both weeks contain recipes (shown in italics) you'll find in Chapter 10. If you have dietary restrictions, substitutions are definitely available, and you will be coached within this meal plan to know what to expect as you continue on your chocolate weight-loss journey. Just make sure to stick to the principles of eating real food—in control—along with your high-cocoa chocolate.

The Principles

Breakfast

If you are not hungry, do not eat. Some people need breakfast, and some don't. How do you know if you need it or not? Not by listening to some arbitrary rule about eating breakfast, but by listening to your own body and attending to its cues. No healthy culture insists that people must eat breakfast. Even in those cultures that do emphasize breakfast, it's often a very little one, consisting of coffee and perhaps a small yogurt, or a piece of fruit, or a bit of bread and cheese, or prosciutto. Need a rule for breakfast? *Go small, if at all.* In keeping with this mantra, each weekday breakfast listing in the meal plan on the following pages provides options for different hunger levels.

If you become hungry and/or hypoglycemic by midmorning, then you should have a little something for breakfast. But you may be very surprised by how quickly you can train your physiology to make it all the way to lunch without even one thought of food. And if you can't do that at first, your body may adapt in that direction over time. Watch for that to happen.

And this will be most likely to occur if you cut out the sugar at breakfast. Lose that, and over time, you will also begin to lose the midmorning cravings. So if you find any sugar in any of your breakfast items, don't eat that food for these 8 weeks. Instead, choose an egg. This is an ideal breakfast, whether you prefer it boiled, poached, scrambled, or fried (in olive oil). In general, it's really, really difficult to mess up an egg. (You *can* mess it up, but you're going to have to work very hard at it!)

Cereals are also good, but only if you include a little fat, fiber, and/or protein. Otherwise, the complex carbohydrates will break down into simple sugars in your bloodstream, overstimulating the insulin response that quickly makes you tired and hungry, which results in moving less and eating more. If you add just a touch of milk or half-and-half to your oats, it will lower the glycemic index of the cereal and slow the rate at which your body absorbs the nutrients, leaving you feeling satisfied longer throughout the morning.

Note that your weekends are going to start with some incredibly leisurely, delicious brunches. For this diet as well as for your weight and health, I want you to relax on the weekends and eat a bit later. And because you'll be having that first meal later in the morning, we will not include a starter for that first meal.

Lunch

One of the biggest challenges you will face if you want to eat chocolate, and eat it in control, is to control the pace of your eating. This is where our typical lunches can totally undermine our efforts at controlling weight. Rushing on a lunch break can lead to the gobbling that—especially with chocolate—creates overconsumption. Creates it! So, to maximize the twin benefits that high-cocoa chocolate can have (controlling portions at the plate and reducing chronic cravings between meals), take as long as you can to finish the chocolate starter and ender. Don't gobble them down.

Here's what to expect after the consumption of chocolate over lunch. First, the natural fiber, fat, and protein that are contained in that rich, wonderful chocolate will increase the time between the offset of your lunch and the onset of your next craving. Next, the extent and duration of any between-meal cravings you do have will be lessened. And you can test both of these outcomes for yourself. If you need help making it from lunch to dinner without starving to death, drink some coffee or tea. When you drink them, always, always, always train your tastes in the direction of the unaltered version. You may not be able to do this at first, but pull back on the amount of sugar and dairy, little by little, and this mid-meal bridge will be as effective as it possibly could be to assist in your weight loss.

So what about dessert for lunch? You can certainly have dessert after lunch, but make it a healthy dessert, such as a piece of fruit or a small piece of delicious cheese. The principle to follow is this: If you have some form of rich chocolate dessert, you cannot also have an ender. However, if your dessert is light—again, such as a piece of fruit—then you may also have an ender.

Dinner

This is important: If you become full while you're in the middle of eating your meal, never, ever finish your dinner. Being full will happen, but it should not be at the end of your meal. You will have a cocoa ender and/or a dessert to complete the meal, and that will help you drift into fullness at that time.

However, if you finish your meal and find that you're full, you won't have the room to eat your ender or dessert. So if you want your ender and/or dessert, you have to "plan on seconds" by putting an amount on your plate that you know is just a bit less than you actually need. The point of the ender or dessert is to finish off your hunger, not to pile onto your fullness.

Also, make time for dinner. It's important for your weight and health. If that means you need to wait until everyone gets home so you can eat together, don't worry. And if you eat alone but work late, don't think you have to hurry up and eat just because you get home at 8:00, 9:00, or 10:00 at night. Healthy cultures eat late; they just don't gobble food down in the process. Bottom line? Eating later in the evening is not a liability for your efforts to control weight. If you enjoy wine, this is the perfect time to share it, in control, with your dining companions.

You will also begin to notice changes over time. For example, when you add the ender to punctuate your dinner, you will begin to be less hungry at breakfast. You will need less food at that meal—and you should honor that feeling in your body and taper back on your breakfast volume. But that's not the only change you'll see! You will also notice that the amount of food you want at dinner will decrease over time as well. Go with that feeling. Encourage it, as this indicates that you are training your physiology in a healthy direction.

Regarding your eating routines, for these next 8 weeks do not eat

Eat Chocolate, Lose Weight

dinner on your feet, in the car, or grazing out of a sack as you walk back to your car. This diet requires you to sit, take your time, and enjoy every bite of your food. This is your recipe for losing weight, and eating chocolate while doing it. Finally, the principle to follow for eating dessert after dinner is the same as it is for lunch: If you are having a light dessert such as a piece of fruit or sorbet, etc., you may also have an ender. If your dessert is one of our wonderful chocolate recipes from Chapter 10, that alone will serve as your ender.

Food Substitutions

Feel free to substitute ingredients if the meal plan features any that you dislike. Just make sure that the new ingredient is real food—not synthetic or modified in any way. For example, if you don't happen to like one kind of fruit, just substitute in another you do enjoy. If you don't care for cilantro, instead use an herb that you do like (perhaps basil). If you are gluten-sensitive, just replace the wheat product with a gluten-free version, such as rice.

In other words, you do not have to eat any specific food, but everything you eat must be real.

Drinks

You can have any drink that is real: tea, coffee, wine, water, juice, beer, carbonated water, or milk. (Note: If you don't or can't consume dairy, feel free to use almond milk as a substitute.) Everything else is off the table, including all sodas (even diet sodas), presweetened teas, and zero-calorie drinks filled with artificial sweeteners.

Reduce the amount of sugar, caramel, and additive flavorings in your coffee and your tea and begin to move in the direction of straight tea and coffee. Keep in mind that your current taste for all the stuff in your coffee or tea has been created by your own consumption of it. The good news is that you can move your tastes into a healthy direction if you desire. And if you lose the sugar, you will lose the weight. Period.

WEEK 1

During the first week, you're just getting started. So expect that your body will adapt over time. For now, though, focus on these two principles as you go:

1. *Your psychology overestimates your physiology.* In other words, the amount your mind thinks you're hungry for is greater than your body's actual need. The chocolate starters allow you to take advantage of this fact. When you pull back on the amount of food you serve yourself at lunch and at dinner, and then take at least 20 to 30 minutes to eat your meal, the starter chocolate will help to generate the satiety signals that will help you control consumption during lunch and dinner.

2. *The ender curtails chronic consumption.* You actually can make it all the way from lunch to dinner without needing to eat. And what you will find is that in addition to your decrease in hunger, your cravings at breakfast will decrease over time as well.

Eat Chocolate, Lose Weight

Breakfast

IF YOU'RE A LITTLE HUNGRY: Handful of walnuts

IF YOU'RE A BIT HUNGRIER: 1 egg made any way you prefer, topped with sliced tomato, balsamic vinegar, olive oil, and salt and pepper

Lunch

STARTER: 1 or 2 thumb-size pieces of high-cocoa chocolate

MEAL: Open-faced ham sandwich with provolone (or similar) cheese and a tomato slice on whole grain bread, served with coleslaw and sliced plum

ENDER: 1 or 2 thumb-size pieces of high-cocoa chocolate

Snack

Small coffee or tea. The more you can train your tastes toward coffee or tea without sweeteners, the better it will be for your health and your weight.

Dinner

STARTER: 1 or 2 thumb-size pieces of high-cocoa chocolate and ½ glass of red wine

MEAL: *Cocoa-Chili Jamaican Fish* (see page 224) served over a bed of rice cooked with a cinnamon stick

ENDER: Your choice of:

- *Earl Grey Hot Chocolate* (see page 246)
- Dessert, which is 2 chocolate-dipped strawberries

Breakfast

IF YOU'RE A LITTLE HUNGRY: Handful of lightly roasted almonds

IF YOU'RE A BIT HUNGRIER: *Black Strappin' Chocolate Smoothie*
(see page 249)

Lunch

STARTER: 1 or 2 thumb-size pieces of high-cocoa chocolate

MEAL: Your choice of:

- *Cocoa-Chili Jamaican Fish* (see page 224) leftovers from last night's dinner
- Salad with garbanzo beans, cocoa nibs, roasted red pepper, and feta cheese

ENDER: 1 or 2 thumb-size pieces of high-cocoa chocolate

Snack

Small coffee or tea

Dinner

STARTER: 1 or 2 thumb-size pieces of high-cocoa chocolate and
½ glass of red wine

MEAL: Broiled salmon fillet with a drizzle of olive oil, white wine vinegar, sesame seeds, and salt and pepper; steamed broccoli florets with a pat of butter, salt and pepper, and a squeeze of lemon

DESSERT: ½ cup raspberry sorbet

ENDER: 1 or 2 thumb-size pieces of high-cocoa chocolate

Breakfast

IF YOU'RE A LITTLE HUNGRY: Handful of walnuts

IF YOU'RE A BIT HUNGRIER: Plain Greek yogurt (2% milk fat or higher) with cut fruit, a drizzle of honey, 1 tablespoon of cocoa, and a little granola (the sweetness of the granola should be all you need for this breakfast)

Lunch

STARTER: 1 or 2 thumb-size pieces of high-cocoa chocolate

MEAL: Mediterranean veggie sandwich (pita with hummus, sliced tomatoes, sliced olives, mozzarella cheese, basil, and roasted red peppers); a few carrot sticks dipped in hummus or peanut butter

ENDER: 1 or 2 thumb-size pieces of high-cocoa chocolate

Snack

Small coffee or tea

Dinner

STARTER: 1 or 2 thumb-size pieces of high-cocoa chocolate and ½ glass of red wine

MEAL: *Slow Cooker Chicken Mole* (see page 220), pinto beans topped with fresh minced onions, and grilled veggies

DESSERT: 1 sliced orange

ENDER: 1 or 2 thumb-size pieces of high-cocoa chocolate

Breakfast

IF YOU'RE A LITTLE HUNGRY: *Chocolate-Citrus Biscotti* (see page 237) with coffee or tea

IF YOU'RE A BIT HUNGRIER: 2 eggs scrambled with goat cheese, diced onions, and a piece of bacon

Lunch

STARTER: 1 or 2 thumb-size pieces of high-cocoa chocolate

MEAL: Your choice of:

- Leftover *Slow Cooker Chicken Mole* (see page 220)
- Open-faced sandwich of sliced turkey, tomato, and avocado on whole wheat bread, served with coleslaw and a piece of sliced fruit

ENDER: 1 or 2 thumb-size pieces of high-cocoa chocolate

Snack

Small coffee or tea

Dinner

STARTER: 1 or 2 thumb-size pieces of high-cocoa chocolate and ½ glass of red wine

MEAL: Grilled pork fillet seasoned with salt and pepper, olive oil or white wine vinegar; black beans seasoned with cocoa, chili powder, salt and pepper, and a dash of ground red pepper; served with rice cooked with a cinnamon stick

ENDER: Your choice of:

- *Gingered Cocoa* (see page 248)
- Dessert: 2" × 2" square of the *Chocolate-Coconut Oat Bars* (see page 234)

Breakfast

IF YOU'RE A LITTLE HUNGRY: Handful of lightly roasted almonds

IF YOU'RE A BIT HUNGRIER: Banana with peanut butter

Lunch

STARTER: 1 or 2 thumb-size pieces of high-cocoa chocolate

MEAL: Your choice of:

- Grilled pork dinner leftovers
- Mediterranean tuna salad (canned tuna in water, dash of extra virgin olive oil, splash of white wine vinegar, tarragon, spicy mustard, capers), served over spinach with a sliced boiled egg and tomato wedges

ENDER: 1 or 2 thumb-size pieces of high-cocoa chocolate

Snack

Small coffee or tea

Dinner

STARTER: 1 or 2 thumb-size pieces of high-cocoa chocolate and ½ glass of red wine

MEAL: Small plates with pieces of cheese, sliced fruit, bread/olive oil with spices, veggies with hummus dip, and walnuts, along with roasted red peppers or smoked salmon

DESSERT: 2 thumb-size pieces of your favorite cheese

ENDER: 1 or 2 thumb-size pieces of high-cocoa chocolate

DAY 6

Brunch

MEAL: *Deconstructed Guacamole Omelet* (see page 206), with salsa and a dollop of sour cream, served with blueberries and cream on the side

ENDER: 1 or 2 thumb-size pieces of high-cocoa chocolate

Snack

Small coffee or tea

Dinner

STARTER: 1 or 2 thumb-size pieces of high-cocoa dark chocolate and ½ glass of red wine

MEAL: *Roasted Beet Salad with Blackstrap Vinaigrette* (see page 209) and *Tuna with Sesame-Soy-Ginger Sauce* (see page 223), served with thin green beans (sautéed with olive oil, sliced almonds, dried cherries, and finished with a squeeze of orange juice over the top)

ENDER: 1 or 2 thumb-size pieces of high-cocoa chocolate

DAY 7

Brunch

MEAL: Eggs bourguignon (eggs poached in a hearty red wine with thyme, thickened with *beurre manié*), served over a garlic-rubbed baguette and followed by a raspberry sorbet to cleanse the palate

ENDER: 1 or 2 thumb-size pieces of high-cocoa dark chocolate

Snack

Small coffee or tea

Dinner

STARTER: 1 or 2 thumb-size pieces of high-cocoa dark chocolate and ½ glass of red wine

MEAL: *Spicy Beef Stew* (see page 216)

DESSERT: 1 plum

ENDER: 1 or 2 thumb-size pieces of high-cocoa chocolate

Eat Chocolate, Lose Weight

WEEK 2

Continue to use chocolate to your advantage during the second week. As long as you take your time while eating, you will notice that the volume you're hungry for at each meal will start to decline. Continue to push that bar lower by training your physiology to expect an amount of food that results in weight control, not weight gain.

You will also notice that your chocolate ender will start reducing the gnawing between-meal cravings you used to have so frequently. Don't feel like you have to eat chocolate. There is nothing at all wrong with taking a break from having your starter or ender.

Breakfast

IF YOU'RE A LITTLE HUNGRY: Handful of walnuts

IF YOU'RE A BIT HUNGRIER: An egg, any style, topped with diced tomato, a little balsamic vinegar, and olive oil

Lunch

STARTER: 1 or 2 thumb-size pieces of high-cocoa chocolate

MEAL: Your choice of:

- Leftover *Spicy Beef Stew* (see page 216)
- Guacamole with whole wheat pita, olives, lightly roasted almonds, a cut crisp apple, and sliced sharp Cheddar cheese

ENDER: 1 or 2 thumb-size pieces of high-cocoa chocolate

Snack

Small coffee or tea

Dinner

STARTER: 1 or 2 thumb-size pieces of high-cocoa chocolate and ½ glass of red wine

MEAL: *Chicken with Cocoa-Tomato Sauce* (see page 221), served with rice cooked with a cinnamon stick

DESSERT: Mango slices

ENDER: 1 or 2 thumb-size pieces of high-cocoa chocolate

DAY 9

Breakfast

IF YOU'RE A LITTLE HUNGRY: 1 boiled egg with salt and pepper

IF YOU'RE A BIT HUNGRIER: *Hot Cocoa Oatmeal* (see page 207)

Lunch

STARTER: 1 or 2 thumb-size pieces of high-cocoa chocolate

MEAL: Your choice of:

- Leftover *Chicken with Cocoa-Tomato Sauce* (see page 221)
- Mediterranean pita: hummus, avocado, feta, and sliced tomato on whole wheat pita, drizzled with olive oil and a dash of white wine vinegar

DESSERT: Apple slices with thinly sliced sharp Cheddar cheese

ENDER: 1 or 2 thumb-size pieces of high-cocoa chocolate

Snack

Small coffee or tea

Dinner

STARTER: 1 or 2 thumb-size pieces of high-cocoa chocolate

MEAL: Broiled salmon fillet with thyme, white beans with rosemary and lemon, and crème fraîche mashed potatoes

ENDER: Your choice of:

- 1 or 2 thumb-size pieces of high-cocoa chocolate
- Dessert: A 2" x 2" square of the *Rich 'n' Nutty Brownies* (see page 238)

Breakfast

IF YOU'RE A LITTLE HUNGRY: Coffee or tea with *Chocolate-Citrus Biscotti* (see page 237)

IF YOU'RE A BIT HUNGRIER: *Black Strappin' Chocolate Smoothie* (see page 249)

Lunch

STARTER: 1 or 2 thumb-size pieces of high-cocoa chocolate

MEAL: Your choice of:

- Leftover salmon fillet dinner
- *Roasted Beet Salad with Blackstrap Vinaigrette* (see page 209)

ENDER: 1 or 2 thumb-size pieces of high-cocoa chocolate

Snack

Small coffee or tea

Dinner

STARTER: 1 or 2 thumb-size pieces of high-cocoa chocolate and ½ glass red wine

MEAL: *Chicken with Spicy Cocoa Rub* (see page 222), served with *Cajun Black Beans* (see page 228) and pineapple grilled in sesame oil

DESSERT: Raspberry sorbet

ENDER: *Cioccolata Calda (Italian Hot Cocoa)* (see page 250)

Breakfast

IF YOU'RE A LITTLE HUNGRY: Handful of walnuts

IF YOU'RE A BIT HUNGRIER: *Black Strappin' Chocolate Smoothie* (see page 249)

Lunch

STARTER: 1 or 2 thumb-size pieces of high-cocoa chocolate

MEAL: Your choice of:

- Leftover *Chicken with Spicy Cocoa Rub* (see page 222) and steamed veggies
- Open-faced sliced turkey, avocado, and bacon sandwich on whole wheat bread, served with Cheddar cheese and sliced apple

ENDER: 1 or 2 thumb-size pieces of high-cocoa chocolate

Snack

Small coffee or tea

Dinner

STARTER: 1 or 2 thumb-size pieces of high-cocoa chocolate and ½ glass of red wine

MEAL: Grilled salmon steak, mashed sweet potatoes, and mango-avocado salsa

ENDER: Your choice of:

- 1 or 2 thumb-size pieces of high-cocoa chocolate
- Dessert, which is *Classic Chocolate Pudding* (see page 242) with raspberries on the side

Breakfast

IF YOU'RE A LITTLE HUNGRY: Handful of lightly roasted almonds

IF YOU'RE A BIT HUNGRIER: *Hot Cocoa Oatmeal* (see page 207)

Lunch

STARTER: 1 or 2 thumb-size pieces of high-cocoa chocolate

MEAL: Mediterranean tuna salad over a small bed of spinach and 1 orange

ENDER: 1 or 2 thumb-size pieces of high-cocoa chocolate

Snack

Small coffee or tea

Dinner

STARTER: 1 or 2 thumb-size pieces of high-cocoa chocolate and ½ glass red wine

MEAL: Baked red snapper with a salsa of diced tomatoes, onions, and olives, served with rosemary-seasoned baby red potatoes and white beans

ENDER: 1 or 2 thumb-size pieces of high-cocoa chocolate

DAY 13

Brunch

MEAL: *Cajun Black Beans* (see page 228) topped with 1 fried egg, salsa, and crumbled feta cheese, served with a side of homemade guacamole

ENDER: 1 or 2 thumb-size pieces of high-cocoa chocolate

Snack

Small coffee or tea

Dinner

STARTER: 1 or 2 thumb-size pieces of high-cocoa chocolate

MEAL: *Cocoa Chili* (see page 218) served with cornbread

ENDER: Chocolate-dipped strawberries

DAY 14

Brunch

MEAL: Toasted bagel with cream cheese, capers, lox, thinly sliced onion, and tomato, topped with salt and pepper and a squeeze of lemon

ENDER: 1 or 2 thumb-size pieces of high-cocoa chocolate

Snack

Small coffee or tea

Dinner

STARTER: 1 or 2 thumb-size pieces of high-cocoa chocolate and ½ glass of red wine

MEAL: *Cuban Cocoa Pork via China* (see page 213)

ENDER: 1 truffle made from *Ganache* (see page 243) infused with Chambord and rolled in cocoa, with a glass of red wine and red fruit of your choosing (raspberries taste amazing with this recipe)

The Eat Chocolate, Lose Weight Meal Plan

Chapter 10

Chocolate-Based Recipes

Chocolate is not candy. Now let's say that together: Chocolate. Is. Not. Candy.

Okay, yes, chocolate is often coated with bizarre oversweetened shellac that turns it into a dietary disaster. But that's not chocolate's fault. We have changed this health food into a sugary engine of weight gain by how we have manufactured it. And the same is true regarding cooking with chocolate.

Right now, wherever you are, conjure in your brain the image of chocolate in the kitchen and the outcome of cooking with chocolate. What likely pops into your mind is invariably some form of fudge, brownie, cookie, truffle, cake, or icing that you eat by the ladleful. You envision these sweets because that's how our culture of health has trained us to think of chocolate.

But I want to emphasize that the reason chocolate is a health food is the same reason that it's awesome to cook with. Not because of the sugar. Not because you can spackle it onto a brownie. And not because it's your favorite flavor of icing. It's great for you because of the cocoa itself. And, believe it or not, that cocoa also happens to be an amazingly nutty and savory addition to a slew of stews and other dishes. In this chapter, I certainly provide the sweet recipes you're expecting, but even better, I also provide recipes that use cocoa to enrich and deepen the flavors of your savory dishes.

Tips for Cooking with Cocoa

When you heat up any food at all, there is a chance the healthy elements can be destroyed by the cooking process. For example, vitamin C is very labile and quickly degrades when cooked under even moderate heat. So tomatoes lose some vitamins when you make that pasta sauce. But don't despair, you marinara mavens, because cooking with tomatoes actually liberates the lycopenes that help you fight both cancer and heart disease. In other words, taking your time to cook your pasta sauce makes the beneficial molecules even more bioavailable.

But what happens when you cook with cocoa? Does it become more bioavailable to your system, or does it degrade into a poof of nutritional pixie dust?

Baking

Of course, research has been conducted to see whether healthy polyphenols and other antioxidants are lost during baking. Three different chocolate cakes were baked: one at 250°F for 110 minutes, another at 300°F for 60 minutes, and the third at 350°F for 35 minutes. In each case, the baking time resulted in a cake that was done—to verify, a toothpick was inserted in each and it came out clean.

The researchers then measured the level of cocoa's antioxidant power in each cake. It turns out that there is zero antioxidant loss regardless of whether you're baking it low and slow or hot and fast.[1] None. In other words, baking does not decrease the healthy nature of your chocolate cake.

However, something that could sap the strength out of your chocolate cake is the leavening. If you use baking soda, the effect of its chemistry is that the pH of your cake batter will increase (becoming more alkaline and less acidic). Back in Chapter 1, we discussed how manufacturers add alkaline to cocoa to make it easier to work with on a mass production level. The effect is a massive loss of the antioxidants in your chocolate. The same thing is just as true for you when you're baking. If you add things that increase the pH of your chocolate and then cook it, you will lose the polyphenols that do so many wonderful things for your health.

The alternative to baking soda is baking powder. Researchers from the Hershey Company determined that chocolate cakes made with baking powder retained essentially all of their antioxidant power during baking.[2] The bottom line is that the healthiest chocolate cake batters will weigh in at a pH right around 6.2 but no higher than 7.25. Rest assured, this doesn't mean that you have to break out your beakers, Bunsen burners, and pocket protectors just to make sure your cake batter stays at a specific pH level. That said, you know the boxed cake mixes you get from the store? Those commercial cakes have pH levels that are quite high (around 8.3 or so) and therefore have zero detectable flavonols after they're baked. So, once you put them in the oven, they lose any antioxidant goodness they might have had. It is better to simply mix up the ingredients yourself. If you're going to make brownies or cake or whatever, just take the extra 2 seconds to mix up your own flour and leavening and cocoa, and you'll get something that's actually not unhealthy for you—until you eat the entire bowl of batter by yourself with a spoon while you're binge-watching *Friends* reruns on Netflix.

A Cocoa-Cooking Energy Boost

You need iron in your diet. You just do. It helps your muscles store and use oxygen, and it's important for enzymatic reactions in your body. Plus, if you don't have enough iron, you can become run down, with low energy.

There's a great deal of healthy iron in chocolate. Normally though, when you think of getting enough iron, your thoughts turn to meats. The form of iron found in meats is attached to the heme molecule in your blood. But there's another form of iron found in vegetables, called nonheme iron. The problem is that your body doesn't absorb this form as well as it does the version found in meats.

To better extract the iron so your body can make use of it, you need vitamin C, which increases your body's ability to absorb non-heme iron.[3] Of course, this doesn't mean you have to douse everything with orange juice. For example, an excellent way to spice up soups, curries, and sauces is to add green chiles. These provide more vitamin C than any other food, with 242.5 milligrams for every 100-gram serving (that's more than 400% of the daily requirement), and 109 milligrams in a single green chile pepper. (Red chiles have almost as much vitamin C as well.)

But is this enough to have an effect? Yes—only 25 milligrams of vitamin C can increase the absorption of iron by up to 23%.[4] So when you're cooking with cocoa, if you add something with this kind of vitamin C content, you'll boost your ability to get the iron out of it and into your body, so you can boost your energy level.

Savory Foods

The most obvious change you'll notice is the rich burgundy color that your savory dishes will become when you add a tablespoon or two of cocoa. But the better change you'll find is in the taste and texture.

Cocoa grains in cocoa powder are very fine. Because of this, they take a little while to get fully incorporated into a dish. I find that when I taste my chili soon after I've added the cocoa, it has a certain graininess, because the cocoa hasn't yet been thoroughly combined. (That also means that the flavor hasn't yet been incorporated either.)

So, when you add cocoa to any savory food, remember that it takes a good 15 to 20 minutes for the full flavor effect to show up. If you want to amp the flavor even more, use natural, un-Dutched cocoa powder instead of the standard stuff. Standard cocoa powder may be easy to find, but the natural cocoa powder is better. That's because it's more acidic than the Dutched version, and that acidity does a couple of things:

- It acts like a flavor enhancer to bring out the tastes in whatever you're making.

- It tenderizes meats by helping to break down connective tissue, whether you allow it to stew in your stew or simply use it as part of a marinade.

Sweet Foods

For desserts like truffles, icing, and ganache, chocolate is cooked in a pan on the stove. Actually, no matter what the recipe says, you will never "cook" solid chocolate. Basically, you have to warm it until it gently turns from a solid into a liquid. Take your time, because if you don't, the chocolate will not have a smooth, shiny finish. Instead, it will become grainy, and once it's grainy, it's very difficult to rescue.

To prevent your chocolate from breaking up and becoming grainy, melt it in a double boiler, with indirect steam heat. If you don't happen to have a double boiler lying about the house, there are other options: You can set the chocolate in a pan over the lowest-heat setting you have, which is what I do when I'm making truffles or ganache. Or you can create your own double boiler by using a big pot and a smaller one that fits into it. In this scenario, you simmer water in the bigger pot and melt the chocolate in the smaller one.

A few other tricks will ensure that you coax the chocolate into melted yumminess without going so far or so fast that you mess it up. First, chop your blocks of chocolate into small pieces. This increases the surface area of the little shards and makes them more likely to melt quickly. Next, if you're making an icing or a ganache, you'll have to add cream to both thin out the chocolate so it's spreadable and to buffer the heat to prevent overcooking. (You can also add a small amount of butter, which contributes a finishing shine to your truffles or cake icing.) Finally, if you're melting chocolate in a pan and it's starting to soften, go ahead and turn off the heat and the remaining solid bits will "coast" into meltness.

Just take your time and be careful not to heat too much too fast, and the pan cooking method will not be a problem.

A Note about Desserts

In this book, I've tried very hard to move us away from that idea that chocolate is only a candy or a sweet by focusing on pulling your sweet tooth, using unsweetened cocoa in cooking, and moving your taste preferences toward high-cocoa chocolate. That said, in my survey of chocolate recipes, there are many desserts. You'll notice, though, that in keeping with the effort of this book to lead you to weight loss, the sugar content is kept low and the cocoa percentage is higher. Still, when you eat these recipes, taste them in very small amounts. The calorie density can quickly catch up to you.

So the bottom line is that while desserts can be good for you, that is true only if you use the lessons you learned in this book, eat small bites, and focus on flavor.

Deconstructed Guacamole Omelet

Total time: 20 minutes
Makes 1 serving

I love it when this happens. Usually it's a late weekend morning, I'm drifting into the end of my first cup of coffee, and the idea of an omelet overtakes my thoughts. There are avocados in the fridge ... and tomatoes ... and onions! Slowly, through the percolating caffeine, comes the idea to "guacamole" an omelet. It's a beautiful thing—and I know you're going to love this, too.

2 eggs, beaten

1 tablespoon milk

Pinch of ground nutmeg

¼ teaspoon salt

¼ teaspoon ground black pepper

Splash of extra virgin olive oil

Pinch of unsweetened cocoa powder

⅓ avocado, sliced

⅓ tomato, diced

1 tablespoon minced onion

Spicy salsa

Sour cream (optional)

Avocado slices (optional)

Diced tomatoes (optional)

In a medium bowl, combine the eggs, milk, nutmeg, salt, and pepper.

In a medium skillet over medium heat, heat the oil. Cook the egg mixture until the bottom begins to firm up a bit.

Sprinkle the omelet with the cocoa powder. Add the avocado, tomato, and onion on top of the omelet. Once the edges of the omelet begin to firm up, grasp the handle of the pan in one hand and a spatula in the other. Put the spatula under the eggs on one side, and tilt the pan so that the omelet slides back onto the spatula even more. Then fold one-half of the omelet over the other half. Once fully cooked, top with salsa to taste and the sour cream, avocado slices, and tomatoes, if using.

Hot Cocoa Oatmeal

Total time: 20 minutes

Makes 4 servings

Oatmeal. You know it's healthy for you, but it has the look and texture of gruel. What you may not know is that it doesn't have to be boring! In fact, this oatmeal has so many unique flavors that you probably won't even recognize it as the health food it is. Yes, it's still oatmeal—only better.

2 cups plain almond milk

2 cups water

2 large bananas, diced

¼ teaspoon vanilla extract

Pinch of salt

2 cups plain rolled oats

2 tablespoons unsweetened cocoa powder

1 tablespoon molasses

2 tablespoons butter

⅓ cup chopped walnuts

Pinch of ground cinnamon

In a large saucepan over medium-high heat, bring the almond milk, water, bananas, vanilla, and salt to a boil.

Stir in the oats, cocoa powder, molasses, and butter. Reduce the heat to medium. Cook, stirring often, until the oats are the desired texture—about 10 minutes. Serve with the walnuts and cinnamon sprinkled over the top.

Island Cacao Nib Salad with Pineapple Vinaigrette

Total time: 20 minutes

Makes 2 servings

You can throw greens together and toss them with olive oil and vinegar, and that would be fine. However, this recipe adds a wonderful twist inspired by Caribbean flavors, fruits, and nuts. The crunchy cacao nibs pop out at you suddenly and balance the sweetness of the pineapple with an earthy, chocolaty pop.

Vinaigrette

1 tablespoon coconut oil

¼ medium pineapple, chopped (about 1½ cups)

1 teaspoon curry powder

½ teaspoon cardamom seeds, freshly crushed

4 tablespoons fresh lime juice, divided

2 tablespoons extra virgin olive oil

1 tablespoon orange juice

¼ teaspoon salt

¼ teaspoon ground black pepper

Salad

1 bag (5 ounces) romaine lettuce

¼ red onion, thinly sliced (about ½ cup)

½ cup roasted cashews

2 tablespoons cacao nibs, lightly crushed

To make the vinaigrette: In a large skillet over high heat, heat the oil. Once hot, add the pineapple and let it caramelize on one side. Add the curry powder and cardamom and stir the pineapple around gently until it's coated.

Remove the skillet from the heat and stir in 2 tablespoons of the lime juice. Remove the pineapple from the liquid. Add the remaining lime juice, olive oil, orange juice, salt, and pepper to the liquid. Whisk together to blend.

To assemble the salad: In a large bowl, mix the lettuce, onion, cashews, and cacao nibs. Add the pineapple and drizzle the vinaigrette over the salad. Toss to coat well and serve.

Eat Chocolate, Lose Weight

Roasted Beet Salad with Blackstrap Vinaigrette

Total time: 1 hour + cooling time

Makes 4 servings

My mom used to eat beets from a can, and it always made me think they tasted like day-old dishwater. Try this beet salad, and you'll learn exactly what beets are supposed to taste like!

Beets

2 tablespoons olive oil

¼ teaspoon salt

¼ teaspoon ground black pepper

6 small beets, washed and peeled

Vinaigrette

¼ cup balsamic vinegar

2 teaspoons unsweetened cocoa powder

2 teaspoons blackstrap molasses

½ teaspoon salt

½ teaspoon ground black pepper

½ cup extra-virgin olive oil

Salad

1 bag (5 ounces) spring mix salad greens

10 mandarin orange slices (about ½ cup)

½ cup chopped walnuts

½ cup crumbled goat cheese

¼ red onion, thinly sliced (about ⅓ cup)

½ cup cacao nibs

To make the beets: Preheat the oven to 400°F.

In a shallow bowl, whisk together the olive oil, salt, and pepper.

Brush the beets with the oil mixture and wrap them together in aluminum foil. Set the foil into a baking pan, and bake for 45 minutes, or until they're tender. Remove the beets from the oven and allow them to cool. Slice the beets and set them aside.

To make the vinaigrette: Meanwhile, in a medium bowl, combine the vinegar, cocoa powder, molasses, salt, and pepper. Whisk until smooth. Slowly add the oil, whisking constantly, until blended.

To assemble the salad: In a large bowl, combine the greens, oranges, walnuts, cheese, onion, and sliced beets. Divide onto 4 serving plates and top each with 2 tablespoons of cacao nibs. Drizzle with the vinaigrette.

Three Cs Grilled Pork

Total time: 1 hour 15 minutes

Makes 8 servings

This is a wonderful spice rub that goes great with cocoa, and it introduces coffee to the palate party you're about to have in your mouth. The savory nature of this combination makes it work very well with the apple-pear chutney.

2 tablespoons chili powder

2 tablespoons unsweetened cocoa powder

2 tablespoons finely ground coffee

½ teaspoon kosher salt

½ teaspoon freshly ground black pepper

1 center-cut pork loin, trimmed (about 2½–3 pounds)

1 tablespoon olive oil

1 tablespoon butter

2 Honey Crisp apples, peeled and diced

2 pears, peeled and diced

½ cup balsamic vinegar

1 tablespoon brown sugar

Salt

Ground black pepper

Juice of ½ orange

Preheat the oven to 375°F and preheat the grill.

In a small bowl, combine the chili powder, cocoa powder, coffee, salt, and pepper. Rub the spice mixture lightly on the pork loin.

In a large ovenproof skillet, heat the oil over medium-high heat.

Sear the pork for 2 minutes on each side, or until browned, and transfer it to the oven. Cook until the internal temperature reaches 145°F.

Meanwhile, place the butter in a medium saucepan over medium heat. Cook the apples and pears, until lightly softened. Add the vinegar and sugar and stir to coat. Cook for 1 minute. Season with salt and pepper to taste.

Thinly slice the pork and top it with the fruit chutney, a squeeze of fresh orange juice, and salt and pepper to taste.

Seared Pork Chops with a Holiday Spice Rub

Total time: 20 minutes

Makes 6 servings

In each of these recipes, I give you different spice combinations to try. All of them go very well with the particular meat of the recipe, but some combinations are more typically found in certain situations—in this case, cinnamon, nutmeg, and cloves give a feel of the holiday season. The cocoa adds to this festive flavor medley.

- 1 tablespoon whole white peppercorns
- 1 tablespoon whole coriander seeds
- 4 tablespoons ground cinnamon
- 2 teaspoons ground nutmeg
- 1 teaspoon ground cloves
- 4 tablespoons unsweetened cocoa powder
- 1 tablespoon salt
- 6 boneless pork chops (5–6 ounces each)
- Splash of extra virgin olive oil

In a large saucepan over medium heat, toast the peppercorns and coriander seeds until they begin to pop. Remove them from the heat and grind them into a powder.

In a small bowl, mix the powder with the cinnamon, nutmeg, cloves, cocoa powder, and salt. Apply the spice rub liberally to the pork chops.

In the same saucepan over medium-high heat, heat the olive oil. Add the pork chops to the pan and sear each side for 3 minutes, or until fully cooked.

Cajun Cocoa Chops

Total time: 25 minutes

Makes 4 servings

When you taste this flavor combination, you'll notice how wonderful it is. But by the second and third time you put this together, you'll start to develop distinctions and preferences for more or less of one spice or another. That's another brilliant part of this dish—you can tailor its abundant flavor to your exact palate preference! But the only way you can get from here to there is to practice preparing and tasting it. Bummer, right?

2 tablespoons packed brown sugar

1 teaspoon ground red pepper

1 teaspoon dried oregano

1 tablespoon unsweetened cocoa powder

1/2 teaspoon ground red-pepper flakes

1/2 teaspoon ground cumin

1/2 teaspoon mustard powder

1 teaspoon salt

1 teaspoon ground black pepper

3 cloves garlic, minced

1 tablespoon extra virgin olive oil

4 pork chops (5–6 ounces each)

Preheat the oven to 350°F.

In a large bowl, combine the sugar, red pepper, oregano, cocoa powder, pepper flakes, cumin, mustard, salt, pepper, and garlic.

Rub the mixture evenly over the pork chops. Swirl the oil into a large cast-iron pan over medium-high heat. Add the pork chops and cook for 2 minutes per side. You can then either set the skillet into the oven and bake, or remove the pork chops to a baking dish. Bake them for 4 minutes, or until they're done.

Transfer the chops to a bed of spiced rice served with a side of red beans.

Cuban Cocoa Pork via China

Total time: 3 hours 30 minutes

Makes 8–10 servings

Whenever we make this, it's an absolute event. "Yum—you're going to make the Cuban Cocoa Pork thingy?" people ask. There's such a wonderful combination of flavors here, and I love the snap that the Sichuan peppercorns give to the overall flavor. If you can't find them, just add regular black pepper instead.

1 tablespoon salt

3 tablespoons unsweetened cocoa powder

1 tablespoon Sichuan peppercorns, ground

1 tablespoon finely ground coffee

5–6 pounds boneless pork butt, trimmed of excess fat

2 tablespoons extra virgin olive oil

1 container (16 ounces) tomatillo salsa

¼ cup white wine vinegar

1 jalapeño chile pepper, seeds and ribs removed and finely minced (optional, wear plastic gloves when handling)

In a small mixing bowl, add the salt, cocoa, Sichuan peppercorns, and coffee. Smear the cocoa rub over the pork. You could either start cooking now or wrap it in plastic and allow it to marinate for a day.

Swirl the oil in a Dutch oven over medium-high heat. Set the pork into the Dutch oven and brown it on all sides. Then add the salsa and the vinegar, and the jalapeño if you like it spicy.

Bring the liquid to a boil, reduce it to a simmer, and cover the pot. Cook it for 3 to 4 hours; every hour or so, peek in and turn the butt over. Once it's falling-apart tender, it's ready to go.

Serve this over a bed of rice topped with black beans. A salsa of mango and avocado goes exceptionally well with this particular meal.

Cocoa-Rubbed Rib Eye
with Bacon-Bourbon Sauce

Total time: 1 hour 5 minutes

Makes 8 servings

This recipe draws flavor from two sources: the sweet, spicy, sultry spices that make up the rub, and also the tangy and smoky bacon-bourbon sauce.

1 tablespoon unsweetened cocoa powder

2 teaspoons ground black pepper + additional

1 teaspoon packed brown sugar

½ teaspoon ground red pepper

2 teaspoons salt + additional

4 thin-cut (¾–1" thick) boneless rib-eye steaks (about 9–10 ounces each)

4 strips bacon, diced

1 medium onion, diced

1 tablespoon all-purpose flour

½ cup bourbon

3 cups chicken stock

2 bay leaves

½ cup half-and-half

1 tablespoon unsalted butter

2 tablespoons chopped parsley

Extra virgin olive oil

In a small bowl, mix together the cocoa powder, 2 teaspoons black pepper, sugar, red pepper, and 2 teaspoons salt. Season the steak on both sides with this dry rub. Cover and let the steak come to room temperature while you're making the sauce.

Meanwhile, heat the bacon in a large skillet over medium heat until crisp, about 5 minutes. Remove the bacon and set aside. Add the onion to the drippings. Once it starts to caramelize (after 10 to 15 minutes), stir in the flour and cook for another minute.

Remove the pan from the heat, add the bourbon, and bring to a simmer over medium heat. Once the sauce starts to thicken, in about 2 minutes, add the chicken stock and bay leaves, and bring to a gentle boil over medium-high heat. Cook until the mixture is reduced by a quarter, about 8 minutes. Whisk in the half-and-half and simmer on medium heat, stirring occasionally, for 7 minutes, or until the sauce coats a spoon. Stir in the butter, bacon, and parsley. Season with additional salt and pepper. Remove the bay leaves and keep the sauce warm.

Heat a large cast-iron skillet over high heat for 2 minutes. Add a swirl of extra virgin olive oil to the pan and sear the steak for 4 minutes per side. Depending on the thickness, this will leave you with a doneness that would be considered "medium-rare" in most restaurants. Once it is done on both sides, transfer it to a plate and let it rest for 5 minutes. Slice each steak in half before serving. Season with a light sprinkle of salt, and serve with the bacon-bourbon sauce on the side.

Spicy Beef Stew

Total time: 2 hours 10 minutes

Makes 4–6 servings

The amazing flavor combinations in this stew can be applied to many recipes. The marriage of cocoa and chili powder, in combination with beef stock, tomato paste, and mushrooms, is unbeatable. You know what? You might even toss in a bit of red wine for good measure!

2 teaspoons + 2 tablespoons unsweetened cocoa powder

1 teaspoon chili powder

1 teaspoon coarsely ground black pepper

1½ teaspoons kosher salt

2 pounds beef stew meat, cut into 1" cubes

1 tablespoon olive oil

2 tablespoons unsalted butter

1 package (8 ounces) sliced mushrooms

1 onion, diced (about 1 cup)

3 tablespoons all-purpose flour

3 cups beef stock

2 tablespoons tomato paste

2 bay leaves

½ teaspoon dried thyme

½ teaspoon dried oregano

¼ teaspoon ground allspice

1 pound small new potatoes

2 carrots, diced (about 1 cup)

2 ribs celery, diced (about 1 cup)

In a shallow bowl, mix together the 2 teaspoons cocoa powder, chili powder, pepper, and salt. Rub the mix onto the beef.

In a large pot over medium-high heat, cook the meat in the oil until all the sides are browned. Remove the beef and set it aside in a bowl.

Turn the heat down to medium and add the butter. After it's softened, add the mushrooms and cook for 5 to 6 minutes, or until they give off fluid, then toss them into the bowl with the beef. Add the onions to the pan and cook for 15 minutes, or until they caramelize, then put them into the beef bowl as well.

You should have leftover oils in the pan that taste like butter and onion and mushroom. Add the flour to that oil, stirring occasionally, until it turns chestnut brown (about 5 to 8 minutes). This is the roux that will flavor the stew.

Add the beef stock and just stir it around to make sure the roux combines with the stock. Then add the tomato paste, 2 tablespoons cocoa powder, bay leaves, thyme, oregano, allspice, and the beef, mushrooms, and caramelized onions from the bowl. Bring the stock to a boil. Reduce the heat to a simmer, cover, and let it stew for 45 minutes. Then add the potatoes, carrots, and celery. Simmer uncovered for another 45 minutes.

Cocoa Chili

Total time: 50 minutes

Makes 6 servings

Cocoa adds depth to chili's flavor, and when used with chili powder and cinnamon, it marries into an amazing combination of spicy, nutty, and sweet.

Seasoning
½ cup unsweetened cocoa powder

2 tablespoons chili powder

2 teaspoons dried oregano

1 teaspoon salt

1 teaspoon ground black pepper

1 teaspoon ground red pepper

1 teaspoon ground cumin

Chili
2 pounds ground beef

1 onion, chopped (about 1 cup)

6 garlic cloves, minced

1 red bell pepper, chopped (about 1 cup)

1 jalapeño chile pepper, ribbed, seeded, and diced (wear gloves when handling)

2 cans (28 ounce each) crushed tomatoes

1 can (6 ounces) tomato paste

2 ounces bittersweet chocolate, chopped

¼ cup lime juice

Sharp Cheddar cheese

Sour cream

To make the seasoning: Put the cocoa powder, chili powder, oregano, salt, black pepper, red pepper, and cumin in a zip-top bag and shake it around until blended. Wet your pinkie, stick it into the mix, and taste to see if there is some flavor that you want more of.

To make the chili: In a large Dutch oven, brown the ground beef over medium-high heat until no longer pink. Remove it from the pan and set aside.

Reduce the heat to medium and add the onions and garlic. Cook until the onions are soft. Then add the bell pepper and jalapeño pepper.

Add the browned beef to the pot, along with the crushed tomatoes, tomato paste, chocolate, lime juice, and the chili-chocolate-spicy seasoning.

Reduce the heat to a simmer and cook for 15 minutes.

Serve with shredded Cheddar cheese and sour cream.

Eat Chocolate, Lose Weight

Chicken Cacciatore

Total time: 40 minutes
Makes 4 servings

In this recipe, herb-infused oils meld into the tomato puree, and this combination is added to chopped dark chocolate. Taste how the chocolate itself deepens the flavor as it melts lovingly into the sauce of herbed tomatoes.

1¼ pounds chicken tenders

¼ teaspoon salt

¼ teaspoon pepper

1 tablespoon unsalted butter

1 tablespoon extra virgin olive oil

1 red onion, chopped

1 green bell pepper, chopped

1 teaspoon Italian seasoning

1 can (14.5 ounces) diced tomatoes

1 cup chicken broth

2 ounces bittersweet chocolate, chopped

Season the chicken tenders with the salt and pepper. In a large skillet over medium heat, add the butter and olive oil. Once the butter has melted, add the chicken and brown lightly, 2 to 3 minutes on each side, working in batches if you have to. Remove the chicken from the pan, set it on a plate, and cover.

In the same skillet, cook the onion, bell pepper, and Italian seasoning and stir for 3 minutes, or until the vegetables begin to soften. Add the tomatoes and stir, deglazing the bottom of the pan and cooking for 5 minutes, or until the mixture begins to thicken slightly. Add the broth, bring to a boil, and then reduce the heat to a simmer.

Cook uncovered for 15 minutes, stirring occasionally, until thickened. Stir in the chocolate, cooking for 5 minutes, or until melted and incorporated.

Set the chicken tenders, along with any accumulated juices, into the sauce and stir gently to cover the pieces. Simmer for 1 to 2 minutes.

Slow Cooker Chicken Mole

Total time: 8 hours 15 minutes

Makes 4 servings

This is a great recipe because it takes something that many people think is too hard or too fussy to make and removes all of those excuses. It's easy: You just dump everything in the pot, leave the house, come back later, and it's all done!

½ large onion, chopped (about 1 cup)

⅓ cup raisins

2 cloves garlic, minced

2 teaspoons chili powder

2 tablespoons toasted sesame seeds

¾ teaspoon ground cumin

¾ teaspoon ground cinnamon

5 teaspoons unsweetened cocoa powder

½ teaspoon hot-pepper sauce

1 can (14½ ounces) diced tomatoes

1 cup tomato sauce

1 cup chicken broth

3 pounds boneless, skinless chicken thighs (5–6 ounces each)

In the morning before you head off to work, throw the onion, raisins, garlic, chili powder, sesame seeds, cumin, cinnamon, cocoa powder, hot sauce, tomatoes, tomato sauce, broth, and chicken in your slow cooker. Stir it all around to make sure the chicken is covered. Cook on the low setting for 8 to 10 hours (put it in at 7 a.m., and it's ready at 5 p.m.). Brilliant.

Chicken with Cocoa-Tomato Sauce

Total time: 1 hour

Makes 4 servings

In this recipe, the cocoa-tomato combination is a little lighter. The flavors are a bit more straightforward, and the cocoa powder pops out more prominently.

6 boneless, skinless chicken breast halves (about 6 ounces each)

½ teaspoon salt, divided

½ teaspoon ground black pepper, divided

3 tablespoons extra virgin olive oil

1 small onion, chopped

1 teaspoon minced garlic

2 cups tomato sauce

3 medium tomatoes, diced (about 1½ cups)

½ cup chicken broth

1 tablespoon unsweetened cocoa powder

1 teaspoon dried oregano

1 teaspoon dried basil

Season the chicken with ¼ teaspoon of the salt and ¼ teaspoon of the pepper. In a cast-iron skillet, heat 2 tablespoons of the olive oil over medium-high heat. Add the chicken and sear both sides, about 3 minutes for each side. Remove the chicken from the pan and set aside.

Add the remaining 1 tablespoon of olive oil, the onion, and the garlic and cook over medium heat for 2 minutes, stirring frequently. Add the tomato sauce, diced tomatoes, chicken broth, cocoa powder, oregano, basil, and the remaining ¼ teaspoon of salt and ¼ teaspoon of pepper. Stir until well blended and allow the flavors to marry, about 5 minutes. Taste to see what it needs, and adjust the seasoning if needed.

Set the chicken in the sauce, cover the pan, and let it simmer for 10 minutes. Flip the chicken pieces and simmer for another 10 minutes. You can serve this with the sauce on the side, but it is also good served over rice.

Chicken with Spicy Cocoa Rub

Total time: 30 minutes

Makes 4 servings

This recipe is prepared like Cajun Cocoa Chops (page 212), but the spices have been changed to suit chicken's taste and texture. The strategy is the same: Quickly sear the outside in a pan (you can also do this on the grill), and then take it off the direct heat to finish cooking the middle. This helps prevent it from drying out.

1 tablespoon chili powder

2 teaspoons unsweetened cocoa powder

1 teaspoon ground cinnamon

½ teaspoon salt

2 tablespoons olive oil

4 boneless, skinless chicken breast halves (about 6 ounces each)

Preheat the oven to 375°F.

In a mixing bowl, combine the chili powder, cocoa powder, cinnamon, and salt.

Heat a large ovenproof skillet over medium heat. Add almost all of the 2 tablespoons of olive oil to the skillet. Brush both sides of the chicken breasts with the remaining oil.

Generously rub the chicken with the rub until it's evenly coated. Place the chicken in the skillet and sear it on both sides. Remove the skillet from the heat and bake it in the oven for 15 minutes, or until the chicken is cooked through.

Tuna with Sesame-Soy-Ginger Sauce

Total time: 25 minutes

Makes 1 serving

This recipe is a total adaptation. Cocoa is completely complementary to the flavor set of this sauce. Served over seared fresh sushi-grade tuna, it's simply amazing.

3 tablespoons ground ginger

2 teaspoons unsweetened cocoa powder

¼ cup soy sauce

⅓ cup sesame oil

½ teaspoon ground red pepper

5 tablespoons rice wine vinegar

¼ cup chicken stock

3 teaspoons sesame seeds

1 tablespoon unsalted butter

1 tuna steak (about 6 ounces)

In a medium saucepan set over medium-low heat, add the ginger, cocoa, soy sauce, sesame oil, pepper, vinegar, chicken stock, and sesame seeds. Whisk to blend, making sure the ginger and the cocoa are fully incorporated. Turn the heat to low and allow these flavors to meld. Then add the butter and let it melt in. Taste this sauce for saltiness. The soy really pops out because of the acidity of the vinegar and the cocoa powder (particularly if you use un-Dutched cocoa powder). If it seems too salty, thin it with additional chicken stock. You want to taste more sesame flavor or more cocoa flavor.

Searing the tuna is pretty simple. First the fish needs to be at room temperature and patted dry with a paper towel. In a dry iron skillet over medium-high heat, cook the tuna steak for 3 to 4 minutes per side, but check the inside to make sure it's done to your preference, keeping in mind that it will continue to cook a bit after you have taken it off the heat.

Place the fish on a plate and spoon a small amount of sauce over it or serve the sauce on the side.

Cocoa-Chili Jamaican Fish

Total time: 1 hour

Makes 4 servings

While in Jamaica with friends and family, I had to choose between going on an afternoon sailing cruise (complete and replete with rum drinks, Jamaican singing, and lots of fun) or attending a cooking demonstration by the resort chef. It's a sickness, I know, but I let my covey of friends go on without me so I could sit in on the Jamaican recipe celebration. In the end, they had fun, but I got this very cool recipe that I can now share with you!

1 large firm white fish steak (such as swordfish), skin removed

Pinch of salt

Pinch + ½ teaspoon freshly ground black pepper

3 tablespoons extra virgin olive oil

¼ onion, chopped (about ½ cup)

½ red bell pepper, chopped (about ½ cup)

1 habañero chile pepper, seeded, ribbed, and finely minced (wear gloves when handling

3 cloves garlic, minced

1 can (6 ounces) tomato paste

2 cups chicken broth

2 tablespoons soy sauce

1 cinnamon stick

1 teaspoon unsweetened cocoa powder

Season the fish with a pinch of salt and pepper. In a cast-iron skillet, heat 2 tablespoons of the oil over medium-high heat. Add the fish and sear both sides, cooking for about 5 minutes on each side. Remove the fish from the pan and set aside.

Add the remaining 1 tablespoon of oil, the onion, bell pepper, chile pepper, and garlic and cook for 2 minutes, stirring frequently. Add the tomato paste, chicken broth, soy sauce, cinnamon stick, cocoa powder, and ½ teaspoon pepper. Stir until the tomato paste is well blended.

At this point, the sauce should be thinner than you want it to be. Over the next 15 minutes, it'll cook down to the consistency you prefer. Thus, if it's already at your desired consistency, it's too thick and you should add more broth.

Cut the fish into bite-size pieces. Set the fish back into the sauce and simmer, uncovered, for 15 minutes. At this point, taste and adjust the sauce for the many overlapping flavors: Saltiness is given by the soy, heat by the chile pepper, savoriness by the cocoa, and the balancing sweetness by the cinnamon.

Once you have the sauce right, serve it and the fish over spiced rice. You make it just like you do regular rice, but you throw in a cinnamon stick at the beginning. You're going to love it.

30-Minute Mole over Polenta

Total time: 30 minutes

Makes 10 servings

This recipe has two benefits. First, you can make it in 30 minutes, so you can get your mole fix even on a weeknight! Second, it introduces you to another flavor combination that is spectacular (and spectacularly simple).

4 dried ancho chile peppers

1 chipotle chile pepper

1 can (14.5 ounces) roasted tomatoes

2 tablespoons extra virgin olive oil

2 large sweet onions, sliced (about 3 cups)

$\frac{1}{4}$ cup slivered almonds

7 cloves garlic, minced

$\frac{1}{2}$ cup raisins

1 tablespoon sesame seeds

$\frac{1}{8}$ teaspoon ground anise

2 corn tortillas, slightly charred under the broiler or over a burner

1 tablespoon chili powder

1 teaspoon ground cinnamon

2 cups chicken stock

2 ounces bittersweet chocolate, chopped

$\frac{1}{2}$ cup cilantro, coarsely chopped

Place the ancho and chipotle chile peppers in a bowl and just barely cover with boiling water. Give them about 30 minutes to soak up the water, at which time you will discard the stems and seeds. Place the softened chile peppers and their soaking water and the roasted tomatoes in a blender.

In a large skillet over medium heat, heat 1 tablespoon of the oil and add half the onions. Stir for 10 minutes, or until they have turned soft and are beginning to caramelize. Add the almonds, garlic, raisins, sesame seeds, and anise and continue stirring until the almonds are lightly browned. Add this mixture to the blender, along with the tortillas, chili powder, and cinnamon. Puree until smooth.

jun Black Beans

time: 10 minutes

s 2 servings

should be a staple side in your world. It's wicked easy, it tastes great, t's incredible for your health! For a quick breakfast, top ½ cup of s with 1 fried egg, salsa, and crumbled feta cheese.

an (15 ounces) black beans, rained and rinsed

easpoon chili powder

easpoon unsweetened cocoa owder

easpoon ground cumin

1 cinnamon stick

1 teaspoon olive oil

1 teaspoon balsamic vinegar

Salt and ground black pepper

is the easiest dish in the world. In a skillet over medium heat, cook the s, chili powder, cocoa powder, cumin, cinnamon stick, olive oil, and bal- c vinegar. Once it begins to simmer, add salt and pepper to taste.

Heat the remaining 1 tablespoon of olive oil in a skillet an
chopped onion. Stir for 5 minutes, or until the onior
colored. Now add the chicken stock, along with the cont
Stir well, reduce to a simmer, cover, and let cook for 10 i

Uncover and stir in the chopped chocolate and the cilant
late has melted and blended into the mole, taste to see i
cinnamon, and chocolate. If the sauce is too thin, cook it
too thick, stir in a bit more stock. The consistency you'i
up to you, but the sauce should lightly coat the back of

Serve this mole over baked, sliced polenta and top it with
Jack cheese.

C

To
Mc
Tl
an
be

1

1

½

½

Thi
be
sar

Black Bean Soup

Total time: 1 hour 10 minutes

Makes 4 servings

Black bean soup is so very good for you. If you're not used to eating beans, this soup is a good one to start with because it has so much flavor and is super simple to throw together. If you like, you can also use dried black beans. Just rinse them, let them soak through the day, then cook them for about an hour, until just tender.

2 tablespoons extra virgin olive oil

1 small sweet onion, diced

3 bay leaves

½ teaspoon sea salt

2 ribs celery, diced

2 carrots, peeled and diced

1 red bell pepper, diced

2 medium tomatoes, chopped in a blender

4 cups chicken broth

1 tablespoon balsamic vinegar

2 cans (15 ounces each) black beans, rinsed and drained

2 tablespoons unsweetened cocoa powder

½ teaspoon chili powder

¼ teaspoon ground cumin

½ teaspoon ground black pepper

Sour cream

In a large pot over medium heat, heat the oil. Cook the onion, bay leaves, and salt. Stir occasionally until the onions are softened, 4 to 5 minutes.

Add the celery, carrots, and bell pepper and continue cooking, stirring occasionally, until all the vegetables are softened, 7 to 8 minutes.

Add the tomatoes, chicken broth, and vinegar. Bring to a boil. Reduce the heat and simmer for 15 minutes.

Stir in the beans, cocoa powder, chili powder, cumin, and black pepper. Simmer for 5 minutes. Remove about ½ cup of the beans, chop them in a blender, and add them back to the soup. Let it simmer for another 10 minutes. Serve topped with a dollop of sour cream.

The Full Monte Mole

Total time: 1 hour 15 minutes

Makes 3 cups

When you make this for the first time, you'll be amazed at how wonderful it is. But know this: Each time you put the chile and cocoa and tomato flavors together, they will get more and more incredible as you learn how they combine from pan to palate. Enjoy the ride!

3 tablespoons extra virgin olive oil, divided

3 dried mulato chile peppers, seeded

3 dried pasilla chile peppers, seeded

1 dried ancho chile pepper, seeded

2 whole plum tomatoes

2 (6") corn tortillas

2 cups chicken stock

¼ onion, chopped (about ¼ cup)

1 ripe plantain, halved lengthwise

¼ cup sliced almonds

4 cloves garlic, minced

1 tablespoon unsweetened cocoa powder

1 tablespoon brown sugar

¾ teaspoon salt

1 teaspoon ground cinnamon

1¼ cups water

2 ounces high-cocoa chocolate, chopped

½ lime, cut into wedges

In a large cast-iron skillet over medium-high heat, heat 1 tablespoon of the oil. Add the mulato, pasilla, and ancho chile peppers and cook until they're brown on each side (about 1 minute per side, if the pan is hot)—be careful not to blacken the peppers or get the pan so hot that the oil smokes, as this will make the mole bitter. Remove the chiles to a bowl and cover them with hot water. Leave them alone for 30 minutes while you do everything else.

Preheat the broiler. Place the tomatoes on a baking sheet and broil them in the oven, directly next to the heat, until singed on all sides (turn them with tongs every 1 to 2 minutes or so). Add the tortillas to a dry pan and cook them over medium heat to brown each side.

Pull the rehydrated chile peppers from the water and place them in a blender. Puree them along with the tomatoes, toasted tortillas, and chicken stock. Leave this in the blender for now, because you're going to add more to it later. At this point, you have a choice to make: If you want your mole to be perfectly smooth, you can run this puree through a sieve to remove the larger particles. However, if you like bits of flotsam and jetsam in the sauce, as I do, save yourself the trouble and use it as is.

Heat the pan over medium-high heat. Add the remaining 2 tablespoons of oil and the onion and sauté for 3 minutes. Add the plantain and sauté until it has browned. Add the almonds and garlic and give them another minute in the pan. Stir in the cocoa powder, brown sugar, salt, and cinnamon. Mix those for another 30 seconds or so. Then add the entire contents of the pan, along with ¼ cup of the water, to the pureed chile mixture in the blender. Process this all into one big, sloppy slurry.

Using a spatula, scrape this back into the pan along with the remaining 1 cup of water and heat it over medium heat. Add the chocolate and cook uncovered for 15 minutes, or until it thickens just enough to cover the back of a spoon. Taste the sauce and correct the flavors as you see fit.

Serve over your meat of choice and have lime wedges at the ready.

Mole Sauce 1.0

Total time: 25 minutes

Makes 2 cups

This is easy to make and brings the flavor marriage of tomatoes and cocoa to a whole new level through the addition of chile peppers. It's not the burn-your-face-off kind of chile, but rather the smoky, husky, dark, and mysterious kind. This recipe is a perfect introduction to how chiles can add to the flavor mix.

2 teaspoons vegetable oil

1/3 onion, minced (about 1/4 cup)

1 tablespoon unsweetened cocoa powder

1 teaspoon ground cumin

1 teaspoon ground coriander

1 clove garlic, minced

2 cups tomato sauce

1 can (4 ounces) diced green chile peppers

Salt and ground black pepper

In a medium saucepan over medium heat, heat the oil. Cook the onions, stirring occasionally, until they soften, about 5 minutes. Mix in the cocoa powder, cumin, coriander, and garlic. Stir in the tomato sauce and the green chile peppers. Bring the mixture to a boil, reduce the heat to low, cover, and simmer for 10 minutes.

What you have at this point is a base, and this is where you can get creative if you like. Add salt and pepper to taste. If you want more spice, ground red pepper is a good addition. Or you can add more cocoa powder or cumin. Once you add in more flavor, let the sauce marry for a little while before you taste it again, so the flavors have matured to their final form.

Cocoa Butter

Total time: 10 minutes

Makes ½ cup

Cocoa butter is the yummy goodness that comes, very naturally, right from the cocoa bean itself. You can throw together this version and refine it on your own. It's actually much like whipped cream in that you have a fat, you add sugar and vanilla to that fat, and suddenly you have something wonderful. The beauty of cocoa-infused butter is that you can use it anytime as a substitute for butter, especially if you want to add a chocolaty savory element to it.

1 stick unsalted butter, softened

1 tablespoon unsweetened cocoa powder

1 tablespoon confectioners' sugar

Dash of vanilla extract

In a medium bowl, blend together the butter, cocoa powder, sugar, and vanilla. Shape the mixture into a log, or a cube, or a dog, or any form you want. Cool in the fridge.

Chocolate-Coconut Oat Bars

Total time: 40 minutes

Makes 12 servings

With a classic macaroon texture, these egg-, dairy-, and gluten-free treats are an adult chocolate indulgence. Kids, of course, will love them, too.

2½ cups rolled oats

1 cup almond meal

1 cup unsweetened shredded coconut

⅓ cup unsweetened cocoa powder

½ cup bittersweet chocolate chips

½ cup coconut oil

¼ cup blackstrap molasses

½ cup brown sugar

Preheat the oven to 300°F.

In a large bowl, thoroughly blend the oats, almond meal, coconut, cocoa powder, and chocolate chips.

In a saucepan, combine the coconut oil, molasses, and sugar over medium heat until the sugar is dissolved and the mixture bubbles a bit.

Pour the sugar mixture over the top of the oatmeal mixture and stir until they are completely combined. Press the mixture into an ungreased 8" x 8" baking pan and bake for 20 minutes. Let it cool, and then cut it into squares.

Easy Cocoa Cookies

Total time: 1 hour 30 minutes

Makes 24 cookies

If you're making cookies, these simple and pure ones are great to start with because they're so straightforward. Do the dry stuff, do the wet stuff, mix together, bake, and eat. Easy peasy.

2¼ cups all-purpose flour + more for dusting

⅓ cup unsweetened cocoa powder

1 teaspoon baking soda

¼ teaspoon salt

2 sticks unsalted butter, softened

¾ cup packed brown sugar

1 large egg

1 teaspoon vanilla extract

In a medium bowl, mix the flour, cocoa powder, baking soda, and salt.

In a large bowl, beat the butter and sugar with a mixer on medium-high speed for 3 to 5 minutes until light and fluffy. Add the egg and vanilla and beat until they're incorporated.

Reduce the mixer speed to low. Add the flour mixture in two batches, beating each until it's just incorporated.

Divide the dough in half, wrap the halves in plastic wrap, and refrigerate until firm—at least 1 hour and up to 1 day.

Preheat the oven to 350°F. Lightly dust your work surface with flour. Using a rolling pin, roll out the dough until it's an even ½" thick. Form the cookies into the shapes of your choice, set them on a baking sheet, and bake for 12 minutes, or until lightly browned. Let them cool a bit.

Chocolate–Peanut Butter Cookies

Total time: 30 minutes

Makes 40 cookies

The great part about cooking is the playful part—adding bits of flavor or texture here or there to change things up a bit. To make these peanut butter and cocoa cookies, you basically tweak the Easy Cocoa Cookies recipe (page 235) and fold in peanut butter to make them that much better.

2 cups all-purpose flour

½ cup unsweetened cocoa powder

1 teaspoon baking powder

½ teaspoon baking soda

¼ teaspoon salt

¾ cup (1½ sticks) unsalted butter, softened

¾ cup all-natural peanut butter (smooth or chunky)

2 cups packed brown sugar

2 large eggs

1 teaspoon vanilla extract

Preheat the oven to 350°F.

In a medium bowl, completely mix the flour, cocoa powder, baking powder, baking soda, and salt.

In a large bowl, beat the butter, peanut butter, and sugar with a mixer on medium-high speed for 3 to 5 minutes until light and fluffy. Add 1 egg at a time and then the vanilla, beating well.

Beat the dry ingredients into the wet ingredients at low speed until they're completely blended. Drop by rounded tablespoonfuls onto a baking sheet, being sure to leave 2" between the cookies, which will spread during baking. Press the top of each cookie with the tines of a fork to form a criss-cross pattern. Bake for 12 minutes, or until lightly browned, and allow to cool on a wire rack.

Chocolate-Citrus Biscotti

Total time: 1 hour 15 minutes

Makes 24 servings

Now that you've mastered the art of making drop cookies with cocoa, try another kind of cookie that you can add chocolate and/or cocoa to: biscotti. *Biscotti* derives from medieval Latin and means "baked twice." Now that you've passed your Latin finals, let's make some, and we'll have an oral (taste) test afterward!

2¼ cups all-purpose flour

½ cup unsweetened cocoa powder

1⅔ cups sugar

1 teaspoon baking powder

3 large eggs

3 large egg yolks

1 tablespoon almond extract

¾ cup chopped walnuts

1 tablespoon orange peel

¾ cup chopped high-cocoa chocolate

Preheat the oven to 350°F.

In a medium bowl, mix the flour, cocoa powder, sugar, and baking powder.

In a large bowl, blend the eggs, egg yolks, and almond extract. Fold the dry ingredients into the wet ingredients, and stir around until they're completely mixed together. At this point, you'll have the basic dough ball in place.

Fold the walnuts, orange peel, and chocolate into the dough, then roll it out into a rectangular loaf that is 6" wide and about 2" tall. Bake the loaf on an ungreased baking sheet for 20 minutes, or until it's golden brown on top. Let it cool on a wire rack.

Once it's cool, cut your biscotti in about ½"-wide slices. Keep these slices standing upright (don't lay them on their sides), but leave some air between the pieces so they can dry out. Then place them back into the oven at the same temperature for 15 minutes, or until they are crisp.

Take them out, let them cool, and you are good to go.

Rich 'n' Nutty Brownies

Total time: 50 minutes

Makes 16–20 servings

Just as we had a "study in cookies" and a "study in cocoa sauces," this is a primer in those classic little rectangles of heaven: brownies.

1¼ sticks unsalted butter

½ cup granulated sugar

½ cup brown sugar

¾ cup unsweetened cocoa powder

¼ teaspoon salt

½ teaspoon vanilla extract

2 large eggs, beaten

½ cup all-purpose flour

⅓ cup pecans, coarsely crushed

Preheat the oven to 325°F. Butter and lightly flour a 13" x 9" baking pan.

In a medium saucepan over medium-low heat, heat the butter until it's just melted. Add the sugars, cocoa powder, and salt and combine until the mixture is smooth. Pour this mixture into a large mixing bowl and let it cool (this will prevent the eggs from scrambling when they are added; it's okay to add the eggs when the mixture is warm, but not hot).

Add the vanilla and eggs, stirring all the while, until they are completely incorporated. Then fold in the flour and mix thoroughly, followed by the nuts. Pour this into the prepared pan and bake for 25 minutes, or until a toothpick comes out clean.

Cocoa Whipped Cream

Total time: 10 minutes

Makes 2 cups

When I tell people that I make my own whipped cream, they respond by exclaiming, "From scratch?!" Yes, if by "from scratch," you mean that I throw ingredients into a bowl and then stand there, beating them for 5 minutes until they thicken up. What a magician, eh?

¼ cup unsweetened cocoa powder

3 tablespoons confectioners' sugar

1 cup heavy cream

½ teaspoon vanilla extract

In a small bowl, blend the cocoa powder and sugar.

In a large bowl, beat the cream and vanilla with an electric mixer. After a few minutes, the cream will form soft peaks. At that point, stir in the cocoa mixture, and beat until the mixture is well blended. Store in an airtight container for up to 1 day.

Flourless Chocolate Cake

Total time: 2 hours

Makes 12–16 servings

You know the phrase "you can't have your cake and eat it, too"? What kind of silliness is this? Of course you can have your cake and eat it, too. First you have it. Then you eat it. See how that works? I know this logic can be confusing, so try it out on this Flourless Chocolate Cake.

2 sticks unsalted butter

1 pound bittersweet chocolate, chopped

¼ cup Kahlua

8 large eggs

¼ cup sugar

1 teaspoon vanilla extract

½ teaspoon salt

Red fruit, such as raspberries

Preheat the oven to 325°F. Butter and flour a 9" springform pan.

In a medium saucepan over the lowest heat possible, heat the butter until just melting. Add the chocolate and Kahlua and stir until the chocolate pieces are almost melted. Then turn off the heat and let the mixture cool. Stir to make sure all the bits are completely melted.

In a large bowl, beat together the eggs, sugar, vanilla, and salt for 10 full minutes. Fold the chocolate mix into this flourless part and stir until thoroughly combined.

Pour the batter into the prepared pan and bake for 45 minutes. You'll notice that the sides will crown a bit. At this point, the outsides will be done and the center will be almost done—a toothpick inserted around the margins will be clean, but the same toothpick inserted in the center will be a bit fudgy.

Remove the cake from the oven and let it sit for at least 30 minutes. At that point it is safe to transfer it to a plate and apply icing, should you choose to use it (this cake is great without it). An excellent garnish for anything deeply chocolate like this is red fruit, such as fresh raspberries or strawberries.

Hot Cocoa Soufflé

Total time: 55 minutes

Makes 6 servings

A soufflé sounds fancy, but it's basically just a cake that has beaten egg whites in it. Just like those egg whites fluff up into a meringue when beaten, they puff up your cake batter when it's baking in the oven. The result is a light taste and very nice texture. Give it a shot and see what you think.

4 eggs, separated

2 tablespoons butter

2 tablespoons all-purpose flour

1 cup whole milk

$\frac{1}{2}$ cup unsweetened cocoa powder

$\frac{3}{4}$ cup sugar, divided

1 teaspoon vanilla extract

Preheat the oven to 400°F. Butter and flour six 8-ounce ramekins (if you don't have ramekins, you can use ovenproof custard cups). Into two separate bowls, separate the egg yolks from the egg whites.

In a medium saucepan over medium heat, melt the butter. Whisk in the flour for 1 minute, or until it forms a smooth paste. Slowly add the milk, whisking so no lumps form. As the sauce thickens, add the cocoa powder and $\frac{1}{2}$ cup of the sugar, whisking constantly. Remove the pan from the heat.

Add a few tablespoons of the hot mixture to the egg yolks and mix until smooth. Add the yolk mixture back into the cocoa sauce and whisk until completely incorporated. Mix in the vanilla and set aside.

In a large bowl, beat the egg whites and the remaining $\frac{1}{4}$ cup sugar with an electric mixer until the peaks are quite firm. Fold the chocolate into the egg whites and mix until completely blended.

Pour the soufflé mixture into the prepared ramekins. Bake for 20 to 25 minutes, or until the tops are lightly browned. You'll note that they puff up substantially. These are best warm, so serve immediately.

Classic Chocolate Pudding

Total time: 30 minutes + 4 hours chill time

Makes 4 servings

There is no substitute for classic chocolate pudding. Though companies tried to make instant chocolate pudding by turning it into a powdered, just-add-[fill-in-the-blank] weirdness, making a generation of people think it actually tastes like that, once you've eaten this base recipe, you'll never go back to the chalky version. Chocolate pudding is wonderful by itself, but it's even better if you whip up some Cocoa Whipped Cream (see page 239) to serve it with.

2 cups whole milk, divided

½ cup sugar

⅓ cup unsweenteed cocoa powder

4 teaspoons cornstarch

¼ teaspoon salt

3 egg yolks

2 teaspoons vanilla extract

In a medium saucepan over medium heat, combine 1½ cups of the milk, the sugar, and the cocoa. Once it starts to steam, turn off the heat.

Meanwhile, in a medium bowl, blend together the remaining milk, the cornstarch, salt, egg yolks, and vanilla.

Very slowly drizzle the hot milk into the egg mixture so that it gets warm but not hot, stirring the entire time. Once all the milk has been incorporated, pour the milk-egg mixture back into the saucepan. Heat it over medium-high heat, whisking all the while, until it begins to simmer. At that point, turn off the heat, still whisking the mixture. In a couple of minutes, it will thicken up.

Pour the pudding into serving cups or ramekins and refrigerate for at least 4 hours, or until it's firm.

Ganache

Total time: 15 minutes

Makes 2 cups

From this standard recipe, you can take ganache any direction you like. Try tweaking the taste by adding flavorings or the thickness by changing the amount of milk you use. The thicker versions are perfect as the filling for chocolate truffles, while the thinner versions are perfect as icing.

1 cup heavy cream, half-and-half, or whole milk	8 ounces bittersweet chocolate, chopped into small pieces

In a medium saucepan, heat the cream over medium heat until it begins to steam. While this is coming to temperature, place the chopped chocolate in a medium bowl.

Once the liquid is steaming, drizzle it over the chopped chocolate. Let these two sit together for a minute or so, then slowly stir the globs of chocolate on the bottom of the bowl until they are completely incorporated. Keep checking the bottom to make sure it's totally smooth.

Let the ganache come to room temperature for 1 hour and then move it to the refrigerator. I have also placed the ganache in a bowl with a lid and then placed that in the freezer. It will keep for weeks in there, and warms very easily after you take it out.

Truffles

Total time: 4 hours, including freezing time

Makes 36 truffles

Truffles used to be a mystery to me. Just as the word *bucolic* sounds like the unholy combination of colic and the bubonic plague, *truffles* remind us of something that pigs root up with their snouts in the dirt. But they also happen to be the delicious extensions of the master Ganache recipe on page 243. Enjoy!

1 cup heavy cream, half-and-half, or whole milk

14 ounces bittersweet chocolate, chopped into small pieces

2 tablespoons vanilla extract, Grand Marnier or another liqueur, or rum

$\frac{1}{3}$ cup unsweetened cocoa powder

In a medium saucepan over medium heat, heat the cream for 5 minutes, or until it begins to steam. While this is coming to temperature, put 8 ounces of the chocolate in a medium bowl.

Once the liquid is steaming, pour it over the chocolate. Let the mixture sit for a minute or so, then gently stir until the ganache is smooth. Add the vanilla and stir to combine. Cool the ganache to room temperature and then put it in the freezer for 3 hours.

Once the ganache is cold, form it into balls with a small melon scooper or a tablespoon. Scoop a 1" portion and then roll it between your palms to form a ball. Place each truffle ball onto a waxed paper–lined baking sheet. If the ganache gets warm, put it back into the freezer for 15 minutes to firm up. Put the truffle balls back into the freezer to cool.

Once the truffles are completely cold, warm the remaining 6 ounces of chopped chocolate in a saucepan over low heat, stirring until completely smooth. Allow it to approach room temperature for 15 minutes.

Place the cocoa powder in a small bowl. Remove the truffle balls from the freezer and, one by one, drop them into the melted chocolate so that they are just barely coated all over. Remove them with a fork, tap off any excess chocolate, and roll them in the cocoa powder so they're well-coated. Transfer the cocoa-coated truffles to a waxed paper–lined baking sheet and let them firm up in the fridge.

Double Chocolate Gelato

Total time: 2 hours

Makes 4–6 servings

What's the difference between gelato and ice cream? Gelato has about half the fat, but it also has half the air whipped into it. Because of these two things, it tastes dense and intense. You make it very much like you do ice cream, but the mixing is slower.

2½ cups whole milk	3 egg yolks
½ cup sugar	2 teaspoons vanilla extract
1 cup unsweetened cocoa powder	½ teaspoon almond extract
2 ounces bittersweet chocolate, chopped	Large pinch of kosher salt

In a large saucepan over medium-high heat, heat the milk and sugar for 5 minutes, or until the sugar dissolves and the milk starts to steam. Sprinkle in the cocoa powder and chocolate. Whisk until smooth.

In a large bowl, beat the egg yolks with an electric mixer on high speed for 3 minutes, or until thickened.

With the beaters on slow speed, drizzle the cocoa liquid into the egg mixture. Once everything has been incorporated, pour this back into the saucepan and set it over medium-low heat, stirring constantly until it has thickened. If it comes close to a simmer, lower the heat.

Remove the pan from the heat and stir in the vanilla, almond extract, and salt. Transfer it to the refrigerator to cool for 30 minutes.

Once it has chilled, transfer the gelato base to a standard ice cream maker and process according to the manufacturer's directions. Voilà!

Earl Grey Hot Chocolate

Total time: 15 minutes

Makes 2 servings

Today we typically drink chocolate with some form of dairy. However, this is not the way the originators of chocolate and cocoa drinks did it. The ancient Mesoamericans drank their cocoa as a frothy "bitter water." You can put cocoa in plain water and froth it, but it's tastier to use flavorful tea, such as Earl Grey.

2 cups water

2 tablespoons Earl Grey
  tea leaves

5 tablespoons unsweetened
  cocoa powder

2 tablespoons brown sugar

In a small saucepan over medium-high heat, bring the water to a boil. Add the tea leaves and let them steep for 3 to 5 minutes. In a small bowl, mix the cocoa powder and brown sugar together. Add to the tea.

Whisk everything together until the cocoa is completely incorporated.

Mint Chocolate Frappé

Total time: 1 hour 15 minutes, including freezing time
Makes 1 serving

This recipe requires a bit of prep work to make the cocoa-infused iced cubes that you'll use for your frigid frappés. But don't worry! You will be very happy with your efforts in the end!

6 ounces bittersweet chocolate, finely chopped

⅓ cup sugar

4 tablespoons water

¼ teaspoon mint extract

¼ teaspoon salt

2 cups whole milk

½ cup whole milk or coffee for serving

In a 4-cup French press coffeemaker, combine the chocolate, sugar, water, mint extract, and salt.

In a medium saucepan over medium-high heat, heat the milk until it begins to simmer. Pour the milk into the French press with the chocolate mixture. Stir until they're well combined. Press the plunger several times to complete the mixing; this will also serve to aerate the broth. Pour the liquid into an ice cube tray and freeze until solid.

To make the frappé, add the cocoa cubes to the milk or coffee and blend. Serve on a hot afternoon when you have time to enjoy the creation you've made!

Gingered Cocoa

Total time: 20 minutes

Makes 1 serving

Ginger isn't typically associated with chocolate, and less so with hot cocoa. But try this neat flavor combination the next time you make cocoa. A ginger infusion sounds fancy, but it's a simple addition and really spices up the drink!

- 8 ounces whole milk
- 2 coins peeled ginger, each about 1" across
- 1 tablespoon unsweetened cocoa powder
- 2 teaspoons brown sugar

In a small saucepan over medium heat, heat the milk and ginger until the liquid starts to steam, about 5 minutes.

While it's warming, remove a couple of tablespoons of milk to a small bowl. Add the cocoa powder and sugar and mix it up until it turns into a paste.

Once the milk is steaming, remove the ginger coins. Then add the chocolate paste and whisk until all the clumps are gone. Done.

Black Strappin' Chocolate Smoothie

Total time: 5 minutes

Makes 1 serving

It's as dark and rich and wonderful as it is great for you! This dark-on-dark combination provides nutrients (potassium, magnesium, iron, calcium) . . . and that's just from the molasses! Add in the peanut butter, banana, and cocoa and you've got a raging superfood on your hands.

- 1 cup whole milk
- 1 tablespoon blackstrap molasses
- 1½ tablespoons unsweetened cocoa powder

- 2 tablespoons peanut butter
- 1 very ripe banana

Put the milk, molasses, cocoa, peanut butter, and banana in a high-powered blender and slurry them together until smooth. The only hitch here is that the cocoa can take a minute or so to completely blend into the milk. So take a little extra time to make sure everything is incorporated.

Cioccolata Calda (Italian Hot Cocoa)

Total time: 15 minutes

Makes 2 servings

I was walking in Perugia, Italy, with my family, and we ducked into a little cafe. I ordered a hot chocolate for my daughter, and when they brought out her frothy cup, I tasted it and immediately ordered my own! This recipe captures its texture and rich flavor, and I hope you enjoy it as much as I did (even if you're not in Perugia)!

5 tablespoons unsweetened cocoa powder

2 tablespoons granulated sugar

2 cups milk, divided

6 ounces dark chocolate (at least 70% cacao solids), finely chopped

In a small saucepan over low heat, combine the cocoa powder, sugar, and 2 tablespoons milk. Heat until the sugar melts and no lumps remain, stirring well. Bring to a low boil, stirring constantly; add the remaining milk. Turn off the heat and add the chopped chocolate, stirring until smooth.

Pour into serving cups and enjoy!

Ricotta Cappuccino

Total time: 1 hour 5 minutes

Makes 1 serving

This classic Italian dessert is a cool treat in the summer and totally addicting. And it's this simple to throw together. Whip it up for yourself or your guests anytime.

½ cup sugar

1 teaspoon vanilla extract

1 container (15 ounces) ricotta cheese

½ tablespoon instant espresso powder

1 teaspoon unsweetened cocoa powder

Pinch of ground cinnamon

Place the sugar in a food processor and start the machine. Add the vanilla, ricotta, espresso powder, and cocoa powder. Blend for 1 minute, then stop the machine and scrape down the sides of the bowl with a rubber spatula. Cover and refrigerate for at least 1 hour and up to 1 day. Serve with a sprinkle of cinnamon.

Chapter 11

The Chocolate Journal

It's a known fact that when reflecting on a meal we've eaten, we typically underestimate the amount we've consumed. When you think back to the past day or week of your own eating habits, however much you think you ate will be an underrepresentation of the actual amount. For example, say you served macaroni and cheese to a group of people every day, and then you randomly made their portions 25% larger on some days. If you asked that group about their portion sizes, two-thirds wouldn't have realized that they were given a larger serving. Shocking, right?

Also, the common motherly wisdom that "your eyes are bigger than your stomach" is actually true (as motherly wisdom usually is). For your body, this means that your mind's sense of how much food you need is actually greater than your body's need. In other words, when you place your food on a plate, your mind tries to estimate how much your body is hungry for. And that estimate is always too high.

Bottom line? When you *overestimate* how much you're hungry for and *underestimate* how much you actually do eat, you're setting yourself up for dietary disaster. A simple solution to this little engine of weight gain is to write things down. Once the information is out of your head and onto a page, you cannot deconstruct and reconstruct it in a way that more closely aligns with *what you wanted to happen.* Instead, you have a written account of *what actually happened.*

This chocolate journal is your link to accountability. And it's critical that you track not only your chocolate consumption but also how that

252

changes what you observe about yourself over time. Even this little bit of self-imposed accountability will keep you from overconsuming your food, so you can enjoy your chocolate without eating so much that you make it bad for you.

How you choose to use this journal is entirely up to you, but to get you started (and to help pull everything together), I've provided some information below on how to address each category listed in the following pages. Make extra copies of these pages so that you can keep a log for the full 8 weeks of the program. And keep them with you at all times to help you stay on track with your chocolate weight-loss journey.

Weight: It's important to keep track of your progress as you embark on this chocolate weight-loss journey. Why? Well, as you see this number go down, your motivation will rise. Whether you want to log your weight daily or weekly is up to you, so determine what helps you stay motivated and then stick to that schedule.

Meals: As we just discussed, we all have a tendency to underestimate our consumption. Keeping a journal of your meals will not only help to ensure you're making healthy choices (and therefore not undermining your efforts) but also hold you accountable for all your dietary choices throughout the day. Make sure to log each starter and ender as well—both what you chose (whether it be one or two thumb-size pieces of high-cocoa chocolate or one of the special recipes from Chapter 10) and how long you took to consume it.

Solve the "Clean Your Plate" Problem: This journal can be your key to reducing the reflexive nature of your emotional eating, because it's going to help you discover that you don't have to eat simply because food is in front of you. Once you make that discovery, you will own those cravings and they will not own you. That, my friend, is a liberating freedom you can apply to your entire life. Keeping this food journal will help you break the psychological reflex. For this entry, you will be answering questions regarding the extra piece of chocolate you've added to your ender. As you answer the questions posed to you, think about how this exercise can apply to your main meals. Do you see this pattern of behavior expanding onto your plate as well?

Lose Your Sweet Tooth: You do not eat sweets because you have a sweet tooth. Actually, the reverse is true: You have a sweet tooth because you eat sweets. Lose that sweet tooth and you will end up choosing darker, healthier chocolates because they'll taste better to you. And even better, you'll end up choosing healthier foods overall. That's a win-win! This journal category provides a coaching structure to make that happen. Do this exercise every third day (or every Tuesday and Friday if you prefer set days). As you complete this entry, keep in mind that you want to move up to a higher percentage of cocoa as soon as you can.

Eat All You Want—Just Want Less: By now, you know that we are coached to drastically overconsume food that is nutritionally bankrupt, leaving us drastically undernourished, overweight, and unhealthy. We can fix this volume problem by lowering the bar on how much your body wants. This journal category helps you get there, so you can train your body to be hungry for an amount that is appropriate for your needs, not greater than them. As you complete this exercise, think back to how you felt before each starter and ender. Did having a starter help you to avoid overeating? And did your ender finish off any hunger that may have been lingering after your meal?

Sculpt Your Tastes: Once you've officially lost your sweet tooth by reaching the benchmark of 70% cocoa, you'll begin sculpting your tastes by practicing sensual eating. It's called sensual eating because you taste all the flavors in your food. When that happens, you align your body's natural knowledge of what healthy flavors are. And when *that* happens, the quality of the food you eat goes up and the quantity comes down. Need a recipe for weight loss? That's it. So once a week, taste two chocolates that have the same cocoa percentage but that come from different places or different brands. Describe the differences you notice—and be detailed. Then, on every third day, compare your current high-quality chocolate with a cheap variety of chocolate (low-cocoa); for this, use the good chocolates you've been testing to lose your sweet tooth but taste them against some cheap chocolate (perhaps one that you used to really like). Again, be as detailed as you want.

Rate Your Overall Mood: Chocolate can modulate your emotional status, or it can make it worse. Whether it takes you in one direction or the other is totally up to you. If you eat chocolate as a way to treat the symptoms of a bad day, it won't help you (and may actually hurt you). But if you use it as a small daily addition to your life, it can prevent the causes of stress from ever popping up. The prevention approach will require many weeks of consistency, however, in order for you to notice a difference. This journal category tracks the impact your high-cocoa chocolate has on your mood over time. As you rate your mood each day, give this special thought: Does your mood improve within 2 hours after eating your chocolate? You may be (pleasantly) surprised at the answer.

Rate Your Overall Energy Level: As you now know, low doses of high-cocoa chocolate can do amazing things for the muscles of your body (and your heart)! They will increase the bloodflow as well as the number and output of the little cellular engines producing energy for you. Higher-cocoa, lower-sugar chocolate is the key to unlocking this energy boost in your daily life. This journal category will track the improvements in your energy level as you continue on your chocolate journey. As you rate your energy level, consider how your stamina (in exercise or just in your daily life) compares with your level before you started on this program.

WEEK:_____ DAY:_____

DATE:_____ WEIGHT:_____

BREAKFAST/BRUNCH: _____
_____

LUNCH

Starter:_____

Meal:_____

Ender:_____

Snack:_____

DINNER

Starter:_____

Meal:_____

Dessert:_____

Ender:_____

SOLVE THE "CLEAN YOUR PLATE" PROBLEM:

Did you add one extra piece of chocolate as an ender to your meal? YES/NO

If you added the extra piece, did you put it away without eating it? YES/NO

How difficult was it to not eat the extra piece of chocolate, on a scale of 1 to 5
(1 being very easy and 5 being very hard)?

　　1　　　　　2　　　　　3　　　　　4　　　　　5

LOSE YOUR SWEET TOOTH:

Cocoa percentage of your current chocolate of choice: _____%

On a scale of 1 to 10, rank the sweetness of this chocolate
(1 being not sweet at all and 10 being very sweet):

　　1　　2　　3　　4　　5　　6　　7　　8　　9　　10

  Eat Chocolate, Lose Weight

Cocoa percentage of your testing chocolate: _____%

On a scale of 1 to 10, rank the sweetness of this chocolate
(1 being not sweet at all and 10 being very sweet):

  1   2   3   4   5   6   7   8   9   1 0

Are you ready to make the testing chocolate your new chocolate of choice? YES/NO

EAT ALL YOU WANT—JUST WANT LESS:
On a scale of 1 to 5, rate your average hunger level after consuming your starter
(1 being not hungry and 5 being very hungry):

  1   2   3   4   5

On a scale of 1 to 5, rate your average hunger level after consuming your ender
(1 being not hungry and 5 being very hungry):

  1   2   3   4   5

SCULPT YOUR TASTES:
Describe the difference in flavors between high-quality chocolate brand #1 and
high-quality chocolate brand #2:_____

_____

_____

_____

_____

Describe the difference in flavors between your current (good) chocolate and the
cheap, low-cocoa chocolate you used to enjoy:_____

_____

_____

_____

_____

RATE YOUR OVERALL MOOD:
(1 being poor and 5 being great)

  1   2   3   4   5

RATE YOUR OVERALL ENERGY LEVEL:
(1 being very low and 5 being very high)

  1   2   3   4   5

Endnotes

Introduction

1. SB Kritchevsky, "A Review of Scientific Research and Recommendations Regarding Eggs," *Journal of the American College of Nutrition* 23, no. suppl. 6 (December 2004): 596S–600S.

2. FB Hu et al., "A Prospective Study of Egg Consumption and Risk of Cardiovascular Disease in Men and Women," *Journal of the American Medical Association* 281 (1999): 1387–94.

3. GP Zaloga et al., "Trans Fatty Acids and Coronary Heart Disease," *Nutrition in Clinical Practice* 21, no. 5 (October 2006): 505–12.

4. B MacMahon et al., "Coffee and Cancer of the Pancreas," *New England Journal of Medicine* 304 (1981): 630–33.

5. Q Li et al., "Coffee Consumption and the Risk of Prostate Cancer: The Ohsaki Cohort Study," *British Journal of Cancer* 108, no. 11 (June 11, 2013): 2381–89.

6. SP Fowler et al., "Fueling the Obesity Epidemic? Artificially Sweetened Beverage Use and Long-Term Weight Gain," *Obesity* (Silver Spring) 8 (August 16, 2008): 1894–900.

Chapter 1

1. AF La Berge, "How the Ideology of Low Fat Conquered America," *Journal of the History of Medicine and Allied Sciences* 63, no. 2 (2008): 139–77.

2. WJ Hurst et al., "Stability of Cocoa Antioxidants and Flavan-3-ols over Time," *Journal of Agricultural Food Chemistry* 57, no. 20 (2009): 9547–50.

3. SD Coe and MD Coe, *The True History of Chocolate,* 2nd ed. (Thames and Hudson, 2007), pp. 99–101.

4. WJ Hurst et al., "Impact of Fermentation, Drying, Roasting and Dutch Processing on Flavan-3-ol Stereochemistry in Cacao Beans and Cocoa Ingredients," *Chemistry Central Journal* 5 (2011): 53.

5. MJ Payne et al., "Impact of Fermentation, Drying, Roasting, and Dutch Processing on Epicatechin and Catechin Content of Cacao Beans and Cocoa Ingredients," *Journal of Agricultural Food Chemistry* 13, no. 19 (October 13, 2010): 10518–27.

6. Ibid.

7. D Taubert et al., "Effects of Low Habitual Cocoa Intake on Blood Pressure and Bioactive Nitric Oxide: A Randomized Controlled Trial," *Journal of the American Medical Association* 298, no. 1 (July 4, 2007): 49–60.

8. M Serafini et al., "Plasma Antioxidants from Chocolate," *Nature* 424, no. 6952 (August 28, 2003): 1013.

9. R Wilson et al., "Overview of the Preparation, Use and Biological Studies on Polyglycerol Polyricinoleate (PGPR)," *Food and Chemical Toxicology* 36, nos. 9–10 (September–October 1998): 711–18.

10. E Roura et al., "Milk Does Not Affect the Bioavailability of Cocoa Powder Flavonoid in Healthy Human," *Annals of Nutrition and Metabolism* 51, no. 6 (2007): 493–98.

11. S Lesser et al., "Bioavailability of Quercetin in Pigs Is Influenced by the Dietary Fat Content," *Journal of Nutrition* 134 (2004): 1508–11.

Chapter 2

1. A Buitrago-Lopez et al., "Chocolate Consumption and Cardiometabolic Disorders: Systematic Review and Meta-Analysis," *British Medical Journal* 343 (August 26, 2011): d4488.

2. D Taubert et al., "Effects of Low Habitual Cocoa Intake on Blood Pressure and Bioactive Nitric Oxide: A Randomized Controlled Trial," *Journal of the American Medical Association* 298, no. 1 (July 4, 2007): 49–60.

3. D Grassi et al., "Blood Pressure Is Reduced and Insulin Sensitivity Increased in Glucose-Intolerant, Hypertensive Subjects after 15 Days of Consuming High-Polyphenol Dark Chocolate," *Journal of Nutrition* 138, no. 9 (September 2008); 1671–76.

4. A Nehlig, "The Neuroprotective Effects of Cocoa Flavanol and Its Influence on Cognitive Performance," *British Journal of Clinical Pharmacology* (July 10, 2012): 716–27.

5. D Vauzour et al., "The Neuroprotective Potential of Flavonoids: A Multiplicity of Effects," *Genes and Nutrition* 3, no. 3–4 (December 3, 2008): 115–26.

6. E Zomer et al., "The Effectiveness and Cost Effectiveness of Dark Chocolate Consumption as Prevention Therapy in People at High Risk of Cardiovascular Disease: Best Case Scenario Analysis Using a Markov Model," *British Medical Journal* 344 (May 30, 2012): e3657.

7. BA Golomb et al., "Association Between More Frequent Chocolate Consumption and Lower Body Mass Index," *Archives of Internal Medicine* 172, no. 6 (March 26, 2012): 519–21.

8. M Jenh et al., "Associations of Daily Walking Activity with Biomarkers Related to Cardiac Distress in Patients with Chronic Obstructive Pulmonary Disease," *Respiration* 85, no. 3 (December 19, 2012): 195–202.

9. M Cuenca-García, et al. "Association Between Chocolate Consumption and Fatness in European Adolescents," *Nutrition* (October 17, 2013).

10. JO Fisher et al., "Children's Bite Size and Intake of an Entrée Are Greater with Large Portions Than with Age-Appropriate or Self-Selected Portions," *American Journal of Clinical Nutrition* 77, no. 5 (May 2003): 1164–70.

11. N Zijlstra et al., "Effect of Bite Size and Oral Processing Time of a Semisolid Food on Satiation," *American Journal of Clinical Nutrition* 90, no. 2 (August 2009): 269–75.

12. FP Martin et al., "Metabolic Effects of Dark Chocolate Consumption on Energy, Gut Microbiota, and Stress-Related Metabolism in Free-Living Subjects," *Journal of Proteome Research* 8, no. 12 (December 2009): 5568–79.

13. ET Massolt et al., "Appetite Suppression through Smelling of Dark Chocolate Correlates with Changes in Ghrelin in Young Women," *Regulatory Peptides* 161, no. 1–3 (April 9, 2010): 81–86.

14. W Clower, *The French Don't Diet Plan: 10 Simple Steps to Stay Thin for Life* (Crown, 2006).

15. KS Burger et al., "Mechanisms behind the Portion Size Effect: Visibility and Bite Size," *Obesity* (Silver Spring) 19, no. 3 (March 2011): 546–51.

16. "Source for Acceptable Macronutrient Distribution Range (AMDR) Reference and RDAs: Institute of Medicine (IOM) Dietary Reference Intakes for Energy, Carbohydrate, Fiber, Fat, Fatty Acids, Cholesterol, Protein, and Amino Acids." http://www.iom.edu/ Global/News%20Announcements/~/media/C5CD2DD7840544979A549EC47E56 A02B.ashx.

17. SJ Long et al., "Effect of Habitual Dietary-Protein Intake on Appetite and Satiety," *Appetite* 35, no. 1 (August 2000): 79–88.

18. MS Westerterp-Plantenga et al., "Dietary Protein: Its Role in Satiety, Energetics, Weight Loss and Health," *British Journal of Nutrition* 1008, suppl. 2 (August 2012): S105–12.

19. AL Sayegh, "The Role of Cholecystokinin Receptors in the Short-Term Control of Food Intake," *Progress in Molecular Biology Translational Science* 114 (2013): 277–316.

20. Dietary Reference Intakes for Energy, Carbohydrate, Fiber, Fat, Fatty Acids, Cholesterol, Protein, and Amino Acids (2002/2005). http://www.iom.edu/Global/News%20 Announcements/~/media/C5CD2DD7840544979A549EC47E56A02B.ashx.

21. D Aune et al., "Dietary Fibre, Whole Grains, and Risk of Colorectal Cancer: Systematic Review and Dose-Response Meta-Analysis of Prospective Studies," *British Medical Journal* 343 (November 10, 2011): d6617.

22. SA Bingham et al., "Dietary Fibre in Food and Protection Against Colorectal Cancer in the European Prospective Investigation into Cancer and Nutrition (EPIC): An Observational Study," *Lancet* 361, no. 9368 (May 3, 2003): 1496–501.

23. MM Perrigue et al., "Added Soluble Fiber Enhances the Satiating Power of Low-Energy-Density Liquid Yogurts," *Journal of the American Dietetic Association* 109, no. 11 (November 2009): 1862–68.

24. NC Howarth et al., "Dietary Fiber and Weight Regulation," *Nutrition Review* 59, no. 5 (May 2001): 129–39.

Chapter 3

1. A Stengel and Y Tache, "Interaction between Gastric and Upper Small Intestinal Hormones in the Regulation of Hunger and Satiety: Ghrelin and Cholecystokinin Take the Central Stage," *Current Protein and Peptide Science* 12, no. 4 (June 2011): 293–304; and A Stengel and Y Tache, "Gastric Peptides and Their Regulation of Hunger and Satiety," *Current Gastroenterology Reports* 14, no. 6 (December 2012): 480–88.

2. D Grassi et al., "Short-Term Administration of Dark Chocolate Is Followed by a Significant Increase in Insulin Sensitivity and a Decrease in Blood Pressure in Healthy Persons," *American Journal of Clinical Nutrition* 81, no. 3 (March 2005): 611–14; and D Grassi et al., "Blood Pressure Is Reduced and Insulin Sensitivity Increased in Glucose-Intolerant, Hypertensive Subjects after 15 Days of Consuming High-Polyphenol Dark Chocolate," *Journal of Nutrition* 139, no. 9 (September 2008): 1671–76.

3. LB Sørensen and A Astrup, "Eating Dark and Milk Chocolate: A Randomized Crossover Study of Effects on Appetite and Energy Intake," *Nutrition and Diabetes* 1 (2011): e21.

4. GK Beauchamp and JA Mennella, "Early Flavor Learning and Its Impact on Later Feeding Behavior," *Journal of Pediatric Gastroenterology and Nutrition* 48, suppl. 1 (March 2009): S25–30.

5. ET Massolt et al., "Appetite Suppression through Smelling of Dark Chocolate Correlates with Changes in Ghrelin in Young Women," *Regulatory Peptides* 161, nos. 1–3 (April 9, 2010): 81–86.

6. S Janssen et al., "Bitter Taste Receptors and α-Gustducin Regulate the Secretion of Ghrelin with Functional Effects on Food Intake and Gastric Emptying," *Proceedings of the National Academy of Sciences* 108, no. 5 (February 1, 2011): 2094–99.

7. V Mani et al., "Bitter Compounds Decrease Gastric Emptying and Influence Intestinal Nutrient Transport," *Animal Industry Report* 2012: AS 658, ASL R2725.

8. SE Swithers, "Artificial Sweeteners Produce the Counterintuitive Effect of Inducing Metabolic Derangements," *Trends in Endocrinology and Metabolism* (July 3, 2013): pii: S1043-2760(13)00087-8, doi: 10.1016/j.tem.2013.05.005 (Epub ahead of print).

Chapter 4

1. HM Heneghan et al., "Influence of Pouch and Stoma Size on Weight Loss after Gastric Bypass," *Surgery for Obesity Related Disorders* 8, no. 4 (July–August 2012): 408–15.

2. E Näslund and PM Hellström, "Appetite Signaling: From Gut Peptides and Enteric Nerves to Brain," *Physiology and Behavior* 92, nos. 1–2 (September 2007): 256–62.

3. DM Small et al., "Changes in Brain Activity Related to Eating Chocolate: From Pleasure to Aversion," *Brain* 124, pt. 9 (September 2001): 1720–33.

4. A Kokkinos et al., "Eating Slowly Increases the Postprandial Response of the Anorexigenic Gut Hormones, Peptide YY and Glucagon-Like Peptide-1," *Journal of Clinical Endocrinology and Metabolism* 95, no. 1 (January 2010): 333–37.

5. A Andrade et al., "Eating Slowly Led to Decreases in Energy Intake within Meals in Healthy Women," *Journal of the American Dietetic Association* 107, no. 7 (2008): 1186–91.

6. LB Sørensen and A Astrup, "Eating Dark and Milk Chocolate: A Randomized Crossover Study of Effects on Appetite and Energy Intake," *Nutrition and Diabetes* 1, e21 (December 5, 2011).

Chapter 5

1. LH Epstein, "The Effects of Calories and Taste on Habituation of the Human Salivary Response," *Addiction and Behavior* 18, no. 2 (March–April 1993): 179–85.

2. C LeDrew, "Cacao Bean Origins Dictate Flavor Variations," *Candy Industry* 173, no. 9 (September 2008): 38.

3. JI Glendinning, "Is the Bitter Rejection Response Always Adaptive?," *Physiology and Behavior* 56 (6): 1217–27.

4. KD Vohs et al., "Rituals Enhance Consumption," *Psychological Science* (July 17, 2013), http://pss.sagepub.com/content/early/2013/07/17/0956797613478949.

Chapter 6

1. DM Small et al., "Changes in Brain Activity Related to Eating Chocolate: From Pleasure to Aversion," *Brain* 124, pt. 9 (September 2001): 1720–33.

2. AN Sokolov et al., "Chocolate and the Brain: Neurobiological Impact of Cocoa Flavanols on Cognition and Behavior," *Neuroscience and Biobehavioral Review* (June 26, 2013) pii: S0149-7634(13)00168-1.

3. V Vicennati et al., "Stress-Related Development of Obesity and Cortisol in Women," *Obesity* (Silver Spring) 9 (September 17, 2009): 1678–83.

4. J Daubenmier et al., "Mindfulness Intervention for Stress Eating to Reduce Cortisol and Abdominal Fat among Overweight and Obese Women: An Exploratory Randomized Controlled Study," *Journal of Obesity* (2011): 651936.

5. R Yoshida et al., "Endocannabinoids Selectively Enhance Sweet Taste," *Proceedings of the National Academy of Sciences of the United States of America* 107, no. 2 (January 12, 2010): 935–39.

6. N Rose et al., "Mood Food: Chocolate and Depressive Symptoms in a Cross-Sectional Analysis," *Archives of Internal Medicine* 170, no. 8 (April 26, 2010): 699–703.

7. JI Macdiarmid and MM Hetherington, "Mood Modulation by Food: An Exploration of Affect and Cravings in 'Chocolate Addicts," *British Journal of Clinical Psychology* 34, pt. 1 (February 1995): 129–38.

8. M Macht and J Mueller, "Immediate Effects of Chocolate on Experimentally Induced Mood States," *Appetite* 49, no 3 (November 2007): 667–74.

9. G Parker et al., "Mood State Effects of Chocolate," *Journal of Affective Disorders* 92 nos. 2–3 (June 2006): 149–59.

10. FP Martin et al., "Metabolic Effects of Dark Chocolate Consumption on Energy, Gut Microbiota, and Stress-Related Metabolism in Free-Living Subjects," *Journal of Proteome Research* 8, no. 12 (December 2009): 5568–79.

11. O Schakman et al., "Glucocorticoid-Induced Skeletal Muscle Atrophy," *International Journal of Biochemistry and Cell Biology* (June 24, 2013), DOI: 10.1016/j.biocel.2013.05.036.

12. MP Pase et al., "Cocoa Polyphenols Enhance Positive Mood States But Not Cognitive Performance: A Randomized, Placebo-Controlled Trial," *Journal of Psychopharmacology* 27, no. 5 (May 2013): 451–58.

13. T Sathyapalan et al., "High Cocoa Polyphenol Rich Chocolate May Reduce the Burden of the Symptoms in Chronic Fatigue Syndrome," *Nutrition Journal* 9 (November 22, 2010): 55.

14. G Desideri et al. "Benefits in Cognitive Function, Blood Pressure, and Insulin Resistance through Cocoa Flavanol Consumption in Elderly Subjects with Mild Cognitive Impairment: The Cocoa, Cognition, and Aging (Cocoa) Study," *Hypertension* 60, no. 3 (September 2012): 794–801.

Chapter 7

1. M Holmstrup et al., "Satiety, But Not Total PYY, Is Increased with Continuous and Intermittent Exercise," *Obesity* (Silver Spring), advance online publication, February 18, 2013, http://www.ncbi.nlm.nih.gov/pubmed/23418154.

2. C Martins et al., "Effects of Exercise on Gut Peptides, Energy Intake and Appetite," *Journal of Endocrinology* 193, no. 2 (May 2007): 251–58.

3. H Kawano et al., "Effects of Different Modes of Exercise on Appetite and Appetite-Regulating Hormones," *Appetite* 66C (February 10, 2013): 26–33.

4. H Oh and AH Taylor, "Brisk Walking Reduces Ad Libitum Snacking in Regular Chocolate Eaters during a Workplace Simulation," *Appetite* 58, no. 1 (February 2012): 387–92.

5. L Nogueira et al., "(-)-Epicatechin Enhances Fatigue Resistance and Oxidative Capacity in Mouse Muscle," *Journal of Physiology* 589, pt. 18 (September 15, 2011): 4615–31.

6. I Ramirez-Sanchez et al., "Stimulatory Effects of the Flavanol (-)-Epicatechin on Cardiac Angiogenesis: Additive Effects with Exercise," *Cardiovascular Pharmacology* 60, no. 5 (November 2012): 429–38.

7. Nogueira et al., "(-)-Epicatechin Enhances Fatigue Resistance."

8. M Huttemann et al., "(-)-Epicatechin Maintains Endurance Training Adaptation in Mice after 14 Days of Detraining," *FASEB Journal* 26, no. 4 (April 2012): 1413–22.

9. PR Taub et al., "Alterations in Skeletal Muscle Indicators of Mitochondrial Structure and Biogenesis in Patients with Type 2 Diabetes and Heart Failure: Effects of Epicatechin Rich Cocoa," *Clinical and Translational Science* 5, no. 1 (February 2012): 43–47.

10. DC Wallace, "Mitochondrial Diseases in Man and Mouse," *Science* 283 (1999): 1482–88.

11. Huttemann et al., "(-)-Epicatechin Maintains Endurance Training Adaptation."

12. C Selmi et al., "Chocolate at Heart: The Anti-Inflammatory Impact of Cocoa Flavanols," *Molecular Nutrition and Food Research* 52, no. 11 (November 2008): 1340–48.

13. G Davidson et al., "The Effect of Acute Pre-Exercise Dark Chocolate Consumption on Plasma Antioxidant Status, Oxidative Stress and Immunoendocrine Responses to Prolonged Exercise," *European Journal of Nutrition* 51, no. 1 (February 2012): 69–79.

14. KJ Spaccarotella and WD Andzel, "The Effects of Low Fat Chocolate Milk on Postexercise Recovery in Collegiate Athletes," *Journal of Strength and Conditioning Research* 25, no. 12 (December 2011): 3456–60.

15. JR Karp et al., "Chocolate Milk as a Post-Exercise Recovery Aid," *International Journal of Sport Nutrition and Exercise Metabolism* 16, no. 1 (February 2006): 78–91.

16. NM McBrier et al., "Cocoa-Based Protein and Carbohydrate Drink Decreases Perceived Soreness after Exhaustive Aerobic Exercise: A Pragmatic Preliminary Analysis," *Journal of Strength and Conditioning Research* 24, no. 8 (August 2010): 2203–10.

17. K Thomas et al., "Improved Endurance Capacity Following Chocolate Milk Consumption Compared with 2 Commercially Available Sport Drinks," *Applied Physiology, Nutrition, and Metabolism* 34, no. 1 (February 2009): 78–82.

Chapter 8

1. S Williams et al., "Eating Chocolate Can Significantly Protect the Skin from UV Light," *Journal of Cosmetic Dermatology* 8, no. 3 (September 2009): 169–73.

2. K Neukam et al., "Consumption of Flavanol-Rich Cocoa Acutely Increases Microcirculation in Human Skin," *European Journal of Nutrition* 46, no. 1 (February 2007): 53–56.

3. U Heinrich et al., "Long-Term Ingestion of High Flavanol Cocoa Provides Photoprotection Against UV-Induced Erythema and Improves Skin Condition in Women," *Journal of Nutrition* 136, no. 6 (June 2006): 1565–69.

4. GF Ferrazzano et al., "Anti-Cariogenic Effects of Polyphenols from Plant Stimulant Beverages (Cocoa, Coffee, Tea)," *Fitoterapia* 80, no. 5 (July 2009): 255–62.

5. RK Srikanth et al., "Chocolate Mouth Rinse: Effect on Plaque Accumulation and Mutans Streptococci Counts When Used by Children," *Journal of the Indian Society of Pedodontics and Preventative Dentistry* 26, no. 2 (June 2008): 67–70.

6. K Ito et al., "Anti-Cariogenic Properties of a Water-Soluble Extract from Cacao," *Bioscience, Biotechnology, and Biochemistry* 67, no. 12 (December 2003): 2567–73.

7. K Osawa et al., "Identification of Cariostatic Substances in the Cacao Bean Husk: Their Anti-Glucosyltransferase and Antibacterial Activities," *Journal of Dental Research* 80, no. 11 (November 2001): 2000–2004.

8. G Waris and H Ahsan, "Reactive Oxygen Species: Role in the Development of Cancer and Various Chronic Conditions," *Journal of Carcinogenesis* 5 (2006): 14.

9. E Ramiro-Puig et al., "Neuroprotective Effect of Cocoa Flavonoids on In Vitro Oxidative Stress," *European Journal of Nutrition* 48, no. 1 (February 2009): 54–61.

10. D Ramljak, "Pentameric Procyanidin from Theobroma Cacao Selectively Inhibits Growth of Human Breast Cancer Cells," *Molecular Cancer Therapeutics* 4, no. 4 (April 2005): 537–46.

11. M Yamagishi et al., "Chemoprevention of Lung Carcinogenesis by Cacao Liquor Proanthocyanidins in a Male Rat Multi-Organ Carcinogenesis Model," *Cancer Letters* 191, no. 1 (February 28, 2003): 49–57.

12. S Carnésecchi et al., "Flavanols and Procyanidins of Cocoa and Chocolate Inhibit Growth and Polyamine Biosynthesis of Human Colonic Cancer Cells," *Cancer Letters* 175, no. 2 (January 25, 2002): 147–55.

13. American Cancer Society, *Cancer Facts and Figures 2013* (Atlanta: American Cancer Society, 2013).

14. DD Mellor et al., "High-Cocoa Polyphenol-Rich Chocolate Improves HDL Cholesterol in Type 2 Diabetes Patients," *Diabetic Medicine* 27, no. 11 (November 2010): 1318–21.

15. J Balzer et al., "Sustained Benefits in Vascular Function through Flavanol-Containing Cocoain Medicated Diabetic Patients: A Double-Masked, Randomized, Controlled Trial," *Journal of the American College of Cardiology.* 3, no. 22 (June 2008): 2141–49.

16. D Grassi, "Short-Term Administration of Dark Chocolate Is Followed by a Significant Increase in Insulin Sensitivity and a Decrease in Blood Pressure in Healthy Persons," *American Journal of Clinical Nutrition,* 81, no. 3 (March 2005): 611–14.

17. I Cordero-Herrera, "Cocoa Flavonoids Improve Insulin Signalling and Modulate Glucose Production Via AKT and AMPK in Hepg2 Cells," *Molecular Nutrition and Food Research* 57, no. 6 (June 2013): 974–85.

18. Mellor et al., "High-Cocoa Polyphenol-Rich Chocolate Improves HDL Cholesterol."

19. JH Weisburger, "Chemopreventive Effects of Cocoa Polyphenols on Chronic Diseases," *Experimental Biology and Medicine* (Maywood) 226, no. 10 (November 2001): 891–77.

20. L Djoussé et al., "Chocolate Consumption Is Inversely Associated with Prevalent Coronary Heart Disease: The National Heart, Lung, and Blood Institute Family Heart Study," *Clinical Nutrition* 30, no. 2 (April 2011): 182–87.

21. Y Gu and JD Lambert, "Modulation of Metabolic Syndrome–Related Inflammation by Cocoa," *Molecular Nutrition and Food Research* 57 (May 2, 2013): 948–61.

22. Djoussé et al., "Chocolate Consumption Is Inversely Associated with Prevalent Coronary Heart Disease."

23. ST Francis et al., "The Effect of Flavanol-Rich Cocoa on the fMRI Response to a Cognitive Task in Healthy Young People," *Journal of Cardiovascular Pharmacology* 47, suppl. 2 (2006): S215–20.

24. C Heiss et al., "Sustained Increase in Flow-Mediated Dilation after Daily Intake of High-Flavanol Cocoa Drink Over 1 Week," *Journal of Cardiovascular Pharmacology* 49, no. 2 (February 2007): 74–80.

25. S Ellinger et al., "Epicatechin Ingested via Cocoa Products Reduces Blood Pressure in Humans: A Nonlinear Regression Model with a Bayesian Approach," *American Journal of Clinical Nutrition* 95, no. 6 (June 2012): 1365–77.

26. A Salonia et al., "Chocolate and Women's Sexual Health: An Intriguing Correlation," *Journal of Sexual Medicine* 3, no. 3 (May 2006): 476–82.

27. N Mondaini et al., "Regular Moderate Intake of Red Wine Is Linked to Better Women's Sexual Health," *Journal of Sexual Medicine* 6, no. 10 (October 2009): 2772–77.

28. D Grassi et al., "Blood Pressure Is Reduced and Insulin Sensitivity Increased in Glucose-Intolerant, Hypertensive Subjects after 15 Days of Consuming High-Polyphenol Dark Chocolate," *Journal of Nutrition* 138, no. 9 (September 2008): 1671–76; and L Hooper et al., "Effects of Chocolate, Cocoa, and Flavan-3-Ols on Cardiovascular Health: A Systematic Review and Meta-Analysis of Randomized Trials," *American Journal of Clinical Nutrition* 95, no. 3 (March 2012): 740–51.

29. N Khan et al., "Regular Consumption of Cocoa Powder with Milk Increases HDL Cholesterol and Reduces Oxidized LDL Levels in Subjects at High Risk of Cardiovascular Disease," *Nutrition, Metabolism, and Cardiovascular Diseases* 22, no. 12 (December 2012): 1046–53; and S Baba et al., "Plasma LDL and HDL Cholesterol and Oxidized LDL Concentrations Are Altered in Normo- and Hypercholesterolemic Humans after Intake of Different Levels of Cocoa Powder," *Journal of Nutrition* 137, no. 6 (June 2007): 1436–41.

Chapter 10

1. L Stahl et al., "Preservation of Cocoa Antioxidant Activity, Total Polyphenols, Flavan-3-ols, and Procyanidin Content in Foods Prepared with Cocoa Powder," *Journal of Food Science* 74, no. 6 (August 2009): C456–61.

2. B Teucher et al., "Enhancers of Iron Absorption: Ascorbic Acid and Other Organic Acids," *International Journal for Vitamin and Nutrition Research* 74, no. 6 (November 2004): 403–19.

3. Ibid.

4. M Diaz et al., "The Efficacy of a Local Ascorbic Acid-Rich Food in Improving Iron Absorption from Mexican Diets: A Field Study Using Stable Isotopes," *American Journal of Clinical Nutrition* 78, no. 3 (September 2003): 436–40.

Index

Underscored page references indicate boxed text. **Boldface** references indicate illustrations.

F

Family, eating with, 118–19
Fat bloom, 104
Fatigue resistance, 149
Favorite foods, 102–3, 115–16
Fennell, Michele, **24**, _24–25_
Fermentation, of cocoa beans, 8
Fiber, 40–41, 52, 156
Fight or flight response, 134–35, 145
Fish
    Cocoa-Chili Jamaican Fish, 224–25
    Tuna with Sesame-Soy-Ginger Sauce, 223
Fitness, 142–43, 154–55. _See also_ Exercise
Flavonols, 167, 169
Flavor accommodation. _See_ Taste adjustment
Flavors
    appreciation of (_see_ Tasting)
    sympathetic, 112
Floral qualities, in tasting, 105, 107
Flow-mediated dilation, 174
Food quality. _See_ Quality
Food substitutions, 184
Fruity qualities, in tasting, 105, 107

G

Ganache
    cooking tips, 204
    Ganache recipe, 243
Garnishes
    Cocoa Butter, 233
    Cocoa Whipped Cream, 239
Gastric bypass surgery, 77
Ghrelin, 58
Ginger
    Gingered Cocoa, 248
    Sesame-Soy-Ginger Sauce, 223
"Goldfish-like" eating behavior, 41–44
Green chiles, 203
Guilt, 127–29
Gustatory habituation. _See_ Taste adjustment

H

Habituation, 78. _See also_ Taste adjustment
HDL, 2, 171, 176
Health foods, viii
Heart health, 169–72, 175, 176
Hershey, Milton, _5_
Horizontal tastings, 113–19
Hume, Donna, _159_
Hunger, exercise and, 144–46. _See also_ Satiety
Hydrogenated oils, _22_
Hyperglycemia, 52, 168
Hypoglycemia, 15, 52, 168

I

Ice cream
    Double Chocolate Gelato, 245
Icing, 204
Insulin levels, 15, 51–52, 59, 170
Invented foods, 22–23
Iron, 202–3
Isoprostanes, 151

J

Jake A., _80_
Journals/journaling
    sample pages, 256–57
    for tastings, 111
    tracking role, 252–55

L

Labeling regulations, _16–17_
Lao-tzu, 73–74
LDL, 2, 171, 176
Leathery qualities, in tasting, _107_
Leavening agents, 201–2
Lecithin, _13_
Lettuce. _See_ Salads
Love, vs. consumption, of food, 97–100

T

Tannins, <u>107</u>
Taoism, 73–74
Taste
    biomechanics of, 56–58
    chew-swallow habits and, 79–80
    sugar effects on, 59–61
Taste adjustment
    Chocolate Challenges for, 18–23,
        113–19
    obstacles to, 102–3
    role of practice in, 104–5
    sweet tooth, losing, 18–21, <u>47</u>, 55, <u>68</u>,
        254, <u>256</u>
    time required for change, <u>118</u>
    tracking of, 254–55, <u>256</u>
Tasting
    comparisons during, 113–19
    flavor changes during, <u>106–7</u>, 116
    procedures for, 109–13
    sensual eating, 102–8
Tea
    additions to, 185
    Earl Grey Hot Chocolate, 246
    as snack, 183
Teeth, health of, 165–66
Temperature effects, 105, 109
Texture, 108–9
Theobromine, <u>173</u>
Thumb, as portion size gauge, <u>35</u>
Timing
    of chocolate consumption, <u>37</u>,
        83–89
    of meals, 184
    taste adjustment, time required for,
        <u>118</u>
Tomatoes
    Deconstructed Guacamole Omelet,
        206
Toppings
    Cocoa Butter, 233
    Cocoa Whipped Cream, 239

Tracking
    journal for, 252–55
    sample pages, 256–57
    during tastings, 111
Treatment, vs. prevention, 125–30
Truffles
    cooking tips, 204
    Truffle recipe, 244
Tuna
    Tuna with Sesame-Soy-Ginger Sauce,
        223
Type 2 diabetes, 168–70

U

Unprocessed foods, <u>23</u>
UV protection, 163

V

Vanilla/vanillin, <u>13</u>, <u>22</u>
Vegetables, iron in, 202–3
Vertical tastings, 29–33, 113–14
Visual appearance, of food, 103–4
Vitamin C, 202–3
"Vitamin Ch," 36–37, 160, 162–72, 174–75
Vitamin supplements, <u>169</u>

W

Walking, 157–58
Want less, 75–79, 81–83, 254, <u>256</u>
Weekends, in meal plan, 183
Weight
    loss, 31, **88**, 128
    tracking of, 253
White chocolate, 11, 53–54
Whole foods, <u>23</u>
Willpower, 76
Wine, 112–13, 139, 175

SUFFRAGIST

THE SUFFRAGIST PLAYBOOK

Your Guide to Changing the World

LUCINDA ROBB
and
REBECCA BOGGS ROBERTS

CANDLEWICK PRESS

First edition 2020

Library of Congress Catalog Card
Number 2020915492
ISBN 978-1-5362-1033-0

20 21 22 23 24 25 LBM 10 9 8 7 6 5 4 3 2 1

Printed in Melrose Park, IL, USA

This book was typeset in
Adobe Garamond Pro.

Candlewick Press
99 Dover Street
Somerville, Massachusetts 02144

www.candlewick.com

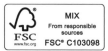

A JUNIOR LIBRARY GUILD SELECTION

To our mothers,
Lynda Robb
and Cokie Roberts,
who taught us
the power of women,
the importance of history,
and the value of friendship

CONTENTS

INTRODUCTION

THIS BOOK IS ABOUT ONE OF THE LARGEST AND LONGEST movements in American history, the story of how women won the right to vote. It took decades to accomplish, and there were many hard setbacks, but when it came, the change was huge and permanent. And it was done almost entirely by women, for the benefit of women.

Because we both grew up learning women's history, we've always been a little shocked at how little most people know about the suffrage movement. Most textbooks devote just a few paragraphs to it, and history classes rush past it (when it is taught at all). There aren't a ton of popular books or movies or other media about it. Unlike famous wars, it involved very little actual fighting, violent societal upheaval, or widespread death, but we think that is EXACTLY the reason we should be studying it! Women's history *is* action packed, just not in a military way.

Chances are you've probably heard about Susan B. Anthony, who was so famous at the end of her life that the Nineteenth Amendment giving women the right to vote was named after her. She's the one pictured on those dollar coins that hardly anyone uses. But what about Lucy Stone, Sojourner Truth, Elizabeth Cady Stanton, Frances Willard, Ida B. Wells, and Alice Paul? After reading this, we hope you will see them as the amazing, brave, resourceful, and often flawed women they were, rather than old-fashioned historical characters wearing itchy lace and judgy expressions. They were far from perfect, and some made decisions we deplore, namely ones that excluded and disrespected women of color. We need to talk about this, because if we ignore racism, past or present, we'll never do better. Instead, we want to look back and show the whole suffrage movement, with all of its accomplishments and failures, starting with the women who led the way.

Why is it important to know about them? Well, for one thing, any version of American history that ignores half the population is simply inaccurate. Also, many of these women leaders are fantastic role models, providing inspiration for girls and boys alike. There is a lot to admire about their accomplishments, and it makes us mad that most Americans have never heard their names.

But most importantly, these women can actually teach us all valuable skills for creating change. The suffragists used just about every tool for political engagement we have today. Petitions? Long before the internet or computers, suffragists gathered millions of signatures to petition for the vote in states around this country. Women's marches at the time of a presidential inauguration? They did that, too, over one hundred years ago. Public speeches, lobbying, raising money, writing articles, advocating? Check, check, check. Publicity stunts? They practically invented them! Trust us when we tell you these women are worth listening to.

Fortunately a lot of great scholarship covers this long movement, but we also know that in this increasingly hectic world, your time is valuable. So just in case you don't have time to read the six-volume *History of Woman Suffrage* (which still left a lot out!), we've made our own quick guide to how the suffragists changed the world. We hope it is useful and fun, and it is definitely irreverent. Most importantly, it highlights the time-tested tactics that they used to achieve their goals, tactics that are still hugely relevant today.

As for us, our friendship actually goes back generations. Lucinda's grandmother Lady Bird Johnson and Rebecca's grandmother Lindy Boggs became friends in the 1940s, when both were young southern political wives in Washington, DC. Both remained involved in politics throughout their long lives. Our mothers, Lynda Robb and Cokie Roberts, were lifelong friends, as well as public figures who actively promoted the contributions of women. They and many other friends and mentors taught us the value of women's history, for which we are deeply thankful.

Susan B. Anthony understood the importance of strategy and marketing and promoting what works. She would also appreciate you and all the potential you have to make the world a better place. She would tell you "Failure is impossible," and we agree.

Lucinda and Rebecca

SUFFRAGIST

1

TELL YOUR STORY

EVERY GREAT CAUSE HAS TO START SOMEWHERE. IN THE beginning, before there are organizations or advocacy groups, there is a story waiting to be told. That's how you get people talking about your idea in the first place. A good story can sway even reluctant listeners. How many times have you resisted a show everyone is watching because it isn't your thing, only to see one episode and get totally sucked in because the story is so compelling? Spoken or written, stories have great power.

It's hard for us to understand just how radical the idea of women voting used to be. But imagine that you lived in America in the early 1800s. Most other countries in the world still had some kind of monarchy or a ruling class. Our republic was just a few decades old. Sure, the idea of democracy and elite men voting had been around since ancient Athens. But minus the occasional queen, there were few examples of women having a say in their own lives, much less their own government. That's why telling a story was so important for the first generation of suffragists. For most Americans, women's suffrage wasn't even on their radar screen.

BE WILLING TO SPEAK UP. One of the first people to speak publicly about women's suffrage was a white woman named Lucy Stone. She was also the first to make it her full-time job. She was born in 1818 in Massachusetts. If you look at the old photographs, Lucy Stone looks totally forgettable. She is usually pictured with that unfortunate middle-part hairdo that covers her ears and makes her look like she's about to lecture you on obscure grammar rules. Don't be fooled. Lucy Stone was a superhero.

Her father helped two of her brothers to go to college but thought it was a bad idea for a girl to get too much education. She was smart and determined to learn, so she took a job as a teacher making less than half the pay of the male teacher she replaced (which, by the way, was completely legal!). She worked for nine years before she could finally afford to pay her own way to Oberlin College, the very first college in America to accept women. While there she cleaned houses for three cents an hour to help pay for her room and board, studying Greek as she washed dishes.

But even the progressive Oberlin had its limits. Her classmates picked her to write a special essay for graduation, but she was forbidden to read it to an audience that included both genders. Rather than have a male faculty member read her words, Stone declined the honor. Not surprisingly, by the time she graduated she was a strong believer that women should be treated as men's equals.

After she graduated from college, most of her family thought she should go back to teaching full time. Instead, at age twenty-nine she followed her conscience and decided to speak out against slavery. This was a time when ministers would preach from the pulpits that wives should be quiet and obey their husbands, so a woman speaking in public was highly controversial. The very few women who did speak publicly drew large, curious, and sometimes angry mobs. If you get nervous about having to give a speech today, be glad you live in the twenty-first century. Back then, lots of men showed up at anti-slavery lectures just to yell insults and throw things, and every once in a while they would burn a building down. (We're looking at you, Philadelphia.)

By all accounts Lucy Stone was a mesmerizing speaker (people were constantly shocked at just how good she was). She was small but had a musical voice that captivated audiences. Originally hired by the Massachusetts Anti-Slavery Society to lecture against slavery, she started adding stories about the injustices women faced, which she knew from her own experience. Her employers at the society wanted her to stick to abolition. But by that time Stone was such a big draw—thousands of people came to hear her—that she eventually worked out a deal to speak about women's rights on the weekdays. She had to take a pay cut, but she didn't care because both issues were hugely important to her. A lot of times you learn to advocate for one cause because of your involvement in another.

In the nineteenth century, listening to speakers was what you did for fun, like going to a blockbuster movie today (yes, entertainment options were pretty limited). Most lecturers at that time gave extremely flowery speeches that went on for hours, but Stone spoke plainly and told deeply personal stories. Newspapers marveled at how she could turn a hostile crowd around by talking directly to her hecklers (who sometimes just happened to be carrying clubs), occasionally shaming them but more often winning them over. Men who came to make trouble by booing and hissing left convinced she was on to something. Women stayed after her speeches to share their own stories, which Stone would weave into her talks. After being ignored for so long, women desperately wanted not just more rights, but to be heard and to make a difference. In 1850, speaking to a packed hall, Stone said:

> We want to be something more than the append-
> ages of Society; we want that Woman should be
> the co-equal and help-meet of Man in all the
> interests and perils and enjoyment of human
> life. . . . We want that when she dies, it may not
> be written on her gravestone that she was the
> "relic" [widow] of somebody.

The crowd ate it up.

Lucy Stone showed that women could speak up for their own rights and that people would want to hear them. Within just a few years of making her first speech for women's rights in 1847, she was getting invitations from all around the country to come speak.

MAKE IT PERSONAL. You can make a story even more effective by sharing your own experiences. From the very beginning of the suffrage movement, a lot of men liked to claim that women didn't need rights because men protected them and looked out for their interests. Sojourner Truth knew better. Unlike Stone, who was white, educated, and middle-class, Truth was Black, enslaved at birth, and literally scarred for life. She didn't have any illusions that men would always be kind.

Sojourner Truth was born 1797 in an area of New York settled by Dutch immigrants. She was given the name Isabella, and after her first owner died, she was taken from her parents. By age thirteen she had already been sold three times. She was eventually purchased by John Dumont, and in his house she worked brutally long days and was sometimes whipped, while his hostile wife made her even more miserable. She was "married" (she had no choice) to an enslaved man named Thomas and had five children. In 1826, after Dumont broke a promise to set her free, she decided she'd had enough. Taking only her baby daughter and the clothes on her back, she walked a few miles down the road to stay with a sympathetic white couple. The next year New York state abolished slavery and she was finally free. But Dumont had illegally sold her five-year-old son to a sadistic owner in Alabama, and she filed a lawsuit to get him back. Against overwhelming odds, she won and they were reunited.

Soon afterward she moved to New York City, and over the next decade she worked as a domestic servant and became involved with a number of popular (and sometimes pretty radical) religious movements. While she had some bad experiences, including a devastating and abusive period with a cult, she also found fellowship and friends, and for the first time she had the opportunity to preach (she was great at it). Although she never learned to read, she memorized the Bible by asking people to read passages several times until she knew them by heart. She particularly liked to have children read to her, because they would do just that, unlike adults who sometimes tried to tell her what to think.

Then on June 1, 1843, she did something absolutely remarkable. Giving her employers an hour's notice, she packed a pillowcase of belongings and went on the road to begin a new life as a traveling preacher. She gave herself the name Sojourner Truth.

In the beginning, most of Truth's public speeches—sermons really—were about finding God and salvation. But many of the people she met in religious communities were involved in the big reform issues of their times—abolitionism, women's rights, temperance, and even vegetarianism—and she listened and paid attention. When it became clear to some of the reformers that she shared their ideals, they recruited her to talk. She began to share the stage with some of the most respected lecturers of the day. That Truth was a Black woman who had once been enslaved made her virtually unique on the speaker circuit. Audiences were fascinated by her and by her story.

Newspapers praised Truth for her wit, wisdom, and common sense, and she certainly knew how to read a crowd. She quoted the Bible extensively to make her arguments against slavery and for women's rights and used humor to take away some of the sting. She sang hymns she wrote herself. As early as 1850, Truth dictated and self-published her autobiography, which she sold for twenty-five cents. It was updated several times, and with the sales from her book and donations from her public speaking, she was able to buy her own house and pay off the mortgage. She even got a glowing review from the author of *Uncle Tom's Cabin*, which was widely believed to be the second-best-selling book in America during the nineteenth century (after the Bible).

In 1851, Truth traveled to Ohio and attended a women's rights convention in Akron. There, in front of a large crowd, she asked if she could say a few words. According to Marius Robinson, editor of the *Anti-Slavery Bugle* (who published an account a month later), she talked about her own personal experience, declaring:

> I am a woman's rights. I have as much muscle as any man, and can do as much work as any man. I have plowed and reaped and husked and chopped and mowed, and can any man do more than that? I have heard much about the sexes being equal; I can carry as much as any man, and can eat as much too, if I can get it.

(We're guessing that if she was alive today she'd have some choice words to stay about the gender pay gap.)

She also knew how to deliver a burn. To those who did not think women should have their own rights, she was happy to make this point: "And how came Jesus into the world? Through God who created him and woman who bore him. Man, where is your part?"

She nailed it. Robinson later admitted, "It is impossible to transfer it to paper, or convey any adequate idea of the effect it produced upon the audience. Those only can appreciate it who saw her powerful form, her whole-souled, earnest gesture, and listened to her strong and truthful tones."

IF YOUR STORY TAKES A LIFE OF ITS OWN, MAKE IT WORK TO YOUR ADVANTAGE. Sometimes the most popular version of a story is not the same as the original. Shocking, right? If this happens, you can either frustrate yourself trying to go for 100 percent accuracy, or you can use your platform to keep getting the word out.

Truth's Akron speech would go on to become far and away her most famous speech and arguably one of the best-known speeches of the entire suffrage movement. But nobody would have predicted that at the time. We don't have a video or audio recording, and Truth didn't write anything down. Robinson's version—created shortly after the convention—was probably pretty close to what she actually said (it also helped that Truth was staying at his house at the time). It went to press a few weeks later, and when it came out, as good as it was, it didn't seem to set the world on fire.

So what changed? In 1863, a white suffragist named Frances Gage wrote an article with her own description of Truth's speech. Gage had presided at the 1851 convention, and twelve years later, capitalizing on Truth's growing fame, she conveniently remembered it well enough to publish a detailed account. Gage couldn't resist making the story even more dramatic. She wrote that the audience jeered when Truth first started talking, but by the end, their eyes filled with tears and hundreds ran forward to congratulate her. But Gage took the most poetic license with the speech itself: she had Truth speaking in a southern accent (Truth was from New York and her first language was Dutch) and claiming to have thirteen enslaved children (she had five). Most memorably, her version included the line "Ain't I a woman?" multiple times. You can compare the two versions online, but here's an excerpt:

> And raising herself to her full height, and her voice to a pitch like rolling thunder, she asked,

"And ain't I a woman? Look at me! Look at my
arm! (and she bared her right arm to the shoulder,
showing her tremendous muscular power). I have
ploughed, and planted, and gathered into barns,
and no man could head me! And ain't I a woman?
I could work as much and eat as much as a man—
when I could get it—and bear de lash as well!
And ain't I a woman?"

Whatever her exact words really were, Truth's message
of equality shines through, but Gage's version is the one
that most people remember today.

We can't be sure how Truth felt about Gage's popular-
ized version. She was proud that she spoke "fairly correct
English" (remember: her second language!) and generally
annoyed when people put words in her mouth. At the
same time, we believe Truth understood the importance
of good publicity. She met some of the most important
people of her day, including two presidents (Lincoln and
Grant). She also used her fame to advocate for freedmen
after the Civil War (probably the cause she cared most
about). On the downside, she ran into the kinds of
problems celebrities have today. Papers would write that

she had died (several years too early) or that she was 110 (not even close). Either way, a later edition of Truth's autobiography, published while she was still alive, included Gage's transcript.

Very few historians (like none) think that George Washington really chopped down a cherry tree. But that well-known legend, true or not, sticks because it gets to something Americans think is fundamentally important about our country. Sojourner Truth was admired in her lifetime and has become an even bigger source of inspiration today (she even had a Mars rover named after her). Then and now, she is a symbol of women's rights.

Before you can change the world, you have to start by telling your story. You can't wait to be invited; you have to be brave and put yourself out there. Make your stories personal so that you can connect with your audience. Be prepared for things to get exaggerated along the way (which they will). That doesn't mean your story is over, so keep talking.

To quote modern-day moms everywhere, use your words.

2

SET A GOAL

ALONG WITH A GREAT STORY THAT GETS EVERYONE
excited, you need to let people know what your goal is,
what success looks like. What, specifically, are you asking
for? But that is only part of it. Most people are pretty
busy with all the things going on in their life, so you will
need to keep your goal statement simple and clear, and
you will probably have to repeat yourself again and again
(and again) to get your message to stick. Advertisers will
tell you that commercials are most effective once people
have seen them multiple times (it is called the rule of
seven), and the same is true for educating people about a
cause. You have to really hammer it home.

As early as 1776, Abigail Adams wrote to John Adams
and asked him to "remember the ladies" and be "more
generous and favorable to them than your ancestors."
We think this is a great idea in general, but it's not quite
a plan. When did the big concept of women's rights come
to be defined in practice as women's suffrage? It all came
together with one of the greatest partnerships in American
history.

BE CLEAR ABOUT WHAT YOU WANT. Elizabeth Cady Stanton was acknowledged by pretty much everyone in her day to be one of the great thinkers and writers of the suffrage movement. Charming and brilliant, she was so sure of herself that later in life she would write her own critique of the Bible, calling out the parts she thought were sexist. This was typical of Stanton. Throughout her long life she was absolutely fearless when it came to taking controversial positions.

Elizabeth Cady Stanton, who was white, was born in 1815, the eighth child of a well-to-do lawyer and judge. Only four of her ten siblings—all girls—lived past twenty, and her father's grief at having no surviving sons (he once told her she should have been a boy) helped shape her belief that the world was unfair to women. By the time she was eleven, she was learning Greek and debating her father's law clerks. Competitive by nature, she hated the fact that even though she was as smart as her male classmates, they went off to college and she got left behind. She wanted excitement and a chance to put her excellent mind to work.

In 1840, she married an abolitionist speaker named Henry Stanton, and on their honeymoon they traveled to the World Anti-Slavery Convention in London. There she met Lucretia Mott, a famous white American abolitionist who had been elected as a delegate to the convention. The British organizers had originally refused to seat her and the other women delegates, but after much debate, they were allowed to sit off to the side (hidden by a curtain), where they were told to remain silent. Stanton, who always loved a good fight, was indignant on Mott's behalf, and the two became friends.

Eight years later, Stanton was living in Seneca Falls, New York, with her growing family. She had seven children, whom she raised in a rather free-range style, but she still had a passion for women's rights. While attending a friendly tea party with female abolitionists, Stanton and a small group of white Quaker women decided on the spur of the moment to hold a women's rights convention, the first one ever. They would hold it in less than two weeks' time so that Lucretia Mott (who was in the neighborhood) could attend, and they put a notice about it in the paper.

They had no idea how popular it would be. It wasn't that women's rights hadn't come up before—it was a buzzy topic in the reform crowd—it just usually took a back seat to issues like slavery. But on July 19, 1848, when Stanton and her group arrived at the Methodist church where the convention would be held, they found a crowd waiting for them. It was mostly women, but also some men and children, and far larger than they expected.

Stanton and another organizer, Elizabeth McClintock, had prepared a document for the convention that they called the Declaration of Sentiments. Based on the Declaration of Independence, it compared the fight for women's rights with the American Revolution. But instead of rebelling against a tyrannical king, they would rebel against the tyranny of men. It started off "We hold these truths to be self-evident: that all men and women are created equal" and then went on to list specific grievances against men, including:

> He has compelled her to submit to laws,
> in the formation of which she had not voice.
> He has made her, if married, in the eyes of
> the law, civilly dead.
> He has taken from her all right in property,
> even to the wages she earns.

Stanton didn't hold back (she never did). Go ahead and read the whole thing. Even with the nineteenth-century language, it is still pretty strong stuff.

On the second day of the convention, the fearless Stanton introduced a resolution calling for the vote for women. This was too much for many of the participants. Even the open-minded Lucretia Mott balked at such a crazy suggestion, saying "Lizzie, thee will make us ridiculous!" (Quakers had mixed feelings about anyone voting.) While the other ten resolutions passed unanimously, the suffrage resolution ("That it is the duty of the women of this country to secure to themselves their sacred right to the elective franchise") only passed after Frederick Douglass, a famous Black abolitionist who had once been enslaved, spoke up in favor of it. Just one hundred of the three hundred people in attendance signed the final document.

The convention and Stanton's Declaration of Sentiments got a lot of press coverage, and Mott was right about the negative reaction. One reporter wrote, "This bolt is the most shocking and unnatural incident ever recorded in the history of womanity. If our ladies will insist on voting and legislating, where, gentlemen, will be our dinners and our elbows? Where our domestic firesides and the holes in our stockings?" (We are not making this up.)

But Stanton's arguments found fans as well, and she got everyone talking about the points she had made (today we would call it driving the news cycle). The idea of conventions on women's rights caught on immediately, and within weeks several more were planned.

Elizabeth Cady Stanton took all the individual wrongs that women had suffered and created a mission statement for the movement. You could agree or disagree with her (and people often disagreed—strongly!), but you were having the debate.

GET YOUR MESSAGE OUT. Probably no one is more associated with the cause of women's suffrage than Susan B. Anthony. Her impressive organizational skills and tireless campaigning for the cause earned her the nicknames "Napoleon" and "General" among her fellow activists. Anthony remains the best-known white suffragist today not because of her great ability as a speaker, although she got pretty good at it during her lifetime. It is because for nearly half a century, Anthony would go anywhere, and at any time, to talk about votes for women. She was nonstop.

Anthony was born in 1820 into a Quaker family. Her father believed in providing a good education for his daughters and, like many Quakers at the time, was active in several reform movements of the day, particularly the abolition of slavery. When the family ran into financial trouble in 1837, Anthony took a job teaching, and like Lucy Stone she was paid way less than the male teacher she replaced (roughly one quarter the salary). As you can probably imagine, she thought this was hugely unfair.

As a young woman, Anthony was much more interested in social reform than suitors. She got involved in the abolitionist movement, as well as the temperance movement to ban alcohol, and attended several teachers' conventions to argue that women teachers should get equal pay. At one convention, the male teachers went on a long public debate (right in front of her!) about whether she should be allowed to say anything at all. This was not OK with Anthony, and she stood up and said so. Over time she became convinced that women's rights—specifi-cally the right to vote—was the cause she wanted to dedicate her life to achieving.

Anthony had been inspired after hearing Lucy Stone speak, and they would go on to become good friends until they had a falling out over the Fifteenth Amendment (more on this later). But Elizabeth Cady Stanton, whom she met by chance on a street corner in 1851, was her true soulmate. They would go on to form one of the most effective partnerships in American political history and a friendship that would last more than fifty years. They made a great team, with Stanton doing most of the writing and Anthony responsible for the organizing. Stanton wrote or cowrote most of the speeches Anthony gave, or as Anthony liked to say, "She forged the thunderbolts and I fired them."

As women's suffrage built up momentum, Anthony hit the road to make speeches. They didn't have planes in her lifetime, but if they did, she would have had platinum status on every major carrier. Instead, Anthony traveled by train, covered wagon, stagecoach, ferry, steamboat, and even sleigh, visiting states and territories across the union to spread the word. Traveling in those days was usually uncomfortable (there were bugs in her mattresses), often risky (her pocket was picked), and generally exhausting (she really missed good coffee). Once she got stuck on a snowbound train for over twenty-four hours in the middle of the Rocky Mountains. But she kept going. In one 1871 diary entry, Anthony recorded that she had given 171 speeches and traveled over 13,000 miles—more than half the circumference of the earth—in that year alone. She would later write to a friend:

> Believe in yourself—and your powers to speak—as well as write! So don't say "no" to a single invitation to speak—but just prepare yourself—and read—if you want to, or when the time comes—drop your paper and talk its contents—tell the story!! That is all I have done these forty years.

Anthony later estimated that she had given anywhere from seventy-five to one hundred speeches a year for well over four decades. She gave her last suffrage speech in 1906 at the age of eighty-six, just a few days before she died.

In the end, when you tell a story often enough, it starts to have a life all of its own. Today, most histories of the women's suffrage movement begin with the Seneca Falls Woman's Rights Convention of 1848. Yet for many years after it happened, it was largely forgotten, even by the women in the movement. But Stanton understood the importance of founding myths, and toward the end of her life she started to promote the anniversary of the convention she helped organize. Most important, when she and Anthony cowrote the history of the suffrage movement, Seneca Falls is where it began. That six-volume, 5,000-plus-page history was the main source historians consulted for years (Anthony, determined to promote the cause, donated free copies to libraries everywhere). So today Seneca Falls is the benchmark we use.

Stone, Truth, Stanton, and Anthony were not the first Americans to talk about women's rights (Google the Grimké sisters or Abby Kelley). But of that first generation of suffragists, they were celebrities—the household names, the voices that stood out, the social influencers of their day. Their commitment to telling their stories and shaping the message made suffrage part of the national conversation, and they laid the groundwork for the next wave of women activists who came after them.

They taught us how important it is to have a measurable goal for success, something that is easy to explain. And once you have your message, tell everyone: in one-on-one conversations, on social media, to some random person you meet at a party. Write a blog, create your own video, use every tool you have. Even if you've told it hundreds of times, keep going—because there are a lot of other things happening, and it takes time for a message to really stick.

NEVER GIVE UP

3

Have you ever put a lot of time and energy into doing something only to have it all fall apart? You wind up depressed that you did all that work for nothing. Or maybe it just seems like success is taking way too long. It's completely normal to want to quit. We get that.

The suffrage campaign had a lot of days like that, years even. One of the most valuable lessons you can learn from the suffragists' long struggle is a sense of perspective. Making big changes is difficult, and there WILL be setbacks (all the best movements have them). Our reason for pointing this out is not to get you super depressed. It is so that when your cause runs into problems, you won't beat yourself up too much. You just need to be ready for the hard times and keep going.

KNOW THAT IT WON'T BE EASY. Sometimes changing the world is going to be tough, and we mean *tough*. Lucy Stone was pelted with trash, rotten eggs, and a hymnal, and once, during the middle of winter, she was sprayed with ice water from a fire hose. A mob interrupted Sojourner Truth and demanded she undress to prove she was a woman. Susan B. Anthony was hung in effigy and arrested and put on trial for voting. Decades later, women picketing in front of the White House were sent to prison, where they were brutally mistreated and force fed when they went on hunger strike. Suffragists were ridiculed in the newspapers and political cartoons, and they put up with an unending stream of verbal abuse. The life of a suffragist was not for the faint of heart.

Even stay-at-home mom Elizabeth Cady Stanton faced challenges, although they were less public. She had to juggle running a busy household and raising her boisterous children (who at one point tied corks to the baby and put him in the river to see if he would float), all the while serving as the intellectual powerhouse of women's rights. In a letter that would sound familiar to any mother today, she wrote:

> To keep a house and grounds in good order,
> purchase every article of clothing for daily use,
> keep the wardrobes of half a dozen human beings
> in proper trim, take the children to dentists,
> shoemakers, and different scholars, or find teachers
> at home, altogether made sufficient work to keep

one brain busy, as well as all the hands I could impress into the service.

You never hear about Jefferson or Madison stressing about childcare.

Then there are the things that happen that are completely beyond your control (also known as bad luck). The suffrage movement was interrupted not once, but twice, by two all-consuming wars. One was the American Civil War, still the most deadly war the US has ever fought. The other was World War I, known then as the Great War, because no one at the time could imagine that there would ever be a bigger war. Not only did these two conflicts sideline the majority of suffrage supporters as the nation's attention was fixated on the wars, but the aftermath of the first war resulted in a significant setback to the cause.

BE READY FOR THE DRAMA. The suffrage movement really stumbled after the Civil War when Congress took up the question of rights for the freed slaves. Most of the first generation of suffragists were also abolitionists, so when the Thirteenth Amendment to the Constitution abolished slavery in 1865, there was great rejoicing all around. Success at last! For a brief time it seemed possible (at least to a small group of clearly idealistic reformers) that both women and former slaves might achieve their goals for equal rights.

Um, no. Their hopes were way too optimistic. When the Fourteenth Amendment was passed a few years later, giving former slaves citizenship and equal rights under the law, it specifically limited the right to vote to male citizens. Believe it or not, this was the first time the word *male* appeared in the Constitution. Then came a push for a Fifteenth Amendment stating that no one could deny a US citizen the right to vote based on "race, color, or previous condition of servitude." Which basically meant that formerly enslaved men could vote (at least theoretically), but still not women. And this is when everything started to fall apart.

The takeaway from this next historical moment is that not all of your problems will come from the outside. Some (and this is especially frustrating) will be self-inflicted wounds. The majority of suffragists reluctantly supported the new amendment, feeling that some progress was better than none. But a minority led by Stanton and Anthony felt abandoned by their fellow activists and were bitterly opposed. When a friend and fellow abolitionist pushed Anthony to support the Fifteenth Amendment, she angrily told him she would sooner cut off her right hand than ask for the ballot for Black men and not for women. She even got into a heated public debate with Frederick Douglass at a rowdy meeting that the *New York World* (in the tradition of tabloid papers) described as "Hisses, Cat-Calls, Yells, and Wild Demonstrations." Their argument was a LOT more dignified than that (and Douglass made a real effort to be gracious), but she was super pissed.

With Black activists and white women suffragists often pitted directly against each other (somehow white men got a pass?!), the already-too-small suffrage movement split. Stanton and Anthony founded the more radical National Woman Suffrage Association (NWSA) in 1869, opposing the Fifteenth Amendment unless it was changed to include women. Only women could join, and thanks to Stanton they highlighted a wide range of controversial issues like divorce and birth control (Anthony was always trying to rein her in). Just a few months later, Lucy Stone founded the more moderate American Woman Suffrage Association (AWSA), which supported the Fifteenth

Amendment as written but was otherwise dedicated to getting women the vote. The NWSA went all in for a constitutional amendment, while the AWSA went for a state-by-state strategy.

The whole mess was especially difficult for Black suffragists, who had to endure twice the prejudice. As Frances Ellen Watkins Harper declared (we'll talk about her more later), "As much as white women need the ballot, colored women need it more." She wound up joining the AWSA, along with prominent women like Josephine St. Pierre Ruffin (the first Black person to graduate from Harvard Law School) and Charlotta Rollin. Others, like Mary Ann Shadd Cary (the first Black woman to edit a newspaper), joined the NWSA. Sojourner Truth was friends with Stanton, Anthony, and Stone and tried hard not to take sides (if you've ever been stuck in the middle, you know what that's like). She mostly went to AWSA conventions but showed up occasionally at NWSA events. From what historians can tell, there were more Black women in the AWSA, but honestly, it is hard be sure from the membership rolls because there weren't many demographic surveys back then.

By the time the Fifteenth Amendment was passed (as

originally written) and then ratified in 1870, the leaders on both sides had dug in, and it was too late. Previously close friends, these strong-willed women—and you could hardly survive as a suffragist in the nineteenth century if you weren't strong willed—criticized and antagonized each other almost to their dying days. Just like the original Founding Fathers, they clashed over matters both political and personal.

Frankly, just reading about it can be depressing. Instead of pulling together in the same direction, the warring camps split what few resources they had. The suffragists delivered a lot of speeches, published countless articles, and spent a mind-boggling amount of time on the road, and it was still mostly loss after soul-crushing loss, with no amendment in sight. This schism lasted for over twenty years.

EXPECT OPPOSITION. This may sound weird, but having organized opposition is a sign you are doing something right. It means your enemies have stopped laughing and are getting worried. When the suffrage movement went mainstream in the late 1890s, two powerful groups rallied against it. The first was the large liquor lobby, which was worried—for good reason—that women would vote to get rid of alcohol (we'll get to that). The second was the anti-suffrage movement, whose sole reason for existing was to campaign against women voting.

There had always been men who were blatantly sexist and thought women were too stupid or fragile or irresponsible to handle the vote. They were dismissive and almost unbearably insufferable. "A woman is nobody. A wife is everything. A pretty girl is equal to ten thousand men" read a condescending editorial against women's rights in a Philadelphia paper (the author probably thought he was being profound). But aside from making fun of the suffragists, they didn't take them too seriously. Instead, by far the most vocal and numerous group of anti-suffragists (not to mention the best organized) were . . . women themselves.

Now you may find it strange that women worked against their own rights (we certainly do), but they had their reasons. The more conservative women felt that a woman's place was in the home and worried they would lose what they viewed as special privileges they already possessed if women entered politics. According to their thinking, their chivalrous male relatives already represented their interests when they voted. They argued that women were so busy running their households that it would be a huge and unwelcome burden if they had to vote as well. Plus, they complained that polling stations were filled with all kinds of rowdy behavior (sort of like a drunken frat house) that made them inappropriate for ladies.

Other women were all for female civic participation, but thought that actually voting would politicize them. "Women now stand outside politics. They are neither Republicans nor Democrats, and therefore their suggestions in matters of education, charity, and reform are welcomed and successful. No suspicions arise that they have partisan ends to serve" read a petition from one state anti-suffrage group. A national anti-suffrage group was much less diplomatic, claiming women voting "would be an official endorsement of nagging as a national policy." (Yes, these are women saying these things.) Ironically, the women in the anti-suffrage movement used the same civic tools available to suffragists, such as petitions, speeches, and lobbying, so their objection to women participating in politics wasn't terribly consistent.

In the course of seventy-plus years, the suffrage movement had to put up with physical hardship, wars, infighting, determined opposition, and, from the very start, the tiresome task of changing public opinion. So how can you avoid these kinds of problems today? The answer is you can't. The big takeaway (blindly obvious but still constantly overlooked) is that changing the world is exhausting. What you can control is how you react to the setbacks, and here is how the suffrage movement survived.

They didn't just form organizations; they formed sisterhoods, with traditions, special symbols, and songs. They looked out after one another and took comfort in the close friendships they made. Susan B. Anthony even did a lot of babysitting of Stanton's children (she referred to them as "our children" in her letters to Stanton), and there was always a special room reserved for Anthony in the various Stanton households. The suffragists wrote the history of their movement, most notably the six-volume *History of Woman Suffrage*, published while it was still in progress. And in the end, the two suffrage organizations reconciled for the good of the cause. In 1890, with the help of Stone's daughter Alice Stone Blackwell, the NWSA and the AWSA merged to become the National American Woman Suffrage Association.

Black suffragists (who kept getting ignored by white suffragists) started their own clubs, which they often named after inspiring women like Harriet Tubman, Sojourner Truth, and the poet Phillis Wheatley. In 1896, they founded the National Association of Colored Women, the first truly national organization for Black women, and in just a few years they had chapters in twenty-six states. Four years later, the newly created Women's Convention—part of the National Baptist Convention—became the largest organization of Black women in the entire country. Along with advocating women's suffrage, the clubs pursued a lot of other goals, like organizing job training programs and day nurseries for working women; raising money for schools, kindergartens, and retirement homes; and talking about issues that were of special importance to women of color, like lynching and Jim Crow transportation laws. These clubs not only improved their communities; they also gave Black women a chance to take important leadership roles. Finally!

The women also took comfort in what they had accomplished. In 1891, Lucy Stone gave a speech titled "The Gains of Forty Years" in which she talked about all the important gains women had made. Among other things, she noted that ducking stools for women who talked sharply to their husbands had (almost) been abolished, married women had more property rights (this was a big deal), more professions and educational opportunities were open to women than ever before, and some voting gains had been made, especially in school elections.

Most of all, despite everything, they kept going. Susan B. Anthony spent decades campaigning for women's suffrage, which she expected to see in her lifetime, but died in 1906 and missed the passage of the amendment named after her by fourteen years. In an 1896 interview with the famous journalist Nellie Bly, she admitted that "our work is exactly like the tide of the ocean. We are swept forward and back." But she remained optimistic. Her final words in her last public speech were "Failure is impossible."

America's Founding Fathers lived to see the birth of a new country, but when we talk about the founding mothers of the suffrage movement, the talk turns to generations. Lucy Stone, Sojourner Truth, Elizabeth Cady Stanton, and Susan B. Anthony all lived to a ripe old age—longer than most of their contemporaries—but each died before suffrage was passed. Of the original signers of the 1848 Declaration of Sentiments, only Charlotte Woodward lived to see the Nineteenth Amendment passed, and she was too ill to vote in the election of 1920 and died before she got another chance. But because of their hard work, because they persevered through tough times, women can vote today.

Be prepared for the fact that it will be hard, that even the best leaders are human and make mistakes, and that there will be heartbreaks and factors beyond your control and really depressing times. If you know what can go wrong and recognize that other successful movements have had similar problems, it will be easier (but not easy) to get past them. Despite these setbacks and against great odds, you can still succeed. Never give up.

IT'S TIME TO TALK ABOUT RACISM

WE HAVE TO TALK.

When we first started writing this book, we wanted to shine a light on some of the successful tactics from the suffrage movement that you can use today to make the world better. So we have tried to showcase positive actions, specifically what you should do. But sadly, one of the most important—and let's be honest, shameful—lessons of the suffrage history is what NOT to do.

Don't be so focused on winning your cause that you lose your soul.

In the case of the suffrage movement, the big ugly issue that constantly came up was racism. And far too often, white suffragists failed to live up to their own ideals.

Don't get us wrong—there were definitely white suffrage supporters who believed in equal rights for both sexes and all races. They talked the talk and walked the walk.

But a lot more wanted to challenge male prejudices against women without ever questioning their own bias against Black people. They bought into the negative stereotypes and even used them for marketing.

Many of the early suffragists saw the vote as a privilege reserved for white, educated women. In those pre–Civil War days, many suffragists were also abolitionists. But the idea of formerly enslaved Americans actually voting seems to have been unimaginable to them. There were no known Black women at Seneca Falls in 1848; the only person of color we know about was Frederick Douglass.

Elizabeth Cady Stanton was particularly lacking in the empathy department. For all the many ways she was willing to challenge the status quo, she was basically the poster child for white privilege. She began writing in favor of "educated suffrage," which—given that it had been illegal to teach enslaved people to read and many new immigrants were illiterate—was pretty much code for white, middle-class suffrage. She was perfectly comfortable throwing others under the bus as long as she got her rights. When the Fifteenth Amendment gave the vote to Black men but not women, Stanton was not just disappointed; she was horrified. This is a verbatim quote: "What will we and our daughters suffer if these degraded black men are allowed to have the rights that would make them even worse than our Saxon [white] fathers?"

As the movement gained followers and spread around

the country, many local suffrage clubs did not admit Black members. Those that did often ignored issues that were important to African Americans, like lynching and the spread of Jim Crow laws. When Black women were included, they were often demeaned or segregated, like when they were told to march at the back of the 1913 parade in Washington, DC (more on that in chapter 6). Even histories of the suffrage movement written well into the twentieth century ignored the contributions of Black women. You can read about some of them, like Frances Ellen Watkins Harper and Mary Church Terrell, in this book, but there were many, many more whose stories remain untold.

Ignoring or demeaning the needs of Black women was bad enough, but some white suffragists went even further. They used openly racist arguments to try to win the vote. In the late 1800s and early 1900s, when the National American Woman Suffrage Association (NAWSA) was trying to win the vote state-by-state, white women regularly made speeches in southern states urging them to give women the vote so white voters would overwhelm Black ones. They weren't subtle about it. Kate Gordon, organizer of the Southern States Woman

Suffrage Conference, said, "The question of white supremacy is one that will only be decided by giving the right of the ballot to the educated, intelligent white women of the South." Belle Kearney, who later became the first woman elected to the Mississippi State Senate, declared, "The enfranchisement of women would insure immediate and durable white supremacy, honestly attained." And Anna Howard Shaw, who would become president of the NAWSA, criticized the men of Louisiana for "putting the ballot into the hands of your black men, thus making them the political superiors of your white women."

(This argument never worked, by the way. White politicians in the South were systematically keeping Black men from the polls with violence and unfair poll taxes, literacy tests, etc. That was working just fine for them. They had no interest in giving the vote to anyone but white men.)

Normally we would caution about judging historical figures by modern norms. But in the case of suffrage, they were specifically talking about fairness. It's just so hypocritical. You would think they would have known better.

It's normal to want your heroes to be good, honorable,

and thoroughly in the right. But the truth is, sometimes your heroes—in this case heroines—will let you down.

It's important to recognize and call out hate when you see it. It's easy to condemn those southern suffragists who were unapologetic white supremacists—they are just so awful. But we also need to take a long, hard look at those who went with the status quo and allowed injustice to thrive. Most of these women would never have considered themselves racists, but their actions (or inactions) had discriminatory, unfair results. We aren't pointing this out so we can feel superior with all of our hindsight, but so we can see the patterns before we repeat them. Obviously racism—and other toxic forms of discrimination—are still huge problems today. They can even seem impossible: too big, too systematic, too entrenched. But we can't stop being on the lookout for them and trying our best to fix them. We can't afford to leave good women, or good people of any kind, behind.

So our advice is this: if you dedicate yourself to a cause, working to make the world a better place, watch out for the tunnel vision that makes you care less about other issues, just because they aren't your issues. And if you do find yourself making mistakes (and let's be honest, you probably will), be strong enough to admit them and figure out how to fix things.

The whole point of being an activist is that you are optimistic that the world can change. And you can start now, by doing politics better.

ENGAGE A WIDER AUDIENCE

SOMETIMES IT'S NOT ENOUGH TO TELL PEOPLE THAT your cause is right; you need to explain why it's right for them. Most people are plenty busy with their own lives, so to get their attention you need to link your cause to popular goals. Give them a reason to care in the first place.

GET AN INFLUENTIAL ENDORSEMENT. Frances Willard was the most famous white suffragist you've never heard of. She was a huge celebrity in her day, arguably the best known and most admired woman in the world after Queen Victoria. For twenty years she was president of the most influential women's organization in the country. She was a celebrated speaker and attracted enormous crowds. She wrote multiple books, including an advice book for young women titled *How to Win* and another on how to ride a bicycle. She was the first woman to have a statue in the United States Capitol, placed there by the state of Illinois in 1905. It would be over fifty years before another other woman would join her there in the halls of Congress.

But in June of 1874, Frances Willard was unemployed and looking for a new direction for her life. In 1871, at the age of thirty-two, she had become the head of the Evanston College for Ladies at Northwestern, the first female college president in the entire country. For three years the students at the college thrived under her leadership, until the new president of Northwestern University (who just happened to be Willard's grudge-holding former fiancé) made her life so miserable she resigned in frustration.

Trying to figure out what she was going to do with her life, she was traveling through Pittsburgh when she witnessed a group of women protesting outside a saloon. Inspired, she joined a new organization dedicated to banning alcohol, the Woman's Christian Temperance Union (WCTU).

Willard was the definition of someone who has their act together. She traveled all over the place to meet people, wrote letters to everyone (sometimes as many as twenty-five a day), and was generally always on top of things. You may know somebody like that, and some-times they are annoying, but just about everyone liked Willard. Within a few months she was elected the corresponding secretary of the WCTU, and five years later she became president. Petite, charismatic, and motherly in her manner, she was an electrifying speaker who talked to her audiences in a conversational tone that had them waving their handkerchiefs wildly (that's how women used to applaud back then).

When she first joined the WCTU, it had just a few thousand members. But largely due to Willard's impressive leadership, by the late 1890s the WCTU had more than 300,000 dues-paying members, making it the largest women's organization in the world. So in 1876, when Willard made the first of several speeches in favor of suffrage, Susan B. Anthony was totally thrilled. Getting Willard's endorsement was a big deal because she already had a huge number of followers, and her fame would only grow in the next two decades.

EXPLAIN WHY IT MATTERS. Frances Willard was a great manager, an amazing organizer, and a popular speaker. But her real genius was her ability to make super-radical ideas acceptable. She did this by explicitly linking them to issues that people—especially women—cared strongly about.

Today the temperance movement is largely dismissed as being unrealistic and joyless. But back in the eighteenth and early nineteenth century, Americans were drinking a

LOT more alcohol, and the alcohol was much stronger. By 1830, estimates had American adults drinking—on average!—ninety bottles of hard alcohol a year. That's just insane. It got so bad that for a while, workers in cities weren't expected to show up on Mondays because employers assumed they'd be hungover. Not surprisingly, that's when temperance groups began to catch on. Even if you didn't drink, alcohol could still mess up your life. By social custom, drinking was largely done by men, usually in saloons that didn't allow women and where the patrons spit on the floor (and worse). Not only did many men drink up all their wages—and often their wives' wages, since husbands could legally take all the money their wives earned—but some became abusive and beat their wives and children (perfectly legal). No wonder women were so dead set against "demon rum"!

Because moms were supposed to be responsible for their children's moral education, it was considered OK for ladies to get involved in temperance reform, which was seen as a moral issue. It became an important gateway cause to get women politically active (Susan B. Anthony and Elizabeth Cady Stanton started off in the temperance movement, and Sojourner Truth was a supporter). But most of the time, that was as far as women went. They signed petitions and raised money and listened to speakers, but only for temperance.

Then Willard linked temperance and the pretty-extreme-sounding idea of women's suffrage. From the beginning, she made a very smart decision. Instead of talking about women's natural rights, she just focused on all the good things that women could do if only they had the vote (she was very specific). She branded it the "home protection ballot" and recruited conservative women by making the argument that "with your vote we can close the saloons that tempt your boys to ruin." Voting wasn't a right but the duty of women, who had to protect their children and country! (She really laid it on thick.)

If you read her long, super-flowery speeches (which could go on for fifty-plus pages), she talks about the home, God, the church, the Sabbath, motherhood, love, virtue, kindness, the Bible, innocent children, and, well, you get the idea. It is so sweet you might get a cavity. But in Willard's day, people ate this kind of talk up. By the time she was done speaking (hours later), the prim Methodist in the front row, who had once been opposed, had started to think suffrage was a pretty good idea! After all, who wanted to be against motherhood? Willard was one of the original influencers and knew how to make something popular (today she would probably have her own YouTube channel).

It is always a good idea to get the moms on your side.

CREATE A PATH FOR SUCCESS. Willard preferred to gradually win people over rather than push too hard and lose people along the way. We know from her private diaries that she was an early convert to women's suffrage. She met Susan B. Anthony right after she joined the WCTU, and a few months later she met Lucy Stone (both would become lifelong friends). In 1876—when Willard was still just the corresponding secretary for the WCTU (although she basically did everything)—she made her first public speech endorsing women's suffrage. There, before an audience of reliable churchgoers, she suggested that this wasn't something she was doing for her own sake, but as a religious duty. She later wrote that she got the call to "speak for woman's ballot" while on her knees, deep in prayer, after a morning of Bible study. This was classic Willard. She rarely admitted to taking an action on her own behalf; it was always for someone else (in this case, God).

A few weeks later, she made a speech at the WCTU national convention supporting the ballot for women. The current president (who was dead set against votes for women) was so pissed off she told Willard publicly, "You might have been a leader, but now you'll only be a scout." (So wrong.) The always good-natured Willard showed no hard feelings and kept going. She knew how to play the long game.

Two years later, Willard led a petition campaign to the Illinois state legislature asking that women be able to vote on the granting of local liquor licenses. Baby steps really, not all that radical. When she presented it to the legislature, the petition was "nearly a quarter of a mile long" and signed by a whopping 180,000 people (men too!). It didn't pass, but it made for great press and got a lot of attention.

In 1880, as the newly elected president of the WCTU (after what might be called a very friendly, very polite coup), Willard introduced a resolution that said "In order to give those who suffer most from the drink curse a power to protect themselves, their homes, and their loved ones, the complete enfranchisement of women should be worked for and welcomed." Nothing too scary, but it didn't go anywhere. But at the next convention it finally passed—unanimously. Even for women who didn't care about women's suffrage, hearing about it so often and in such unthreatening language made it seem more normal. For the first time since its introduction, the idea of votes for women was going mainstream.

Willard worked openly and behind the scenes with suffrage leaders like Anthony and invited her to attend the 1881 WCTU national convention in Washington, DC. She made Anthony's niece, Lucy Anthony, the head of the WCTU lecture bureau. Willard even went so far as to (reluctantly) move the site for the 1896 WCTU convention from California to St. Louis at Anthony's request. Women's suffrage was on the ballot that year in California, and Anthony was afraid that if men saw how many women were working for temperance, they would be even more likely to vote against it (the referendum failed anyway).

Despite being team suffrage all the way, Willard was careful to never get too far ahead of what her mostly white evangelical members could be convinced to support, believing it was better to compromise and make some progress than hold out for the best outcome and make none at all. Willard also created a "Do Everything" philosophy that allowed each individual WCTU chapter to decide which specific causes they supported. Some chapters just did temperance. Other chapters got involved in issues like women's suffrage, public health, education, labor conditions, anti-polygamy laws, prison reform, and banning tobacco. This flexibility allowed the organization to grow without splintering along ideological lines.

"Do Everything" also meant that women should do everything they could to promote those causes: petitioning, testifying before state legislatures, making public speeches, protesting at saloons, and writing articles— anything that might sway popular opinion. She even encouraged her members to wear small white ribbons on their clothing that would identify them as temperance supporters (sound familiar?).

Willard was president of the WCTU for nearly twenty years, until 1898, when she died suddenly of flu while in New York. Her body was carried home to Illinois by a special train, and thousands of mourners lined up alongside the route to pay their respects. Her coffin lay in state in Chicago, where over 30,000 people came to say their final goodbye.

Frances Willard rarely gets the credit she deserves for advancing women's suffrage. In part this is because the temperance movement is seen as a failed experiment, but she is also a victim of her own success. Because she made activism look so easy and conventional, it is hard to remember just how radical she was. Willard permanently changed the game for women's suffrage, recruiting an entire army of women for the cause by convincing them they could use it to do a lot of good things. This is an important point to remember. For a movement to gain widespread acceptance, it needs to be seen as beneficial for society as a whole, not just one group.

If you are having trouble getting people to support your cause, try to get an influential endorsement. Look at what people already want and make direct connections to popular goals. You don't have to ask people to support your entire cause immediately; give them an option to go halfway. You can persuade people to gradually change their minds over time just by exposing them to the concept. They might even think it was their own idea!

5

BE BOLD WHEN YOU GET STUCK

SOMETIMES, EVEN THE MOST PASSIONATE ADVOCATES can get burnt out. Maybe you've had a long, dull stretch where nothing much has happened. Maybe the routine organizing, planning, and fundraising is feeling tedious, even a little pointless. We're not judging. It can happen to anyone.

It definitely happened to plenty of suffragists right around the beginning of the twentieth century. Elizabeth Cady Stanton died in 1902. Susan B. Anthony died in 1906. The women who took over leadership of the National American Woman Suffrage Association (NAWSA), Carrie Chapman Catt and Anna Howard Shaw, both white, were incredibly smart, effective advocates. But they weren't the fire-breathing dragons Stanton and Anthony had been, and they didn't get new recruits as fired up about the suffrage cause.

To be honest, there wasn't that much to be fired up about in the early 1900s. In 1890, Wyoming became the first state to allow women to vote. Colorado passed suffrage in 1893, and Idaho and Utah followed in 1896. Then . . . nothing. For fourteen years, not a single new state passed suffrage. Throughout the first decade of the new century, the number of states where women could vote was stuck at four, and they were all western states with small voting populations. It was hard to believe that one more petition drive, one more sidewalk speech, one more visit to a lawmaker was going to make any difference. You can imagine it was a challenge to get a new generation of young women excited about suffrage when the movement looked so tired and ineffective.

One of those apathetic young white women was Alice Paul. She grew up Quaker in New Jersey, believing in equal rights, but never feeling inspired to get involved in women's issues herself. Then in 1907, when she was twenty-two, she moved to England for graduate school. The British suffragists had their staid and steady advocates, too. But they also had the Pankhursts (mother Emmeline and daughters Sylvia and Christabel), who were willing to break windows, set fires, send letter bombs, and even slap police officers to get attention for women's rights. Now, let's be clear that we are not advocating the use of these tactics. And Alice Paul didn't agree with all of them, either. But she was excited and energized by the boldness of the British movement. She was arrested several times. When she was sent to jail, she went on a hunger strike, as Emmeline Pankhurst taught all her followers to do. Paul was a tiny, pale woman, and prison officials were terrified that she would get really sick or even die, winning huge sympathy for the cause. So they decided to force feed her. This is just as horrible as it sounds; she was held down, and a tube was forced down her throat. If she refused to open her mouth, the tube was sent down her nose. Liquid nutrition was poured through the tube directly into her stomach, then the tube was ripped out. It was painful, bloody, and humiliating.

When Paul returned to the United States, she wasn't particularly eager to repeat her experience in prison. But she was willing to take bold steps to kick-start the American suffrage movement back into gear. When her friend Lucy Burns moved back to the US, Paul had a partner who was willing to take some risks with her. Lucy Burns was also a young white American woman who went to Europe for graduate school and was arrested for fighting for suffrage. In fact, Burns and Paul met in a police station. They both knew an important truth: it is easier to take a bold step when you have at least one person you can count on to be right there with you.

Try something totally new. Together, Alice Paul and Lucy Burns convinced the leaders of the NAWSA to let them plan a huge parade on March 3, 1913. There had been suffrage parades before, but this one was different for a few important reasons. For one thing, it was in Washington, DC, starting at the US Capitol and marching right down Pennsylvania Avenue to the White House. Now we hear about marches on Washington all the time, for all kinds of causes and commemorations. But the 1913 suffrage march was the very first march on Washington. Also, March 3, 1913, was the day before Woodrow Wilson's inauguration as America's twenty-eighth president. President Wilson opposed women's suffrage. Over the years he gave a lot of reasons for his opposition. Some of them were pretty lame ("I haven't really thought about it"), and some of them were a little more understandable ("I really need to pay more attention to World War I right now"). But all his excuses boiled down to the simple truth that he didn't want women to vote. There was definitely a racist subtext to this objection, by the way—President Wilson, like many southerners, *really* didn't want Black women to vote. So a huge suffrage march in Washington the day before he officially became president would definitely get his attention.

The march was also a great way to get people interested in the suffrage movement again. Newspapers wanted photos of the floats and bands and banners as they processed down Pennsylvania Avenue. Even the usually anti-suffrage *New York Times* called it "one of the most impressively beautiful spectacles ever staged in this country." Young women who had never been involved in the movement before wanted to help organize and plan and participate. After years of incremental progress and constant frustration, suffragists felt like they were finally *doing* something.

Make it work when everything goes wrong.
As it happened, the 1913 march did not go at all according to plan. A huge crowd gathered to watch, so huge, in fact, that people spilled into the street and blocked the parade route. Pennsylvania Avenue was, and still is, a very broad street with wide sidewalks. But so many people showed up that in many of the pictures from that day you can't see a single inch of pavement; it's just all humans,

shoulder to shoulder. And the humans are almost all men. They weren't there to support the suffrage parade—they were in town for the Wilson inauguration the next day. And not all of them were friendly. They tripped the women as they marched, spit on them, called them names. About one hundred marchers were taken to the hospital with injuries. The police did very little to control the crowd, and in some cases they even joined in the tripping and the spitting and the name calling. It took the marchers hours of pushing and shouting and a little help from soldiers on horseback to finally get to the end of the parade route.

Alice Paul recognized right away that it was the best thing that could have happened. All those newspaper reporters who were there for beautiful photos now wrote long articles about how the crowd had been violent and rude, but the women had bravely marched on. People across the country read those articles and were disgusted that women were treated so badly simply for demanding the right to vote. Young women who had never seen the need to get involved in suffrage started to see that this was a movement that mattered and they could help accomplish its goals. That one day in 1913 gave a languishing cause a much-needed shot in the arm and really marked the beginning of the final push for the Nineteenth Amendment.

Paul and Burns, flush with the success of their march, wanted to continue to use bold, attention-getting tactics to keep the suffrage cause energized. This made the leaders at the NAWSA very nervous. They had worked for years to get the men in power to respect them as smart, reasonable advocates. They worried that more aggressive stunts borrowed from the British movement would undermine their credibility and make more enemies than allies. Paul and Burns didn't want to break the law and pursue violence and destruction, but they didn't want to be quiet and polite all the time either. Finally they split from the NAWSA organization and formed their own group, eventually known as the National Woman's Party. For the next several years, they planned headline-grabbing activities, including building a booth at the 1915 World's Fair in San Francisco, creating a national petition some claimed was several miles long, and taking a cross-country road trip in a car they called the Suffrage Flier. And between 1910 and 1915, seven more states gave women the right to vote: Washington, California, Arizona, Kansas, Oregon,

Montana, and Nevada. Illinois allowed women to vote for president only.

But 1916 was disappointing. Woodrow Wilson was re-elected despite his continued opposition to a constitutional amendment allowing women to vote. Several states had suffrage on the ballot in 1916, but not a single one of them passed it. And Inez Milholland, one of the National Woman's Party's brightest leaders and its boldest public speaker, collapsed onstage while giving a suffrage speech in California. She died a few weeks later. The movement had hit another frustrating impasse.

TAKE RISKS—AND BE WILLING TO PAY THE CONSEQUENCES. It was once again time to do something bold. Harriot Stanton Blatch, who was just as fearless as her mother, Elizabeth Cady Stanton, proposed a daring and terrifying idea. The women would stand every day at the White House gate, not marching, not making speeches, just standing there with banners that said things like "Mr. President, how long must women wait for liberty?" and "Mr. President, what will you do for woman suffrage?" Today, this idea does not seem that radical. If you go visit the White House now, you are guaranteed to see a few protesters with provocative signs. But this was the very first time anyone had picketed the White House. Starting in January 1917, the National Woman's Party sent out picketers every day, no matter the weather, to stand at the gates and remind President Wilson that women still could not vote in most of the nation.

The pickets certainly succeeded in getting attention for the suffrage cause. For the first few months, the crowds passing by were more or less supportive, if a little confused. Women came from all over the country to take their turns as "Silent Sentinels." With some critical exceptions, the newspapers loved it and ran long articles with excellent photographs. The police more or less ignored the pickets.

But as 1917 progressed, and the US became more and more involved in World War I, some women thought it was time for the pickets to end. Criticizing the president so publicly was bound to make people mad in wartime, when it would be seen as un-American, even treasonous. But the pickets kept going. One of the main reasons Wilson gave for involving the US in WWI was that we had to fight to ensure democracy around the globe. The women found this totally hypocritical—how could

President Wilson talk about the importance of democracy abroad while ignoring the fact that half of the US population couldn't participate in democracy at home?

Public opinion started to turn against the picketers. Now the crowds passing by were less friendly—some even tore the picket signs from the women's hands and knocked them to the ground. The police didn't bother to stop them. The women responded by making more signs, including ones that criticized President Wilson even more directly. Finally President Wilson had enough and asked the police to get the women off the sidewalk in front of his house. The problem was, they weren't breaking any laws. They were standing on a public street corner with signs, which is totally legal. Eventually the police made up a charge: obstructing the traffic on the sidewalk. They started arresting the women and sending them to jail. The pickets kept up, day after day. The jail sentences got longer. The women kept picketing. Just as Alice Paul had done in England, the women who were in jail the longest went on hunger strikes and eventually were brutally force fed.

Then one night in November 1917, a group of suffragists was arrested and sent to the Occoquan Workhouse in Virginia. The guards there threw them into concrete jail cells. One woman slammed her head and passed out. Her cellmate thought she was dead and, in her panic, had a heart attack. Lucy Burns, who was among the group, started calling out names in the dark, checking to see if everyone was all right. She refused to stop when the guards ordered her to be quiet, so they chained her with her arms above her head all night. All of that, just for standing on the sidewalk with signs.

Being bold is not easy, and you have to be willing to take the risk. Sometimes being bold means doing something pretty scary, like picketing the White House and going to jail. Less dramatically, sometimes being bold means a huge amount of work, like the 1913 parade. You have to have a realistic sense of what you're getting into. But if your cause is stuck, and you are getting bored and frustrated, it can be exactly what you have to do to get the energy and attention you need.

DON'T ALWAYS DO WHAT YOU'RE TOLD

IF YOU'RE LUCKY, YOU WILL LIKE AND RESPECT YOUR fellow activists. There might also be times when they drive you crazy. There will be small disagreements, perhaps over how to set up an event. And medium disagreements; for example, maybe over the best way to work with a partner organization. Those kinds of disputes are common, and if you have decent judgment and some willingness to compromise, we are confident you can work them out. But every so often, you might find yourself fundamentally disagreeing with decisions being made by others in your cause. And then you have to decide: Do you make a clear argument for your point of view but then let it go? Do you ignore your colleagues and do what you think is right? Or do you leave?

If reform movements worked like professional sports teams, Frances Ellen Watkins Harper would get drafted in the first round. A famous writer and author of protest poetry, she was also a dynamic speaker and all-around workhorse. Like most of the great women activists of her age, she started as an abolitionist before moving on to temperance and suffrage work. Harper was easily one of the most influential Black women of the nineteenth century, essentially the Godmother of Black Feminism. But because there were no national Black women's organizations when she was in her prime (local for sure, but not national), she spent much of her life belonging to organizations primarily composed of white women. It was definitely a balancing act.

Born free in Maryland in 1825 and orphaned at age three, she was sent to live with her uncle William Watkins, who ran one of the most prestigious academies for freedmen in the state. While there she studied mathematics, Greek, Latin, and rhetoric, which taught her how to win in a fight with words. She wrote her first book of poetry at age twenty, and her second volume was so popular that it went through numerous editions, with over 10,000 copies in print.

From an early age, Harper was passionate about reform issues. She helped out for a brief time on the Underground Railroad before taking a job in 1854 as an anti-slavery speaker, traveling for six years through the free states and Midwest. Young and whip smart, she left audiences in awe everywhere she went. One journalist wrote, "Seldom have we heard a more cogent, forcible, and eloquent lecture upon any subject, especially from a woman." Her powerful essays and poems like "Bury Me in a Free Land" and "The Slave Mother" helped build her reputation with both Black and white audiences as a persuasive and important thinker.

Figure out how to make changes from the inside. After the Civil War, Harper joined the American Woman Suffrage Association and the Woman's Christian Temperance Union. She was an officer and prized member in both organizations, but despite her clear talents she didn't break through into the very top leadership ranks. Still, Harper didn't give up, and because of her reputation she was invited to a lot of important conferences. In rooms filled with mostly white women, Harper spoke passionately about the impact of race and issues affecting Black women. It wasn't easy to do (then or now), but she was convinced that representation was important. She encouraged young Black women to become more visible, even suggesting they attend the fortieth anniversary of Seneca Falls.

Harper was especially active in the WCTU. She was a member for over thirty years, ten of those as an elected superintendent. Unfortunately her title didn't come with a salary, so she supported herself in part with her earnings as a writer (it is estimated that at one point she had over 100,000 books in print). She traveled extensively through the South talking to freedmen and saw firsthand how hard their lives were. Since most women's clubs in the South were strictly segregated by race, Harper lobbied Willard to look into the integration of WCTU chapters. At the same time, she defended the creation of separate auxiliary chapters for African American women, where they could hold leadership positions and endorse issues that were especially important to the Black community. Many of the local groups she worked with became eager supporters of women's suffrage. It was during this time that she wrote the humorous poem "John and Jacob— A Dialogue on Woman's Rights," which featured two African American men debating whether women should be able to vote.

JACOB

But, John, I think for women's feet
The poll's a dreadful place;
To vote with rough and brutal men
Seems like a deep disgrace.

JOHN

But, Jacob, if the polls are vile
Where women shouldn't be seen
Why not invite them in to help
Us men to make them clean?

Over time, however, Harper found it harder and
harder to get her voice heard in primarily white organizations. She was unsuccessful in her effort to get the
national WCTU to condemn lynching and come out in
favor of suffrage for African American women. In 1890,
when the WCTU reorganized, Harper's high-profile
position disappeared. And as more suffrage groups tried
to win over white southerners to the cause, they ignored
or actively erased the contributions of Black women. Soon,
however, a new generation of Black women activists was
ready to take over.

**DON'T WAIT FOR PERMISSION; DO WHAT YOU THINK IS
RIGHT.** Younger Black suffragists respected Harper, but
they were tired of waiting for change, especially Ida B.
Wells. She was tiny—not even five feet tall—but Wells
was *fierce.* Her grandson once said, "She didn't suffer fools

and she saw fools everywhere." She was born into slavery in 1862, less than one year before emancipation. Both her parents died of yellow fever when Ida was just a teenager, and she had to take care of her siblings. But she managed to find time to take classes at Fisk University, and she supported the family by working as a teacher. As a Black woman, she faced discrimination everywhere. Generations before Rosa Parks refused to give up her seat on the bus, Wells refused to move to the "Colored" section of a train from Memphis to Nashville. She even bit the conductor's hand. She was kicked off the train. She sued the train company and won, but the verdict was overturned. Furious with the injustice, she wrote blistering anti-racism articles in local newspapers, eventually becoming editor and part owner of a newspaper in Memphis.

In 1892, Wells started writing articles about lynching, a form of violence used to terrorize Black communities. White mobs murdered African Americans in public spectacles, often targeting people who were accused of minor social transgressions or who simply asserted their rights. She became very well known, earning praise, criticism, and alarmingly regular death threats. Wells got into a heated public exchange with Frances Willard, criticizing the WCTU for invoking racist stereotypes about Black men. She eventually prevailed and shamed Willard and the WCTU into passing an anti-lynching resolution.

Like a lot of female activists, Wells realized women needed the vote if male politicians were ever going to take them seriously. Because the existing suffrage groups were not always welcoming to Black members, Wells formed the Alpha Suffrage Club for African Americans in Chicago in 1913. One of the first actions Wells took as club president was to travel to Washington to march in the 1913 suffrage parade alongside dozens of other women from Illinois.

Meanwhile, some women at Howard University were trying to figure out how to become more politically active. Then as now, Howard was a very well-respected historically Black university in Washington, DC. A group of female undergraduates there was frustrated that the biggest sorority on campus focused more on social parties than on political ones. In January 1913, the women formed Delta Sigma Theta, a new sorority dedicated to women's advancement and public service. One of their advisors was Mary Church Terrell, an activist and teacher in Washington, DC. Like Wells, Terrell helped form the National Association of Colored Women and the National Association for the Advancement of Colored People. Terrell was born into a wealthy family; in fact, some say her father was the first Black millionaire in America. At a time when few Americans had a college degree, Terrell had a master's degree. She spoke several languages fluently (she once gave a speech in Berlin three times in succession, first in German, then in English, and finally in French). She firmly believed suffrage was the best way to elevate the status of Black women in America. White suffragists, many of whom were very attuned to distinctions of race and class, found Terrell "acceptable" because of her education and wealth. She was often the only woman of color invited to NAWSA meetings. Terrell would use these opportunities to remind her fellow activists to keep the needs of Black women on the suffrage agenda. As their very first public act, Terrell and the Deltas wanted to march with the other college women in the 1913 parade.

When Alice Paul heard about this plan, she panicked. Ida B. Wells marching with the Illinois delegation was alarming enough, but now a whole sorority from Howard? Paul was convinced she'd lose the support of hundreds of white women if Black women were allowed to march alongside them. Although the movement had reunited under the NAWSA banner in 1890, the compromise was still tenuous, and race was the underlying issue in their split. Would holding an integrated parade expose all those rifts lying just below the surface? She waffled. She made excuses. She didn't even write back to the Delta Sigma Theta women for a week, which was highly unusual for the prompt and organized Paul. Finally the word came down from NAWSA headquarters: all women are welcome to participate in this parade.

So Paul issued what she thought was a compromise: Black women could march, but only in a segregated group at the back. Ida B. Wells was incensed, as were Mary Church Terrell and the Deltas. But they did not quit. Instead, they did what they wanted to all along. Ida B. Wells joined the audience of spectators on Pennsylvania Avenue. When the Illinois delegation marched past, she slipped out of the crowd and took her place with them, between two white friends. Apparently the Deltas, too, elbowed their way into the march with the other college students. All of these women remained dedicated to the suffrage cause. Wells continued to fight for suffrage and organized Black women across the Midwest. Terrell joined the White House pickets in 1917. And in 2013, the Deltas led the parade to commemorate the hundredth anniversary of the suffrage march.

KNOW WHEN IT IS TIME TO LEAVE. After the success of the 1913 parade in Washington, DC, Alice Paul and Lucy Burns wanted to plan more large, attention-grabbing events. They also wanted to focus on getting a constitutional amendment passed, instead of the slow, steady state-by-state strategy the movement had been following for years. The leaders of the NAWSA were not on board. They worried too many public stunts would hurt their credibility. They fretted that the amendment campaign would alienate southern states, where local politicians were still mad about the amendments passed after the Civil War. Alice Paul and Lucy Burns tried to change the leaders' minds, but ran into a brick wall. Finally, they decided they had to leave the NAWSA to pursue their goals. The NAWSA was more than happy to see them go. They formed their own organization, which would eventually be known as the National Woman's Party (NWP). The NAWSA and the NWP competed with each other for members, funding, and national attention. They even criticized each other in the press, despite working toward the same goal.

It hurts our Girl Power hearts to read about these women fighting with one another, but looking back, this split might have actually helped the cause. A political movement needs both radical and mainstream voices to move forward. The activists on the fringes of a movement take risks, push the agenda, and grab attention while the mainstream majority does the constant, steady work to pass legislation, recruit supporters, and sway public opinion. Plus, a radical edge always serves to make the rest of the movement look more reasonable by comparison. During the suffrage fight, congressmen could say, "I'd never talk to that crazy Alice Paul, but Carrie Chapman Catt seems like a nice lady." NAWSA lobbyists got to meet with many male leaders by promising not to act like those militant NWP women.

And the advantage works both ways. The NWP was free to take huge risks like picketing the White House and criticizing the president because the NAWSA continued to build support and goodwill. The NAWSA was always the much bigger and better funded of the two groups. If they weren't there, fighting state by state for voting rights and women's equality, the NWP would look like just a tiny fringe group of women pushing controversial tactics. No movement will survive with just a radical or just a moderate branch. To change the world, you need both.

It's never easy or comfortable when you find yourself disagreeing with the leaders of your cause. Ask yourself some basic questions, starting with "How much do I care about winning this argument?" The answer might be "Not very much." But if your answer is "I care a whole lot—I am willing to die on this hill" (metaphorically, we hope), then you have some decisions to make. Can you let your fellow activists know how you feel but accept their decision? Is this worth leaving over? Or maybe you can steal a secret from the suffragists and find a way to support your cause wholeheartedly while you do what you think is right.

PAY ATTENTION TO HOW THINGS LOOK

A PICTURE IS WORTH A THOUSAND WORDS. OK, THIS IS incredibly clichéd and we're almost embarrassed to write it, but that doesn't make it any less true. With so many things competing for our attention, sometimes a few seconds is all you get to make an impression. This is where the right image can make a huge difference for your cause. If you want good TV coverage, or a lot of attention on social media, you have to consider how things look.

The optics of your cause may seem like a concern of the digital age, something that previous activists didn't have to consider. And it is true that images have never traveled as quickly or as widely as they do now. But they have always been vital, and many of the suffragists were masters at constructing the perfect visual.

PUT ON A GOOD SHOW. Take, again, the 1913 suffrage parade in Washington, DC. Every little bit of that parade was designed to look impressive to the live audience, from the purple-and-gold banners to the splendid, if slightly odd, allegorical floats to the matching costumes worn by nurses, teachers, and writers. But the crowds of people on Pennsylvania Avenue were only a small fraction of the ultimate audience for the suffragists' message. Many more people would see photographs of the parade in the nation's newspapers. Photographs then were all black and white; those gorgeous purple-and-gold banners wouldn't look very impressive. In crowd shots of marching women, each figure would be too small for the details of her costume to be visible. For the newspapers, there had to be a few striking close-up shots of dramatic, eye-catching sights.

Alice Paul knew this very well and made sure the photographers had plenty of subjects. There was an elaborate pageant on the steps of the US Treasury Building. It represented a somewhat awkward allegory that didn't have much to do with suffrage, and very little of the crowd actually got to see it. But the women performing the pageant—some in togas, some in armor, some surrounded by children and balloons and at least one live dove—featured prominently in the newspaper coverage.

KNOW YOUR AUDIENCE. One of the most famous pictures from that day shows Inez Milholland, a white woman, atop a white horse as she prepares to lead the parade. She wears a flowing white cape and a starred crown, Wonder Woman style. Now, Inez Milholland was a labor lawyer and a very accomplished professional. But the male reporters at the time never failed to mention how pretty she was. They routinely called her "the most beautiful suffragist." Alice Paul decided to use this to the advantage of the cause. The press insisted on talking about how attractive Inez was instead of how smart she was, so maybe if she wore a white cape on a white horse, stuck a star on her forehead, and led the parade, everyone would take her picture. Years later, when Inez Milholland collapsed during a suffrage speech and died a martyr to the cause, the image of her on horseback would be romanticized on posters and pamphlets until it took on an almost holy aspect.

MAKE YOUR MESSAGE EASY TO READ AND UNDERSTAND.
As you can imagine, visuals were a huge part of the National Woman's Party strategy to picket the White House in 1917. A small group of women, bundled up in winter coats, with the grand home of the president rising up above the fence behind them—it makes a pretty good picture. But the women also carried banners with dark

letters on a light background, in easy-to-read fonts, that would not only be visible to passersby in Washington, but look clear and bold in photographs.

When Russian diplomats met with President Wilson in June 1917, NWP picketers stood by with a special banner addressed "To the Russian Envoys." It was probably far too wordy for the Russians to read as they drove through the White House gates, even if their English skills were excellent. It was even a little hard to read if you were standing a few feet away. But it was exactly the kind of message—new, provocative—that would go viral on social media today. Instead it did the twentieth-century equivalent and showed up in photos on the front pages of newspapers across the country.

CRAFT YOUR OWN IMAGE, OR OTHERS WILL DO IT FOR YOU. Even back in the 1800s, Sojourner Truth was extremely careful about the image she presented. In the course of her life, she sat for at least fourteen studio photographs (which, pre iPhone, was a LOT of photos), and she put a great deal of thought into how she was portrayed. Unfortunately, abolitionist societies tended to depict enslaved African Americans kneeling and half naked (the more pitiful-looking the better). In her photographic portraits, Truth was always well dressed and formally posed, frequently with knitting or a book as a prop. While Truth didn't accept money in speaking fees, she did sell her photos as souvenirs to help support herself and her preaching. This helped her image become more widely known, both in her lifetime and long after.

Photography wasn't the only visual medium the suffragists exploited. Both sides made great use of editorial cartoons. The anti-suffragists drew women's rights activists as old, wart-faced battle-axes. They published a whole slew of cartoons predicting inevitable doom for the American family if women got the vote. These are generally some variation on a wailing baby and a wide-eyed husband looking overwhelmed by a mountain of laundry and dishes while the selfish mother leaves them behind to go to the polls.

But the suffrage cause had several very talented artists on their side, most notably Nina Allender. Allender joined the NAWSA as an organizer and speaker. But she was also a talented painter and found she could use art, specifically cartooning, to promote the cause in a new way. When the NWP started publishing their newsletter,

The Suffragist, Allender's cartoons appeared on the cover of almost every issue. She created a figure known as the "Allender Girl," a vibrant American woman who represented what a modern suffragist could be. Suffragists had been mocked for years as old maids in fussy blouses. The Allender Girl was completely different—young, stylish, and modern, she was someone readers actually wanted to be like. Nina Allender's drawings went a long way toward replacing the public image of the suffragist from the tired, graying earlier generation to a new one that was optimistic and ready to change the world.

SOMETIMES A LITTLE STAGECRAFT IS CALLED FOR.
In 1872, Susan B. Anthony was arrested for voting. She wasn't the only woman to go to the polls that presidential election—quite a few did, including Sojourner Truth—although most women were turned away (not always nicely). But inspectors in Rochester had actually allowed Anthony to vote (for which they were later sent to jail). Her actions made the papers, and she was soon summoned by a United States commissioner. When she deliberately ignored his "invitation," a clearly embarrassed deputy marshal showed up at her house to arrest her.

Despite her best efforts, Anthony couldn't get him to put handcuffs on her, although she stretched out her hands in front of her.

At her trial, the judge refused to give Anthony a chance to speak in her defense and told the jury that they had to find her guilty. He then asked Anthony if she had any reason why the sentence should not be pronounced. Predictably, she had quite a few things she was determined to say, despite his interrupting her (six times) and ordering her to stop talking and to sit down. At last he fined her $100, which she promptly announced she had no intention of paying. Now normally, if you don't pay a court fine, you go to jail, but the judge stated that she would not serve her time until she paid. Not very logical, but he probably wanted to avoid generating more publicity (too late) and keep her from being able to take the case to the Supreme Court (in this he succeeded). After the trial, she printed out thousands of copies of the proceedings, some of which she sent to members of Congress. For the rest of her life, she would often begin her speeches by saying "I stand before you as a convicted criminal!" The fact that she was a middle-aged woman with spectacles (and later an elderly woman with white hair) and hardly looked threatening would have only made the whole affair more ridiculous. She never paid a dime.

When NWP members were arrested for picketing the White House, many of them were sent to serve their time at the workhouse in Occoquan, Virginia. There was a lot to hate about the workhouse, including worm-ridden food, freezing buildings, and a superintendent known for his cruelty. But the women really hated the itchy, ill-fitting uniforms they were forced to wear. In her memoir *Jailed for Freedom,* NWP activist Doris Stevens wrote, "The thick unbleached muslin undergarments are of designs never to be forgotten! And the thick stockings and forlorn shoes!" The women saw those horrible uniforms as a symbol of their unfair treatment, a power-ful sign that they were treated like criminals despite the fact (and we can't say this enough) that *they broke no laws.* After they were released from jail, the women went on a speaking tour around the country to tell their stories. They called it the "Prison Special." They traveled the nation giving speeches and recruiting new activists to their cause. And they wore, you guessed it, replicas of those awful prison uniforms. Presumably with better shoes. Suffragists who had been to jail were also allowed to wear a special pin, designed by Nina Allender, which looked like a jail cell door.

When you spend a lot of time crafting your message and marshalling your best arguments, it can be easy to forget the visual part of your story. Intentional imagery isn't an extra—it's not something added on to your message. *It is a vital part of your message.* And if you want people to pay attention, especially people who aren't focused on you, the right visual can catch even the most distracted eye. So pay attention to how things look, and make sure the visuals work in your favor.

DO YOUR HOMEWORK

WE LIKE A GOOD PROTEST MARCH AS MUCH AS ANYONE, and bold, attention-grabbing moves are essential. But you can't have a movement made up only of publicity stunts. They are not a substitute for clear and thorough organization, effective management, and impeccable research. You have to do your homework.

The National Woman's Party was known for its aggressive tactics. Plenty of critics dismissed the group as all style and no substance. But almost everything the NWP did was based on invaluable research. Over the years, they steadily amassed a huge database of information, kept on meticulously maintained index cards, about every member of Congress. This card index listed where each man stood on suffrage and quoted anything he said on the subject. The cards listed information like the names of his wife and children, where he went to college, organizations he belonged to, whether any of his relatives were suffragists, and any relevant personal qualities. For instance, a card might note that a certain senator always arrived at work early, and 7:30 was the best time to find him at his desk. Here's a typical entry, written for Congressman

James Covington of Maryland in 1915: "Morals above reproach. He loves his home. His weak points are that he is selfish, cold and afraid to take a stand."

With over twenty cards for each member of Congress, the index eventually filled a small room at NWP headquarters, where it was updated every time someone died, retired, lost his election, or changed his mind. Rumors even started that the women had hired detectives to ferret out dirt on elected officials. But the truth was much less scandalous and much more exhausting: the details came from countless phone calls, meetings, parties, speeches, and lobbying trips throughout the long years of the push for a federal amendment.

All that work paid off in 1918 and 1919 as the federal amendment finally came up for a real vote in Congress (several votes, as it turned out). NWP members used the information they had gathered on those cards to get just a few politicians to change their minds—and that was, ultimately, all it took. Even the *New York Times*, which had been unapologetically anti-suffrage for years, had to give the Congressional Card Index its due. "To the index, and the machinery it sets to work, chief credit is given for the gains in votes in favor of the amendment," the *Times* sniffed in early 1919.

LEARN HOW TO ASK FOR MONEY. Organization is also vital when it comes to fundraising. Every cause needs money. It doesn't solve all your problems, but it really helps. Unfortunately, asking people for money is many activists' absolute least favorite task. Susan B. Anthony spent a huge amount of time fundraising, including six years paying off the debt from the failed newspaper *The Revolution.* She sought out very small contributions from anyone she could. The whole time she hated it. "More than half of my spiritual, intellectual, and physical strength has been expended in the anxiety over getting the money to pay for the Herculean work that has been done in our movement," she complained. The constant lack of funds made life for the first generation of suffragists so much harder and forced them into some dicey moral compromises.

Years later, Alice Paul also exhausted herself raising contributions a few dollars at a time. She had all kinds of strategies for attracting new donors. She knew people were most likely to give money if they could see what their money was being used for. In 1915, she told one national organizer not to spend any money on a telephone, but instead to make a big production of what a pain it was to use a public call box. She reasoned that when local supporters understood the inconvenience, they might be willing to chip in. Dollar by hard-fought dollar, the money added up.

While a lot of small contributions can make a movement look popular and broad, the suffrage movement learned pretty quickly that cultivating a few big donors made a lot of difference. The NAWSA was well funded by Katharine McCormick, while the NWP received the majority of its budget from Alva Belmont. Neither woman was content to be a hands-off donor who simply wrote the occasional check. Both demanded a voice in strategy and leadership decisions, sometimes in opposition to the organizations' actual leaders. It must have been a relief for Carrie Chapman Catt and the NAWSA when their biggest donor, Miriam Folline Peacock Squier Leslie Wilde, died and left them her entire $2 million estate. Finally they were free from worrying about money, and their donor had the good grace to be too dead to meddle.

TRAIN YOUR VOLUNTEERS. Another worthwhile, if not very exciting, investment of your time is to train your fellow activists thoroughly. We know, it sounds tedious, but it is incredibly important. In later years, as the numbers of suffragists grew, new generations of volunteers would be taught to speak on street corners where they could attract a crowd. Along the way, they learned how to deal with troublemakers too. One suffragist was being heckled by a man in the crowd who yelled out to her, "How would you like to be a man?" "Not much" was her quick reply. "How would you?"

Frances Willard created manuals for local WCTU chapters (titled *Hints and Helps in our Temperance Work*) and later ones for girls and boys explaining how to become politically active. She cloaked her advice in comforting, familiar language and covered all the details—these are the flowers you should use to decorate your meeting, this is how to send an invitation to your pastor to attend your temperance gathering. Her user-friendly instructions brought a whole new group of women into political activism.

In the 1917 White House pickets, for instance, nothing was left to chance. The women knew what to wear, which order to walk in, how to stand, and who was in charge. They practiced what to do if the police gave them a hard time. They rehearsed statements to the press and decided who would deliver them. Everyone agreed in advance that if they were arrested, they would seek maximum public sympathy by taking jail time instead of paying a fine. As their jail sentences got longer and longer, they learned how to demand political prisoner status and when to go on hunger strikes. Not all of this came easily. There were women who dreaded public speaking or were terrified of spending even a minute in jail. But with careful preparation and training, each had their talking points and plans to cover whatever came their way. The NWP tried very hard to never send a woman out to do something she feared without preparation and support.

STEAL IDEAS THAT WORK. This thorough preparation was something Alice Paul had learned as a young activist in England from Emmeline Pankhurst and her militant suffragettes. (By the way, "suffragette" was a term embraced by some British activists. The American women were "suffragists.") Stealing good ideas from other movements or other people you think are smart and effective is also often worthwhile. Alice Paul took lots of effective ideas from Emmeline Pankhurst, including wearing white in parades to look great in pictures, wearing prison uniforms with pride, seeking political prisoner status, and going on hunger strikes.

Paul also swiped some ideas that didn't work that well, most notably opposing all Democrats, even pro-suffrage Democrats, in the 1914 and 1916 elections. The idea was that since the Democrats controlled the presidency, the House of Representatives, and the US Senate, they should take responsibility for making their leaders pass suffrage nationwide. This "party in power" strategy made much more sense when Pankhurst tried it in England's parliamentary system. In the representative democracy of the United States, it made many more enemies than friends. If you are going to steal an idea from someone else, make sure it actually works for you.

BUILD YOUR NETWORKS. Excellent training and organization were certainly not limited to the NWP. Once the federal amendment finally passed both houses of Congress in June of 1919, it went to the states for ratification. That's when the organizational strength of the NAWSA took over, with its vast network of state organizations all over the country. The driving force behind this massive network was the supremely confident Carrie Chapman Catt, who had been handpicked by Susan B. Anthony to take over as president of the NAWSA. Anthony had been compared to Napoleon by her peers because of her ability to strategize and see the big picture, and Anthony knew the importance of finding a great general.

Back in 1916, Catt revealed her "Winning Plan" for women's suffrage, which she insisted that at least thirty-six state NAWSA chapters adopt. She didn't pull that number out of thin air—thirty-six was the minimum number of states needed to ratify an eventual federal amendment. Thanks to Catt's foresight, by the summer of 1920, all those state chapters had offices on the ground, filled with leaders, networks, political knowledge, favors owed, goodwill, bank accounts, and even the phone numbers of dozens of reporters. And it's a good thing she had them all in place by the summer of 1919 because they were in for the fight of their lives when ratification rolled around.

Taking the time for research, training, and building networks can feel really boring and pointless. It can feel, in other words, just like homework. But whenever you are tempted to skip it, picture yourself face-to-face with someone who doesn't support your cause. This person makes a cogent, reasonable argument against you. And you don't know what to say. You haven't rehearsed those arguments. You stand there feeling embarrassed and foolish, kicking yourself for not being better prepared. It feels, in other words, like being called on by the teacher when you didn't do your homework. If you want to be a successful activist, do your homework. Trust us, it matters.

RECRUIT THE ALLIES YOU NEED

No matter how hard you are willing to work for change, sometimes you can't do it all by yourself. Especially if you want to do big things and you want to do them peacefully (as opposed to violent revolution, which we aren't recommending), at some point you need the cooperation of those in power. This is not only true for women's suffrage— most American movements to expand civil rights have eventually had to work together with the people in charge.

Here is an important truth. Women could never have gotten the Nineteenth Amendment passed without men. Period. Women worked for decades to get the right to vote, but at the end of the day they couldn't just give it to themselves. They had to convince men, especially the overwhelmingly white elected representatives who passed the laws, but also the mostly white male voters who had put those guys in office.

While men didn't take the lead roles in the suffrage story, at key times and in the final hour they made a big difference. We don't think their involvement is something to be downplayed; we think it makes the final outcome even more impressive.

START WITH THE PEOPLE YOU KNOW. From the beginning, men got involved for the same reason that most people get involved in a cause—they had a personal connection. To be sure, a lot of them thought it was the right thing to do. Absolutely. But they also signed on because it was important to the women they knew—their wives, sisters, mothers, sweethearts, daughters, friends, and fellow activists. This is true throughout the entire history of the suffrage movement.

Going all the way back to 1848, there were men at the first Woman's Rights Convention in Seneca Falls. Originally it was supposed to be ladies only, but quite a few husbands had tagged along with their wives, and when the women saw that the men were sympathetic, they were allowed in. Lucretia Mott's husband, James Mott, even helped chair the meeting. On the first day of the convention, only the women participated in the discussion (probably a new experience for the men). On the second day, the men were allowed to comment as well, which turned out to be important because of what one man said.

Frederick Douglass came to the gathering because he was a friend of one of the women organizers. He had been enslaved and knew what it was like to be powerless.

He was also friends with Lucretia Mott and other women abolitionists, and he had seen how effective they were and how unfairly they were treated. When it looked like Elizabeth Cady Stanton's "ridiculous" suffrage resolution would fail, he stood up. Women, he declared, were born equal to men. No custom or law could change that. Any rights men could claim women should have as well. As he would later write, "Seeing that the male governments of the world have failed, it can do no harm to try the experiment of a government by man and woman united." His powerful speech swayed the crowd, and the resolution passed (just barely), ultimately making history. In the end, of the one hundred original signers of the Declaration of Sentiments, thirty-two of them were male.

Douglass was proud to be an ally and said, "When I advocated for emancipation, it was for my people. But when I stood up for the rights of women, self was out of the question, and I found a little nobility in the act." For the rest of his life he championed the rights of women, lending his words—and star power—to the cause. He supported it with editorials in his paper, the *North Star*. He gave public speeches in favor of women's suffrage. He showed up for almost every national women's rights convention for the next fifty years. At the International Council of Women in 1888, he told the audience:

> She is her own best representative. We can neither speak for her, nor vote for her, nor act for her, nor be responsible for her; and the thing for men to do in the premises is just to get out of her way and give her the fullest opportunity to exercise all the powers inherent in her individual personality, and allow her to do it as she herself shall elect to exercise them. Her right to be and to do is as full, complete and perfect as the right of any man on earth. I say of her, as I say of the colored people, "Give her fair play, and hands off."

Even after his (extremely) painful split with Stanton and Anthony over the issue of Black male suffrage and the Fifteenth Amendment, Douglass later reconciled with his friends. Douglass and Stanton had a deep respect for each other, and a portrait of her hung in his private study at his home at Cedar Hill. And on February 20, 1895, in his last public appearance, he attended a meeting of the

National Council of Women in Washington, DC, where he was welcomed warmly to the stage by his old friend Susan B. Anthony and given a standing ovation by the crowd. He died later that night at home.

Some men were inspired to join the suffrage movement by their families. This was the case with a white man named Henry Blackwell, who was already comfortable with strong women. His five remarkable sisters were all professionals, including Elizabeth Blackwell, the first woman to graduate from medical school in the United States. And when Blackwell heard Lucy Stone speak for the first time, he was captivated. Stone, on the other hand, never intended to get married and was committed to a life of lecturing on abolition and suffrage. Blackwell pursued her patiently for nearly two years. Stone wasn't interested in flowers or gifts, so as part of his wooing he helped arrange a speaking tour. Finally, when he rescued a child from slavery, Stone realized she had found someone who felt as strongly about justice as she did.

As Stone's focus turned from abolition to women's equality, Blackwell followed her lead, starting with the vows he and Stone made at their wedding in 1855. In front of a small audience, he read a protest rejecting all legal "rights" he had to her body and property. No couple had ever done anything like this before, and papers across the country printed their vows. Stone became the first American woman to legally keep her own name after marrying. Together, she and Blackwell became role models for other couples who wanted to have an equal marriage. For a while, women who kept their names after marriage were known as "Lucy Stoners."

Blackwell also helped edit the *Woman's Journal*, the longest running women's suffrage paper, campaigned cross-country, and wrote pamphlets such as *Objections to Woman Suffrage Answered*. There were a lot of points in it—here are just a few:

> *Suffrage is not a right of anybody.*
> To say so is to deny the principles of the Declaration of Independence and the Bill of Rights. "Governments derive their just powers from the consent of the governed"—women are governed. "Taxation without representation is tyranny"—women are taxed. "Political power inheres in the people"—women are people.

It would diminish respect for women.
Voting is power. Power always commands respect.
To be weak is to be miserable. How many men
are tolerated in society only because they are rich
and powerful! Woman armed with the ballot will
be stronger and more respected than ever before.

It is contrary to the Bible.
Nowhere is it said in the Bible to women, "Thou
shalt not vote."

After Lucy Stone died in 1893, Blackwell spent the rest
of his life working for women's suffrage and, along with
daughter Alice Stone Blackwell, served as an officer of the
National American Woman Suffrage Association.

PUT YOUR FRIENDS TO WORK. At the turn of the
twentieth century, a new wave of men came along who
had grown up hearing about equal rights for women from
their mothers. Oswald Villard was the white publisher of
two major New York papers and came from a family of
activist royalty. His mother was the suffragist and peace
activist Fanny Garrison Villard, and his grandfather was

the famous abolitionist William Lloyd Garrison. In 1908 (after a strong hint from his mom), Villard started the Men's League for Woman Suffrage and recruited Max Eastman, who was also white, to organize the group. Eastman had even more ties to suffragists, including his mother, his sister, and his glamorous girlfriend, Inez Milholland (who rode the white horse in the 1913 parade).

Eastman got to work right away and recruited some of the most influential men in New York, the A-list of high society. Figuring (correctly) that they would be ridiculed for their stand, he promised not to release the names until he had over one hundred supporters. The league's mission statement noted, "There are many men who inwardly feel the justice of equal suffrage, but who are not ready to acknowledge it publicly, unless backed by numbers. There are other men who are not even ready to give the subject consideration until they see that a large number of men are willing to be counted in favor of it." Soon chapters sprung up in big cities such as Chicago and New York. The *Woman's Journal* published a plan to recruit more men. "Every man . . . should be personally asked to join the league by some woman he respects and esteems." By 1912, there were 20,000 members in the league nationally.

At first, Eastman and Villard didn't expect much from the Men's League. The idea was that the socially prominent New Yorkers would lend their names to the cause, but they wouldn't actually have to *do* anything. But to everyone's surprise, the men started to make a real difference. They held fundraisers, lobbied politicians, and spoke out for suffrage in public alongside their wives. Those who were publishers encouraged their papers to be more pro-suffrage, while those who were lawyers represented women who wound up in court. In 1912, over a thousand men marched at the end of a New York City suffrage parade, where they were mocked mercilessly by the crowds (in an anonymous article, one male marcher wrote about "the over 11,863" hecklers who told him to go wash dishes). But the men's presence inspired even more men to join the league. The growth of the league in New York and the social acceptance it represented was one of the reasons that the New York legislature passed women's suffrage for New York in 1917, a major victory for the movement!

Use your influence. As the suffragists inched closer to their goal, the fight became even harder. This is where they had to call on every connection and every friend they had in the final battle. As early as 1878, an amendment for women's suffrage had been introduced to Congress by Senator Aaron Sargent of California. His wife was a suffrage supporter, and they became friends with Susan B. Anthony when they were stranded together on a train. But amending the Constitution has always been unbelievably difficult, and although it would be introduced every year for the next forty years, it never went anywhere. But after the end of World War I, things were starting to look up. On January 10, 1918, after a special appeal by President Wilson (a reluctant convert to say the least), the House of Representatives was ready to try once again. To pass, it needed a two-thirds majority in both the House and Senate, and the suffragists were up in the galleries counting every vote.

The tension was high. Jeannette Rankin of Montana, the first woman elected to Congress, argued in favor of the amendment to much applause. Three congressmen came from their hospital beds to vote "aye" (one was actually carried in on a stretcher), and another from Tennessee arrived in horrible pain with an unset broken shoulder, determined to vote yes and to stay till the end to persuade any other members who might need encouragement. In perhaps the most moving case of all, Congressman Frederick Hicks from New York traveled from the bedside of his dying wife, who wanted him to vote for suffrage. It passed with one vote to spare, and when it reached the magic number needed (274), the women present started to sing out "*Praise God, from whom all blessings flow . . .*"

But after all the drama, the amendment failed in the Senate. It fell short by only one vote in May of 1918, and short by just two in February 1919. But Wilson, wanting to pass suffrage (and desperate to have it all over with), called a special session of Congress in May of 1919. Once again, after all their struggles, it was up to the legislators (this time all male, since Jeannette Rankin had left office). Finally on May 21, 1919, the House voted once again, and it passed with forty-two votes to spare. Two weeks later, it passed in the Senate with fifty-six for and twenty-five against. Now it was on to the states!

In 1919, there were forty-eight states in the Union, so thirty-six of them had to ratify the amendment for it to become law. At the start, states raced to see who could be the first to ratify (go Wisconsin!), but as time went on, it was clear that it would come down to the wire. Month by month, more states were added to the list, until finally, they needed just one more state. And then after March 1920, the momentum stopped with thirty-five states. There weren't many states left to decide, since many southern states had already rejected ratification. Then Tennessee agreed to hold a special session in August of 1920 to vote on the issue.

From the beginning, it was very close. People wore roses on their jackets to show who they supported— yellow roses for the suffragists, red roses for the anti-suffragists. There was intense lobbying on both sides and accusations that the liquor lobby was bribing elected officials with booze to get them to vote against ratification. Carrie Chapman Catt later wrote about legislators "reeling through the hall in a state of advanced intoxication." Several representatives who had previously been for ratification mysteriously changed their minds. The Tennessee Senate had quickly voted for it, so it was up to the House, where they only needed a majority of votes— but would they get it?

In the end, it all came down to the kind of dramatic

conclusion that wouldn't be out of place in a Hollywood movie. On August 18, the roll for a vote was called one last time, and it looked like it might be a tie. After all this time, and all these fights, down to the last chamber in the last state, and it's a TIE? That wouldn't be enough to ratify it, and suffrage would fail.

But at the very last minute, the youngest member of the all-white, all-male delegation, twenty-four-year-old Harry Burn, changed his mind. He was still wearing the red rose of the anti-suffrage supporters when he voted "Aye." What swayed this one crucial vote? Well, he had a letter from his mother, Febb Burn, which said, "Hurrah and vote for suffrage. And don't keep them in doubt." He later gave her all the credit, saying "I knew that a mother's advice is always safest for a boy to follow, and my mother wanted me to vote for ratification."

On August 26, 1920, the official results from Tennessee arrived in Washington. The suffrage amendment, exactly as written by Anthony and Stanton so many years ago, was now part of the United States Constitution. And it made it over the finish line because a mother wrote her son at the right time.

While men weren't the major players in the suffrage

story, at key times and in the final hour they made a big difference.

Given that women have been left out of so many of the histories written by men, you might still wonder (as some of our friends do), why give men space here?

For two reasons. First, we think it is important to remember that even people who don't obviously benefit from a cause can be moved to support it. When you are planning your strategy, don't overlook allies you will need because you assume they'll be against you. Find those that are sympathetic and do the work to get them on your side.

Also, everyone needs examples of how to behave and what to do, and we hope that these men will be role models not just for boys, but for everyone, in how to be a supportive ally. There are big challenges on the horizon that can't be solved alone. Now more than ever, we think it is important to look outside of our "own" interest and work together.

If you want to make a change, you need help from the people with power. Start recruiting influential allies using your own personal connections and then build from there. Get your partners actively involved so that it becomes their cause too. Let them know what you need from them and don't be afraid to call in favors. The suffrage movement was filled with people who weren't interested in the issue until they met someone who asked them to help. You can do that too.

CONCLUSION

IN THE END, VOTING ISN'T EVERYTHING.

Wait a minute. You've just read an entire book about all the heroic work that women did to get the right to vote, only to be told at the end that voting isn't everything? How can that possibly be true?

Don't get us wrong. Obviously, you should exercise your right to vote in every election you are qualified to vote in, and we mean EVERY. SINGLE. ELECTION. Yes, even the minor off-year school board ones. It is your responsibility if you are a citizen over eighteen and the least you can do to support our great shared experiment in democracy. Even if you aren't old enough to vote, you can still canvass for candidates and encourage eligible voters to head to the polls on election day.

That said, for all the work involved in passing the Nineteenth Amendment, having the right to vote isn't the whole story. It is just the first step.

When the Nineteenth Amendment officially became part of the Constitution on August 26, 1920, the suffragists celebrated like they'd been waiting for it their entire lives (they had). Carrie Chapman Catt of the NAWSA returned home to New York from Tennessee to a hero's welcome, with parades and congratulations from the governor and other dignitaries. At noon on August 28, the first Saturday after ratification, church bells rang, train whistles blew, and car horns honked around the nation. Men in Chicago were invited to tip their hats to welcome their new fellow voters. In the summer of 1919, Alice Paul had started sewing stars on a special banner each time a new state ratified the amendment, and when the word arrived about the thirty-sixth state, she sewed her last star and hung it from the balcony of NWP headquarters in Washington, DC, while a jubilant group of supporters cheered below.

The upcoming presidential election, just two months away, would be the first time that women everywhere in the country could vote—at least in theory—and no one knew quite what to expect. Would the country become a much better, more moral place like the suffragists hoped? Or would the anti-suffragists' predictions come true, and all of a sudden the divorce rate would soar and men would have to stay home doing laundry?

In November 1920, roughly 33 percent of the women

who could vote actually voted. As far as anyone could tell, they didn't vote all that differently from men. It was anything but earth shattering. The general reaction was something along the lines of "meh."

There were a lot of explanations for the disappointing numbers. Women weren't in the habit of voting (and this is true—it IS a habit). A significant minority of women didn't believe women should vote in the first place, so they probably didn't. And in a disturbing sign of the civil rights fight to come, women in Mississippi and Georgia deliberately weren't given enough time to register, basically to make sure Black women didn't vote. Making voting easy has rarely been a political priority. In fact, at times a LOT of effort has been put into making it difficult (almost impossible) for some groups to vote.

But low turnout isn't enough to explain why that first election didn't live up to the hype. Women still represented a significant expansion of the voting pool. So why didn't they have more of an impact?

A deeper reason, which is often overlooked, is that that simply voting isn't enough. Voting is only one tool of many that you can use to create change. You don't get to use it very often, usually just one Tuesday in November.

And as tools go, it is a pretty blunt because you don't get to attach a note saying "I voted this way because _____."

Believe it or not, most politicians are pretty responsive to what their constituents want because they (like most of us) want to keep their jobs. But when there are hundreds of different issues at stake, it isn't always clear what is most important to their voters. To have your vote be effective for change, you not only need to vote; you need to connect your vote LOUDLY and CLEARLY to the issues you care most about.

Right after the Nineteenth Amendment passed, both major political parties wanted the support of the new women voters. Just to be on the safe side, Congress reacted to this possible game change by quickly passing important laws that women had been lobbying for, such as the Sheppard-Towner Act, which provided federal money for maternity and child care. The act led to a significant decrease in the number of babies who died in childbirth. But it became obvious in the next few years that women weren't voting anyone in or out of office based on this kind of legislation; in fact, it appeared they were voting just like men. Congress took note and promptly lost interest in funding the Sheppard-Towner

Act. Despite having saved thousands of lives, it was repealed in 1929.

But there is a more positive reason why the political landscape after the election of 1920 didn't seem all that different. In the decades leading up to the Nineteenth Amendment, women—first a handful, then an army—had been flexing their political muscles. They had already begun to change things by speaking in public, lobbying and petitioning their elected representatives, giving interviews in the press, publishing their own newspapers, influencing public opinion, suggesting new laws, and (in those states that had suffrage before 1920) voting. Women's suffrage wasn't a giant leap; it was a hard-won next step—one with great potential.

But as gradual as the year-to-year changes may have seemed, the differences between 1848 and 1920 were huge—you just had to look back. As Anthony noted in a letter she wrote to Stanton in 1902, just days before Stanton died:

> We little dreamed when we began this contest, optimistic with the hope and buoyancy of youth, that half a century later we would be compelled to

leave the finish of the battle to another generation of women. But our hearts are filled with joy to know that they enter upon this task equipped with a college education, with business experience, with the fully admitted right to speak in public—all of which were denied to women fifty years ago. They have practically but one point to gain—the suffrage; we had all. These strong, courageous, capable young women will take our place and complete our work. There is an army of them where we were but a handful. Ancient prejudice has become so softened, public sentiment so liberalized and women have so thoroughly demonstrated their ability as to leave not a shadow of doubt that they will carry our cause to victory.

Just as the various suffrage groups chose different strategies to winning the vote, they went in different directions afterward. Ida B. Wells's Alpha Suffrage Club concentrated on registering Black voters and electing Black candidates in Illinois. Carrie Chapman Catt helped transform the NAWSA into the nonpartisan League of Women Voters, an organization that is still around today.

Their goal was to train and mobilize women to vote so they could have an impact on legislation. It took time, and it wasn't until the election of 1980 that the percentage of women voting was higher than the percentage of men voting. Today, women regularly vote in higher numbers than men, and in the presidential election of 2016, almost 10 million more women voted than men. Black women have become some of the most consistent voters of any ethnic group, defying decades of racism and voter suppression to participate at a rate 6 percent higher than the national average in 2018.

The National Woman's Party had a more specific goal. After ratification, they considered several options for their future (they did, after all, finally have the vote!), but instead they doubled down on getting equal rights for women across the board. In 1921, Alice Paul and Crystal Eastman followed the example of Susan B. Anthony and Elizabeth Cady Stanton and wrote a proposed amendment to the Constitution, the Equal Rights Amendment. But it is still waiting to pass. In 1972, it passed both the House and Senate and was sent to the states for ratification. Over the next five years, it was ratified by thirty-five states, but then stalled short of the required thirty-eight as opposition grew. Despite the recently renewed efforts today, it is still not part of the US Constitution.

If you really want to make change, you have to know what it is you want to accomplish. Don't depend on your vote to change everything, and don't think you have to wait for an election to make things happen. Use all your tools. By using your other rights guaranteed to you in the Constitution, namely your First Amendment right to free speech and a free press, to peaceably assemble, and to petition your government, you can actually get quite a bit done! You can make people aware of problems, shape public opinion, and convince lawmakers to pass new laws. You don't even have to be old enough to vote. You can get started now.

SOURCE NOTES

INTRODUCTION

p. xii: "Failure is impossible": quoted in Lynn Sherr, *Failure Is Impossible: Susan B. Anthony in Her Own Words* (New York: Times Books, 1995), 324.

CHAPTER 1

p. 7: "We want to . . . of somebody": quoted in Andrea Moore Kerr, *Lucy Stone: Speaking Out for Equality* (New Brunswick, NJ: Rutgers University Press, 1992), 60.

p. 11: "I am . . . can get it": Sojourner Truth, "Women's Rights Convention," *Anti-Slavery Bugle*, June 21, 1851, Chronicling America: Historic American Newspapers, Library of Congress, https://chroniclingamerica.loc.gov/lccn/sn83035487/1851-06-21 /ed-1/seq-4/.

p. 11: "And how came . . . your part?": ibid.

pp. 11–12: "It is impossible . . . truthful tones": quoted in Alison Piepmeier, *Out in Public: Configurations of Women's Bodies in Nineteenth-Century America* (Chapel Hill: University of North Carolina Press, 2004), 124.

p. 13: "And raising herself . . . ain't I a woman?" Frances Gage, "Ain't I a Woman?" *New York Independent*, April 23, 1863, quoted in the Sojourner Truth Project, https://www.thesojournertruthproject.com /compare-the-speeches/.

CHAPTER 2

p. 17: "remember the ladies": Abigail Adams to John Adams,

31 March–5 April 1776, Adams Family Papers: An Electronic Archive, Massachusetts Historical Society, https://www.masshist.org /digitaladams/archive/doc?id=L17760331aa.

p. 17: "more generous and favorable to them than your ancestors": ibid.

p. 20: "We hold these . . . created equal": *The First Convention Ever Called to Discuss the Civil and Political Rights of Women, Seneca Falls, N.Y., July 19, 20, 1848*, National American Woman Suffrage Association Collection, Library of Congress, https://www.loc.gov/item/27007548/.

p. 20: "He has compelled . . . wages she earns": ibid.

p. 21: "Lizzie, thee will make us ridiculous!": quoted in Sally McMillen, *Seneca Falls and the Origins of the Women's Rights Movement* (New York: Oxford University Press, 2009), 93.

p. 21: "That it is . . . elective franchise": *The First Convention Ever Called*.

pp. 21–22: "This bolt is . . . in our stockings?": quoted in Joe Starita, *A Warrior of the People: How Susan La Flesche Overcame Racial and Gender Inequality to Become America's First Indian Doctor* (New York: St. Martin's, 2016), 112.

p. 24: "She forged the thunderbolts and I fired them": quoted in "Tribute from Miss Anthony," *New York Times*, October 27, 1902, https://timesmachine.nytimes.com/timesmachine/1902/10/27 /101293533.html?pageNumber=1.

p. 25: "Believe in yourself . . . these forty years": quoted in Lynn Sherr, *Failure Is Impossible: Susan B. Anthony in Her Own Words* (New York: Times Books, 1995), 136.

CHAPTER 3

pp. 30–31: "to keep a house . . . into the service": Elizabeth Cady
Stanton, *Eighty Years and More: Reminiscences 1815–1897* (New York:
European Publishing Company, 1898), 145.

p. 32: "race, color, or previous condition of servitude": House Joint
Resolution proposing the 15th amendment to the Constitution,
December 7, 1868, Enrolled Acts and Resolutions of Congress,
1789–1999. General Records of the United States Government, RG 11,
National Archives.

p. 33: "Hisses, Cat-Calls, Yells, and Wild Demonstrations": quoted in
Geoffrey C. Ward and Ken Burns, *Not for Ourselves Alone: The Story
of Elizabeth Cady Stanton and Susan B. Anthony* (New York: Knopf,
1999), 118.

p. 34: "As much as white women need the ballot, colored women need
it more": quoted in Rosalyn Terborg-Penn, *African American Women
in the Struggle for the Vote, 1850–1920* (Bloomington: Indiana University
Press, 1998), 47.

p. 36: "A woman is . . . ten thousand men": quoted in Elizabeth Cady
Stanton, Susan B. Anthony, and Matilda Joslyn Gage, eds., *History of
Woman Suffrage, Volume I* (New York: Fowler & Wells, 1881), 804.

p. 37: "Women now stand . . . ends to serve": Massachusetts
Association Opposed to the Further Extension of Suffrage to Women
to Representative Edwin Y. Webb, April 12, 1910. Committee on
the Judiciary, Papers Accompanying Specific Bills and Resolutions,
HR61A-D8 (Folder HJ RES 151), 61st Congress. Records of the US
House of Representatives, RG 233, National Archives.

p. 37: "would be . . . a national policy": quoted in James H. Hutson, *To Make All Laws: The Congress of the United States, 1789–1989* (Washington, DC: Library of Congress, 1989), 70.

p. 40: "our work is . . . forward and back": Ann D. Gordon, ed., *The Selected Papers of Elizabeth Cady Stanton and Susan B. Anthony: An Awful Hush, 1895 to 1906* (New Brunswick, NJ: Rutgers University Press, 2013), 31.

p. 40: "Failure is impossible": quoted in Lynn Sherr, *Failure Is Impossible: Susan B. Anthony in Her Own Words* (New York: Times Books, 1995), 324.

It's Time to Talk About Racism

p. 44: "What will we . . . fathers?": quoted in Jerry Mikorenda, *America's First Freedom Rider: Elizabeth Jennings, Chester A. Arthur, and the Early Fight for Civil Rights* (Lanham, MD: Rowman & Littlefield, 2019), 204.

p. 46: "The question . . . of the South": quoted in Elna C. Green, *Southern Strategies: Southern Women and the Woman Suffrage Question* (Chapel Hill: University of North Carolina Press, 1997), 131.

p. 46: "The enfranchisement . . . honestly attained": quoted in Ida Husted Harper, ed., *History of Woman Suffrage: 1900–1920* (New York: Little & Ives, 1922), 5:82.

p. 46: "putting the ballot . . . your white women": quoted in Marjorie Spruill Wheeler, *New Women of the New South: The Leaders of the Woman Suffrage Movement in the Southern States* (New York: Oxford University Press, 1993), 118.

Chapter 4

p. 55: "with your vote . . . boys to ruin": Frances Elizabeth Willard, *Woman and Temperance: Or, The Work and Workers of the Woman's Christian Temperance Union* (Chicago: Woman's Temperance Publication Association, 1886), 355.

p. 56: "speak for woman's ballot": Frances E. Willard, *Glimpses of Fifty Years: The Autobiography of an American Woman* (Chicago: Woman's Temperance Publication Association, 1889), 351.

p. 57: "You might have . . . only be a scout": quoted in Ruth Bordin, *Frances Willard: A Biography* (Chapel Hill: University of North Carolina Press, 1986), 103.

p. 57: "nearly a quarter of a mile long": Willard, *Glimpses of Fifty Years,* 364.

pp. 57–58: "In order to . . . for and welcomed": quoted in "Frances E. Willard," *Literature: An Illustrated Weekly Magazine* 1, no. 28 (September 1888): 267.

Chapter 5

p. 67: "one of the . . . in this country": "Told the Story of the Ages," *New York Times*, March 4, 1913, https://timesmachine.nytimes.com /timesmachine/1913/03/04/100390355.html?pageNumber=5.

Chapter 6

pp. 76–77: "Seldom have we . . . from a woman" quoted in Ann D. Gordon et al, eds., *African American Women and the Vote, 1837–1965* (Amherst: University of Massachusetts Press, 1997), 48.

pp. 77–78: "But, John, I . . . make them clean?": quoted in Mary

Chapman and Angela Mills, *Treacherous Texts: U.S. Suffrage Literature, 1846–1946* (New Brunswick, NJ: Rutgers University Press, 2011), 48–50.

pp. 79–80: "She didn't suffer . . . saw fools everywhere": quoted in Caitlin Dickerson, "Ida B. Wells," *New York Times*, last updated March 9, 2018, https://www.nytimes.com/interactive/2018/obituaries/overlooked-ida-b-wells.html.

CHAPTER 7

p. 95: "I stand before you as a convicted criminal": quoted in Jean H. Baker, *Sisters: The Lives of America's Suffragists* (New York: Farrar, Straus and Giroux, 2006), 84.

p. 96: "The thick unbleached muslin undergarments . . . and forlorn shoes!": Doris Stevens, *Jailed for Freedom* (New York: Boni and Liveright, 1920), 108.

CHAPTER 8

p. 100: "Morals above reproach . . . take a stand": "James Harry Covington of Maryland Reputation," 1915, National Woman's Party Congressional Voting Card Collection, https://nationalwomansparty.pastperfectonline.com/archive/4AE7C629-A614-4A2C-9B9B-282042770160.

pp. 100–101: "To the index . . . the amendment": "Her Pressure on Congress," *New York Times*, March 2, 1919, https://timesmachine.nytimes.com/timesmachine/1919/03/02/98279494.html?pageNumber=71.

p. 101: "More than half . . . in our movement": Ann D. Gordon, ed., *The Selected Papers of Elizabeth Cady Stanton and Susan B. Anthony: An Awful Hush, 1895 to 1906* (New Brunswick, NJ: Rutgers University Press, 2013), 211.

p. 103: "How would you . . . would you?": quoted in Elizabeth Gurley Flynn, "The Rebel Girl," *Masses & Mainstream* 7, no. 1 (1954): 26.

CHAPTER 9

p. 111: "Seeing that the . . . and woman united": Frederick Douglass, *The Life and Times of Frederick Douglass, from 1817 to 1882,* ed. John Lobb, F.R.G.S. (London: Christian Age Office, 1882), 424.

p. 111: "When I advocated . . . nobility in the act": quoted in *Report of the International Council of Women: Assembled by the National Woman Suffrage Association, Washington, D.C., U.S. of America, March 25 to April 1, 1888, Volume 1* (Washington, DC: R. H. Darby, 1888), 329.

p. 112: "She is her . . . and hands off": "Frederick Douglass on Woman Suffrage: 1888," Virginia Commonwealth University Social Welfare History Project, accessed March 17, 2020, https://socialwelfare.library .vcu.edu/woman-suffrage/frederick-douglass-woman-suffrage-1888/.

p. 114: "Suffrage is not a right of anybody": Henry B. Blackwell, "Objections to Woman Suffrage Answered," Broadsides and Ephemera Collection, Duke University, accessed March 11, 2020, https:// repository.duke.edu/dc/broadsides/bdsma30834.

p. 114: "To say so is . . . women are people": ibid.

p. 115: "It would diminish respect for women": ibid.

p. 115: "Voting is power . . . than ever before": ibid.

p. 115: "It is contrary to the Bible": ibid.

p. 115: "Nowhere is it said in the Bible to women, 'Thou shalt not vote'": ibid.

p. 116: "There are many . . . favor of it": quoted in Brooke Kroeger,

The Suffragents: How Women Used Men to Get the Vote (Albany: State University of New York Press, 2017), 102.

pp. 116–117: "Every man . . . respects and esteems": ibid, 30.

p. 117: "the over 11,863": quoted in Johanna Neuman, *Gilded Suffragists: The New York Socialites who Fought for Women's Right to Vote* (New York: New York University Press, 2019), 93.

p. 120: "reeling through the hall in a state of advanced intoxication": Carrie Chapman Catt and Nettie Rogers Shuler, *Woman Suffrage and Politics: The Inner Story of the Suffrage Movement* (New York: Scribner's, 1923), 442.

p. 121: "Hurrah and vote for suffrage. And don't keep them in doubt": Letter to Harry Burn from Mother, August 1920, Harry T. Burn Papers, C.M. McClung Historical Collection, Knox County Public Library, http://cmdc.knoxlib.org/cdm/ref/collection/p265301coll8/id/699.

p. 121: "I knew that . . . vote for ratification": quoted in Elaine Weiss, *The Woman's Hour: The Great Fight to Win the Vote* (New York: Penguin, 2018), 315.

Conclusion

pp. 129–130: "We little dreamed . . . cause to victory": Ann D. Gordon, ed., *The Selected Papers of Elizabeth Cady Stanton and Susan B. Anthony: An Awful Hush, 1895 to 1906* (New Brunswick, NJ: Rutgers University Press, 2013), 217.

ABOUT THE AUTHORS

REBECCA BOGGS ROBERTS is the author of *Suffragists in Washington, DC: The 1913 Parade and the Fight for the Vote* and the coauthor of *Historic Congressional Cemetery.* She has been many things, including a journalist, producer, tour guide, forensic anthropologist, event planner, political consultant, jazz singer, and radio talk show host. Currently she is a curator of programming at Planet Word Museum, a new museum whose mission is to inspire a love of language and literature. She has made it a personal mission to highlight the history of our capital city, Washington, DC, where she lives with her husband, three sons, and a big fat dog.

LUCINDA ROBB was project director for *Our Mothers Before Us: Women and Democracy, 1789–1920* at the Center for Legislative Archives. The project rediscovered thousands of overlooked original documents and produced a traveling exhibit and education program highlighting the role of women in American democracy. She also helped organize the National Archives' celebration of the seventy-fifth anniversary of the Nineteenth Amendment in 1995 and is on the board of Running Start, a bipartisan group that trains young women to run for office. She lives in Virginia with her husband, three children, one dog, and more than five hundred PEZ dispensers.

ACKNOWLEDGMENTS

First, and most important, we must express our gratitude and admiration for the spectacular women of Candlewick Press: Karen Lotz, Lydia Abel, Olivia Swomley, Jackie Houton, and Cibby Acosta. Every chance they got, they made our work smarter, more inclusive, more thoughtful, and more important. This book quite literally would not exist without them.

Huge thanks to our early readers, who gave us invaluable feedback when we needed it most: Cokie Roberts, Lynda, Catherine, and Jennifer Robb, Madeline and Austin Florio, Ann Waigand, Teri Hlavacs, Brigid McDermott, Michele Rubenstein, Elizabeth Seay, Heather Gordon Schloss, Solange Brown, Susan Chi, and Rebecca Morrison. And special gratitude to Michelle Moyd, who wisely advised us to look at systematic racism in the movement and how to do politics better.

And big love to our families, Lars, Madeline, Austin, and Lawrence Florio and Dan, Jack, Cal, and Roland Hartman, who supported our grand plans for this little book and helped keep us sane(ish) while we made them happen.